Advanced Orthodontics: Fixed Functional Appliances

Advanced Orthodontics: Fixed Functional Appliances

Editor: Tyler Diego

AMERICAN
MEDICAL PUBLISHERS
www.americanmedicalpublishers.com

AMERICAN
MEDICAL PUBLISHERS
www.americanmedicalpublishers.com

Cataloging-in-Publication Data

Advanced orthodontics : fixed functional appliances / edited by Tyler Diego.
p. cm.
Includes bibliographical references and index.
ISBN 978-1-63927-050-7
1. Orthodontic appliances. 2. Dental instruments and apparatus. 3. Malocclusion--Treatment. 4. Dentistry.
5. Orthodontics. 6. Orthodontists--Guidebooks. I. Diego, Tyler.
RK527 .F59 2022
617.643--dc23

American Medical Publishers,
41 Flatbush Avenue,
1st Floor, New York,
NY 11217, USA

ISBN 978-1-63927-050-7 (Hardback)

Contents

Preface

This book has been an outcome of determined endeavour from a group of educationists in the field. The primary objective was to involve a broad spectrum of professionals from diverse cultural background involved in the field for developing new researches. The book not only targets students but also scholars pursuing higher research for further enhancement of the theoretical and practical applications of the subject.

Orthodontic appliances are the appliances created by orthodontic technology that is used for the treatment of malocclusions. There are two main types of orthodontic appliances: active and functional. They can either be fixed or removable appliances. The active appliance is the tool that is used to apply forces to the teeth in order to change its relation. Some examples of fixed orthodontic appliances are begg light wire appliances, bi helix, self-ligating edgewise appliances, tri helix, pre-adjusted edgewise appliances etc. The functional orthodontic appliance is used to produce orthodontic forces by utilizing the muscle action of the patient and responses of the nervous system. Some examples of fixed orthodontic functional appliances are herbst appliance and twin block appliance. This book provides comprehensive insights into the field of fixed orthodontic appliances. It covers in detail some existent theories and innovative concepts revolving around this domain. Researchers and students in this field will be assisted by this book.

It was an honour to edit such a profound book and also a challenging task to compile and examine all the relevant data for accuracy and originality. I wish to acknowledge the efforts of the contributors for submitting such brilliant and diverse chapters in the field and for endlessly working for the completion of the book. Last, but not the least; I thank my family for being a constant source of support in all my research endeavours.

Editor

1

Evaluation of an alternative technique to optimize direct bonding of orthodontic brackets to temporary crowns

Francilena Maria Campos Santos Dias[1], Célia Regina Maio Pinzan-Vercelino[2], Rudys Rodolfo de Jesus Tavares[3], Júlio de Araújo Gurgel[4], Fausto Silva Bramante[5], Melissa Nogueira Proença Fialho[6]

Objective: To compare shear bond strength of different direct bonding techniques of orthodontic brackets to acrylic resin surfaces. **Methods:** The sample comprised 64 discs of chemically activated acrylic resin (CAAR) randomly divided into four groups: discs in group 1 were bonded by means of light-cured composite resin (conventional adhesive); discs in group 2 had surfaces roughened with a diamond bur followed by conventional direct bonding by means of light-cured composite resin; discs in group 3 were bonded by means of CAAR (alternative adhesive); and discs in group 4 had surfaces roughened with a diamond bur followed by direct bonding by means of CAAR. Shear bond strength values were determined after 24 hours by means of a universal testing machine at a speed of 0.5 mm/min, and compared by analysis of variance followed by post-hoc Tukey test. Adhesive remnant index (ARI) was measured and compared among groups by means of Kruskal-Wallis and Dunn tests. **Results:** Groups 3 and 4 had significantly greater shear bond strength values in comparison to groups 1 and 2. Groups 3 and 4 yielded similar results. Group 2 showed better results when compared to group 1. In ARI analyses, groups 1 and 2 predominantly exhibited a score equal to 0, whereas groups 3 and 4 predominantly exhibited a score equal to 3. **Conclusions:** Direct bonding of brackets to acrylic resin surfaces using CAAR yielded better results than light-cured composite resin. Surface preparation with diamond bur only increased shear bond strength in group 2.

Keywords: Orthodontic brackets. Dental bonding. Shear bond strength. Temporary dental restoration.

[1] MSc in Orthodontics, Universidade Ceuma, São Luís, Maranhão, Brazil.
[2] Assistant professor, Universidade Ceuma, Department of Orthodontics, São Luís, Maranhão, Brazil.
[3] PhD in Oral Rehabilitation, Universidade de São Paulo (USP), School of Dentistry, Bauru, São Paulo, Brazil.
[4] PhD in Orthodontics, Universidade Ceuma, São Luís, Maranhão, Brazil.
[5] Associate Professor, Master's Program in Odontology, Universidade Ceuma, São Luís, Maranhão, Brazil.
[6] MSc in Orthodontics, Universidade Ceuma, São Luís, Maranhão, Brazil.

» The authors report no commercial, proprietary or financial interest in the products or companies described in this article.

Francilena Maria Campos Santos Dias
Rua Duque Bacelar, casa 20, quadra 22 - Quintas do Calhau. São Luís/MA, Brazil
E-mail: francilenasantos@yahoo.com.br

INTRODUCTION

In recent decades, there has been a growing concern for esthetics, in addition to increased life expectancy of individuals. As a result, the number of adult patients seeking orthodontic treatment has significantly increased.[1] Patients seek orthodontists for personal reasons, including esthetic or functional improvements of occlusion, or because other dentists refer them to have dental movements carried in order to aid different restorative procedures.

In many cases, adult patients use definitive or temporary crowns.[2] Temporary crowns are commonly used to protect tissues and render dental position stable before definitive crown manufacture.[3] Additionally, they also contribute to reestablish both esthetics and function during rehabilitation treatment.

Whenever a patient has temporary crowns, definitive restoration before orthodontic treatment is not recommended due to occlusal changes resulting from dental movement. In these cases, the orthodontist must bond or band the accessories on the surface of temporary material. Banding is recommended for posterior teeth; however, in the anterior region, direct bonding of accessories is used due to the poor esthetic aspect of bands.

During orthodontic movement of healthy teeth, bracket bonding on tooth enamel is part of orthodontic routine. However, bonding brackets on acrylic surfaces of temporary crowns is critical and presents high bonding failure rates. Frequent rebonding procedures hinders the advance of mechanotherapy, thereby contributing to increase treatment time, costs and chairside time.[4] Therefore, these procedures are undesirable for both orthodontist and patient.

Among the different types of material available to manufacture temporary crowns, chemically activated acrylic resin (CAAR) is the most commonly used[5] due to being inexpensive, easily manipulated and allowing repair, adjustment and relining, all of which may prove necessary during treatment. Additionally, this resin is resistant to oral function, including mastication; supports orthodontic forces and does not damage dental crown surface during debonding.

Despite the advantages of using CAAR as a temporary restorative material, its surface has lower bond strength values in comparison to what is clinically acceptable, when testing orthodontic accessories bonding.[5] Various studies have compared different types of material used to manufacture temporary crowns,[6-10] different methods of preparing the provisional material surface before direct bracket bonding[5,11,12] and different adhesives.[7] However, studies assessing the use of CAAR as a material for direct bonding of orthodontic brackets are scarce.

Composite resin is a common adhesive used for direct bracket bonding regardless of the surface (tooth or restoration). However, this type of material yields results lower than what is clinically acceptable when brackets are bonded to provisional acrylic resin material.[5] Thus, it has been speculated that the use of an alternative adhesive could optimize the results. Therefore, the objective of this study was to test the following null hypothesis: there is no difference in shear bond strength values of different direct bonding techniques (varying adhesive material and surface treatment) of orthodontic brackets to acrylic resin surfaces.

MATERIAL AND METHODS

Sample size calculation was carried out by means of the statistical program SAS, version 9.1.3. (SAS Institute Inc., Cary, USA). The following parameters were adopted: shear bond strength value of 5.3 ± 3.3 MPa;[6] significance level set at 5%; power of test of 80%; and effect size equal to 1. A sample size (n) of 12 specimens in each group was then determined. As a precaution, n = 16 was adopted.

Sixty-four CAAR Duralay discs (Dental Mfg. Co, Worth, USA) were prepared using rigid polyvinyl chloride (PVC) cylinders as matrix. Resin was prepared following the manufacturer's instructions (volume ratio of 3:1). After manipulation, the material was poured into the PVC rings until 3-mm thickness was reached. The remaining space in the PVC ring was filled with colorless CAAR also prepared according to the manufacturer's instructions (volume ratio of 2.5:1). To homogenize the bonding surfaces, CAAR surfaces were finished and polished with silicon carbide sandpaper in decreasing order of roughness (400 and 600). Specimens were then randomly divided into four groups (Table 1).

In group 1 (conventional adhesive without surface treatment = control group), surface was polished for 10 seconds with extra-fine pumice and rubber prophylactic cups with the aid of a low-speed hand piece. It was then rinsed with water and dried with oil-free air spray for 30 seconds. Subsequently, 37% gel phosphoric acid was applied for 30 seconds, followed by copious washing for

30 seconds and drying with oil-free air spray for 15 seconds. A thin coat of Transbond XT primer (3M Unitek, Monrovia, Calif., USA) was applied, followed by drying with a brief air spray and light-curing for 20 seconds. Stainless steel 14.79-mm^2 brackets (Standard Edgewise maxillary central incisors, Morelli Ortodontia, Sorocaba, SP, Brazil) were bonded to the surface prepared with Transbond XT light-cured composite resin (3M Unitek , Monrovia, Calif). Brackets remained in the manufacturer's package until immediately before bonding and were handled with bonding tweezers to avoid contamination of the bonding base.

Brackets were positioned at the center of specimens and then firmly pressed during 5 seconds, so as to obtain a fine layer of bonding material.[13] Excess material was carefully removed by means of an exploratory probe. Light curing was performed with a light intensity of 450 mW/cm^2 measured by a radiometer. The duration of light incidence was 20 seconds, 10 seconds on each side (mesial and distal), following the manufacturer's instructions.

In group 2 (conventional adhesive with surface treatment), surface was initially roughened with a cylindrical diamond bur, medium granulation (PM 82. Vortex; São Paulo, Brazil). The bur was positioned parallel to the surface of the specimen with a rotation speed of 4,000 rpm (Fig 1). Brushing movements were made with the bur over the specimens, using a device for standardization. Subsequently, prophylaxis, acid etching and direct bracket bonding were performed as described for group 1.

In group 3 (alternative adhesive without surface treatment), after prophylaxis, 37% gel phosphoric acid was applied for 30 seconds, followed by copious rinsing for 30 seconds and drying with oil-free air spray for 15 seconds. Afterwards, CAAR monomer was applied with the aid of a brush, and direct bracket bonding was performed with Duralay resin applied to the base of brackets with a brush, according to the powder/liquid technique; subsequently, brackets were positioned. After excess material removal, self-curing of CAAR was carried out.

Group 4 (alternative adhesive with surface treatment) was subjected to the same roughening procedure described for group 2. The direct bonding procedure was carried out as described for group 3.

After the bonding procedure, specimens were immediately stored in distilled water, in a bacteriological incubator at 37 ± 1 °C. Tests were performed after 24 hours.[14] Shear bond strength was assessed by means of a universal testing machine, with a 50-kg load cell, operating at a speed of 0.5 mm/min[15] (Fig 2).

A single previously calibrated operator performed all bonding procedures. Laboratory tests were conducted by another operator who was blind with respect to the technique used for bonding.

After bracket debonding, the surfaces were analyzed by two examiners using a magnifying glass under 5 x magnification (Illuminated Magnifier, Fujian, China), so as to determine the adhesive remnant index (ARI). Scores recommended by Artur and Bergland were used.[16] They range from 0 to 3, as follows: 0 = no adhesive left on dental enamel; 1 = less than half adhesive left on dental enamel; 2 = more than half adhesive left on dental enamel; and 3 = all adhesive left on dental

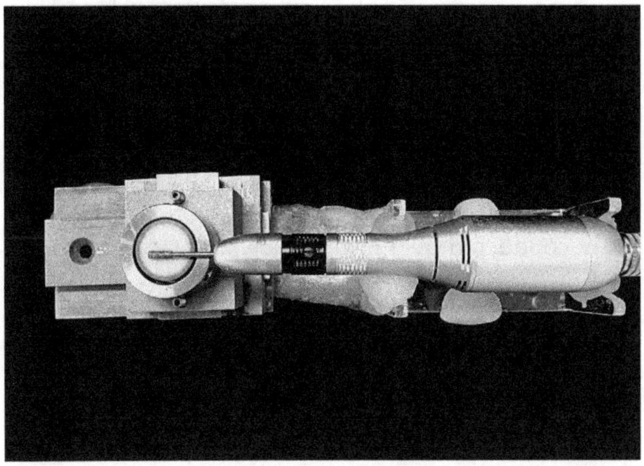

Figure 1 - Surface preparation with a diamond bur.

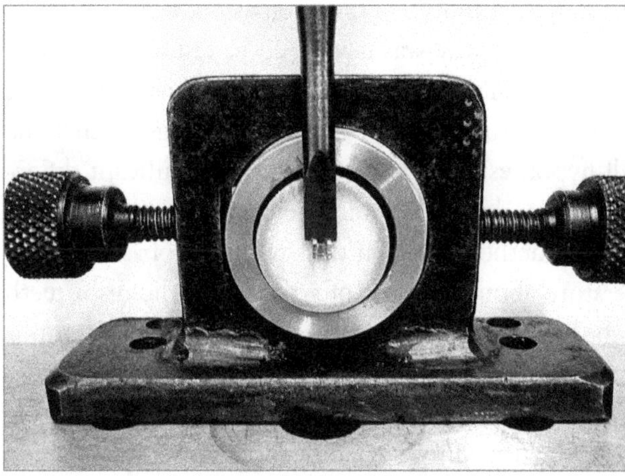

Figure 2 - Specimen ready to be tested.

enamel, including impression of the bracket mesh. Although they were developed to assess the enamel surface, in the present study, these scores were applied to assess acrylic resin surface.[17,18]

Shapiro-Wilk test confirmed that data followed normal distribution. Analysis of variance (ANOVA) and post-hoc Tukey test were used to compare groups. Data regarding ARI were analyzed by means of Kruskal-Wallis and Dunn tests for multiple comparisons. Significance level was set at $p < 0.05$. Statistical analyses were performed with SAS software version 9.1.3 (SAS Institute Inc., Cary, USA).

RESULTS

Results revealed that groups 3 and 4, in which brackets were bonded by means of CAAR, had significantly greater shear bond strength values than groups 1 and 2, in which brackets were bonded with light-cured composite resin. Groups 3 and 4 yielded similar results (Table 2).

The surface prepared with diamond bur yielded better bonding only for the group bonded with light-cured composite resin (Table 2).

Regarding ARI, groups 1 and 2 predominantly exhibited a score equal to 0, whereas groups 3 and 4 predominantly exhibited a score equal to 3. Multiple comparisons demonstrated that groups 1 and 2 and groups 3 and 4 were similar. However, ARI differed significantly when comparing groups 1 and 2 with groups 3 and 4 (Table 3).

Table 1 - Description of groups.

Groups	Surface preparation and adhesive agent
1	Acid etching, application of primer and bracket bonding using light-cured composite resin.
2	Surface roughened with diamond bur, acid etching, application of primer and bracket bonding using light-cured composite resin.
3	Acid etching, application of monomer and bracket bonding using CAAR.
4	Surface roughened with diamond bur, acid etching, application of monomer and bracket bonding using CAAR.

Table 2 - Means, standard deviation (SD), minimum and maximum values in MPa and comparison between groups.

Groups	Mean ± SD*	Min. value	Max. value
Group 1	1.38 ± 0.40[a]	0.82	2.14
Group 2	4.37 ± 1.14[b]	2.55	6.61
Group 3	12.19 ± 1.58[c]	9.7	15.2
Group 4	12.41 ± 1.96[c]	10.19	16.22

*Different letter suggest statistically significant difference (Tukey test).

Table 3 - ARI scores and comparison between groups.

Groups	Scores				Median*
	0	1	2	3	
Group 1	16	0	0	0	0[a]
Group 2	13	1	0	2	0[a]
Group 3	0	0	2	14	3[b]
Group 4	0	0	0	16	3[b]

*Different letter suggest statistically significant difference.

DISCUSSION

Direct bracket bonding to temporary material must be of good quality to support orthodontic forces applied during dental movement, as well as masticatory forces. The present study was developed to test an alternative technique using CAAR as adhesive to improve shear bond strength in these cases. Results suggest that the null hypothesis was rejected because significant differences were observed among the techniques analyzed.

The methods used in this study were based on the literature about bonding of artificial acrylic resin teeth to the base of complete dentures[9] and surfaces of temporary material bonded by means of light-cured composite resin[6,7,11,12] due to shortage of studies on this subject.

Before the direct bonding procedure was carried out, specimens had their surfaces treated with 37% phosphoric acid. Phosphoric acid is a bactericidal agent that increases the energy of dental enamel surface by removing non-reactive hydroxyapatite crystals and the acquired pellicle, thereby transforming the surface into a highly porous tissue.[19] Although the acid does not alter the original topography of acrylic resin, this substance was used to promote cleaning of debris generated during the preparation of the bonding surfaces.[7,12] A previous study conducted by Thean, Chew and Goh[20] reported that removal of contaminants, such as saliva and material residues, was more important than the mechanical preparation of surfaces. Bonding failure can occur if the surface is contaminated before the bonding procedures.

In the present study, groups 3 and 4 yielded the best shear bond strength values. The results obtained for the alternative technique using CAAR as adhesive showed values that could be considered as clinically acceptable.[21] Studies demonstrating satisfactory bonding forces between orthodontic brackets and temporary crowns are scarce in the literature. Various studies assessing direct bonding of brackets onto temporary material have reported bond strength values below what is clinically acceptable.[11,12]

Shear bond strength values for groups 3 and 4 were greater than those obtained by Chay et al,[5] Maryanchik et al,[6] Blakey and Mah[11] and Masioli et al.[12] The main difference between our study and the aforementioned ones was the adhesive used to bond brackets to provisional crowns. However, when compared to group 1, the values reported by certain authors[5,11] were greater. This result is most likely related to the use of different procedures in the preparation of the tested surfaces.

In groups 3 and 4, it is believed that moistening the test surface with monomer provided an additional measure to improve effectiveness of the acrylic resin/acrylic resin chemical interaction.[10]

Despite the high values obtained for groups 3 and 4, it is important to emphasize that *in vivo* and *in vitro* studies comparing bond strength demonstrate that the values obtained *in vivo* are significantly lower than those obtained *in vitro*.[22]

Orthodontists commonly use diamond burs to prepare bonding surfaces on provisional crowns.[5] As in a previous study,[7] surface preparation with burs was performed following a systematic protocol conducted by a single operator. Minor differences in the surfaces, if present, most likely did not affect the results obtained. Masioli et al[12] assessed roughness of surfaces prepared with burs and demonstrated reasonable uniformity with a variation coefficient below 30%.

When the groups were compared in terms of surface treatment, results revealed that shear bond strength values differed significantly between groups 1 and 2, with group 2 exhibiting higher values than group 1. It is speculated that this result occurred because, after curing, the composite resin requires macromechanical retentions to become attached to other material. Composite resin does not chemically react with the acrylic resin of temporary crowns, which gives support to the better bonding values yielded by roughened surfaces compared with surfaces without preparation.[12] It is further speculated that the tertiary amines present in CAAR composition can inhibit adequate polymerization of light-cured composite resins, thereby impairing bonding between different types of material. Inhibition could also explain the lower bond strength values observed in groups 1 and 2 compared with the values observed in groups 3 and 4. It is emphasized that the strength values obtained for groups 1 and 2 were lower than what is considered as clinically acceptable.[21]

Groups 3 and 4, bonded with CAAR, exhibited similar strength values. It is speculated that this result occurred because the test surface had a short aging time, and the mechanical properties of the material were not altered after bonding.[5]

The predominant ARI score for groups 1 and 2 was 0. This result indicates that when light-cured composite resin was used as adhesive, there was no effective bond between the bracket and the tested surface. In groups 3 and 4, in which CAAR was used as bonding material, the predominant ARI score was 3, which can be explained by the fact that CAAR underwent chemical interaction with a new material of the same composition after being moistened with the monomer.[10] These findings suggest that groups 3 and 4 exhibited adequate bonding between the specimen and CAAR used as bonding material.

Results suggest that when there is a need to bond accessories to acrylic resin surfaces, the orthodontist can effectively use CAAR as adhesive and monomer before the procedure.

CONCLUSIONS

Direct bonding of orthodontic brackets to acrylic resin surfaces using CAAR was effective in increasing shear bond strength.

Surface preparation by means of a diamond bur increased shear bond strength only in the group bonded with light-cured composite resin; however, the values obtained for this group were lower than what is clinically acceptable.

Author contributions

Conceived and designed the study: FMCSD, CRMPV. Performed experiments: FMCSD, CRMPV, RRJT, MNPF. Data analysis: FMCSD, CRMPV, RRJT, JAG, FSB. Contributed with reagents/materials/analysis tools: CRMPV. Wrote the article: FMCSD, CRMPV, RRJT, JAG, FSB, MNPF.

REFERENCES

1. Pabari S, Moles DR, Cunningham SJ. Assessment of motivation and psychological characteristics of adult orthodontic patients. Am J Orthod Dentofacial Orthop. 2011;140(6):e263-72.
2. Wassell RW, Steele JG, Welsh G. Considerations when planning occlusal rehabilitation: a review of the literature. Int Dent J. 1998;48(6):571-81.
3. Yannikakis SA, Zissis AJ, Polyzois GL, Caroni C. Color stability of provisional resin restorative materials. J Prosthet Dent. 1998;80(5):533-9.
4. Pasquale A, Weinstein M, Borislow AJ, Braitman LE. In-vivo prospective comparison of bond failure rates of 2 self-etching primer/adhesive systems. Am J Orthod Dentofacial Orthop. 2007;132(5):671-4.
5. Chay SH, Wong SL, Mohamed N, Chia A, Yap AUJ. Effects of surface treatment and aging on the bond strength of orthodontic brackets to provisional materials. Am J Orthod Dentofacial Orthop. 2007;132(5):577.e7-11.
6. Maryanchik I, Brendlinger EJ, Fallis DW, Vandewalle KS. Shear bond strength of orthodontic brackets bonded to various aesthetic pontic materials. Am J Orthod Dentofacial Orthop. 2010;137(5):684-9.
7. Rambhia S, Heshmati R, Dhuru V, Lacopino A. Shear bond strength of orthodontic brackets bonded to provisional crown materials utilizing two different adhesives. Angle Orthod. 2009;79(4):784-9.
8. Cardash HS, Applebaum B, Baharav H, Liberman R. Effect of retention grooves on tooth-denture base bond. J Prosthet Dent. 1990;64(4):492-6.
9. Chung RWC, Stanford JW, Serio A. Properties of self-curing denture base resins. J Adv Prosthodont. 2011;3(3):136-9.
10. Cunningham JL, Benington IC. An investigation of variables that may affect the bond between plastic teeth and denture base resin. J Dent. 1999;27(2):129-35.
11. Blakey R, Mah J. Effects of surface conditioning on the shear bond strength of orthodontic brackets bonded to temporary polycarbonate crowns. Am J Orthod Dentofacial Orthop. 2010;138(1):72-8.
12. Masioli DLC, Almeida MAO, Masioli MA, Almeida JRM. Assessment of the effect of different surface treatments on the bond strength of brackets bonded to acrylic resin. Dental Press J Orthod. 2011;16(1): 37-47.
13. Machado CT, Borges BCD, Araujo GJR, Santos AJS, Dametto FR, Pinheiro FHSL. Influence of adhesion promoters and curing-light sources on the shear bond strength of orthodontic brackets. Indian J Dent Res. 2012;23(6):747-52.
14. Endo T, Ozoe R, Shinkai K, Aoyagi M, Kurokawa H, Katoh Y, et al. Shear bond strength of brackets rebonded with a fluoride-releasing and recharging adhesive system. Angle Orthod. 2009;79(3):564-70.
15. Isber H, Ambrosio AR, Carvalho PEG, Valle-Corotti KM, Siqueira DF. Comparative in vitro study of the shear bond strength of brackets bonded with restorative and orthodontic resins. Braz Oral Res. 2011;25(1):49-55.
16. Artun J, Bergland S. Clinical trials with crystal growth conditioning as an alternative to acid-etch enamel pretreatment. Am J Orthod. 1984;85(4):333-40.
17. Northup RG, Berzins DW, Bradley TG, Schuckit W. Shear bond strength comparison between two orthodontic adhesives and self-ligating and conventional brackets. Angle Orthod. 2007;77(4):701-6.
18. Bishara SE, Soliman MM, Oonsombat C, Laffoon JF, Ajlouni R. The effect of variation in mesh-base design on the shear bond strength of orthodontic brackets. Angle Orthod. 2004;74(3):400-4.
19. Vieira TI, Valença AMG, Santiago BM, Gondim BLC. Antimicrobial activity of phosphoric acid associated or not associated with 2% chlorhexidine over dental biofilm bacteria. Int J Dent. 2011;10:143-7.
20. Thean HP, Chew CL, Goh KI. Shear bond strength of denture teeth to base: a comparative study. Quintessence Int. 1996;27(6):425-8.
21. Reynolds PR. A review of direct orthodontic bonding. Br J Orthod. 1975;2:171-8.
22. Hajrassie MKA, Khier SE. In-vivo and in-vitro comparison of bond strengths of orthodontic brackets bonded to enamel and debonded at various times. Am J Orthod Dentofacial Orthop. 2007;131(3):384-90.

2

Comparative study of torque expression among active and passive self-ligating and conventional brackets

Érika Mendonça Fernandes Franco[1], Fabrício Pinelli Valarelli[2], João Batista Fernandes[3], Rodrigo Hermont Cançado[2], Karina Maria Salvatore de Freitas[2]

Objective: The aim of this study was to compare torque expression in active and passive self-ligating and conventional brackets. **Methods:** A total of 300 segments of stainless steel wire 0.019 x 0.025-in and six different brands of brackets (Damon 3MX, Portia, In-Ovation R, Bioquick, Roth SLI and Roth Max) were used. Torque moments were measured at 12°, 24°, 36° and 48°, using a wire torsion device associated with a universal testing machine. The data obtained were compared by analysis of variance followed by Tukey test for multiple comparisons. Regression analysis was performed by the least-squares method to generate the mathematical equation of the optimal curve for each brand of bracket. **Results:** Statistically significant differences were observed in the expression of torque among all evaluated bracket brands in all evaluated torsions ($p < 0.05$). It was found that Bioquick presented the lowest torque expression in all tested torsions; in contrast, Damon 3MX bracket presented the highest torque expression up to 36° torsion. **Conclusions:** The connection system between wire/bracket (active, passive self-ligating or conventional with elastic ligature) seems not to interfere in the final torque expression, the latter being probably dependent on the interaction between the wire and the bracket chosen for orthodontic mechanics.

Keywords: Torque. Orthodontic appliance design.

[1] Graduate student, Faculdade Ingá (UNINGÁ), Department of Orthodontics, Maringá, Paraná, Brazil.
[2] Professor, Faculdade Ingá (UNINGÁ), Department of Orthodontics, Maringá, Paraná, Brazil.
[3] Mechanical Engineer, Universidade Federal de Itajubá (UNIFEI), Itajubá, Minas Gerais, Brazil.

Karina Maria Salvatore Freitas
Department of Orthodontics - Ingá Faculty - Rodovia PR 317, n° 6114
Maringá, PR - Brazil - CEP: 87035-510 - E-mail: kmsf@uol.com.br

INTRODUCTION

Torque is a moment generated by the torsion of a rectangular wire in the bracket slot. In Orthodontics, it represents the buccolingual inclination of a tooth's root/crown and it is an orthodontic adaptation used to describe the rotation around the X-axis.[1]

Theoretically, third-order moments can be calculated from the nominal dimensions of arches and brackets. It has been shown that there is a significant discrepancy between what has been accomplished in theory and what is seen clinically between bracket/wire. These variations in torque can be attributed to many factors, such as bracket design, clearance (or play) between the wire and the slot, slot dimension, ligature mode, bracket deformation, wire stiffness, torsion magnitude and wire size.[2-5] Other factors also have an impact on third-order moments, including bracket bonding errors[6] and irregularities in the morphology of tooth crown.[7,8]

Some studies have found only minor differences among the various systems of brackets, active and passive self-ligating brackets as well as conventional ones, with respect to their effectiveness in relation to torque expression and correction.[9] It was also found that self-ligating brackets are not superior in relation to conventional ones; particularly to what concerns their biomechanical characteristics, there are no statistically significant differences between them.[10,11]

Whereas some of these systems seem to have less friction *in vitro*, their torque characteristics have not yet been studied in detail.[12] Due to the complexity of the experimental setup, there have been only small studies conducted to evaluate torque expression, and numerical analyses have not been carried out for the expression of torque in various types of self-ligating brackets.[7,13]

Thus, the objective of the present study was to compare the expression of torque in active and passive self-ligating as well as conventional brackets, generated at different torsion angles of the wire. Comparisons regarding torque expression among brackets of different brands were also performed. Furthermore, it was found the range of torsion angles corresponding to the torque ranges considered clinically effective.

MATERIAL AND METHODS

The sample used in this *in vitro* study comprised 30 maxillary right central incisor brackets of six distinct brands (five self-ligating and one conventional). Among the self-ligating brackets tested (5 of each brand), Damon 3MX (Standard torque, Ormco, USA) and Portia (3M, Abzil, Brazil) were considered by the manufacturers as passive; while In-Ovation R (GAC, USA), Bioquick (Forestadent, Germany) and Roth SLI (Morelli, Brazil) were considered as active. The conventional bracket tested (n = 5) was Roth Max (Morelli, Brazil), used as a control. The ligation method used in conventional brackets was the elastomer. Slot size of all brackets was 0.022 x 0.028-in. The tested brackets were purchased randomly, instead of being donated, in order to avoid potential influence from manufacturers in the final results.

Three hundred stainless steel wire segments were used (Morelli, Sorocaba, SP, Brazil), each one 3.5 cm in length; and a rectangular section of 0.019 x 0.025-in, so that, for each test, a different segment of wire was used.

Stainless steel metal cylinders were manufactured, each one 4 cm in length and approximately 1 cm in diameter, in order to have accessories bonded to them. Grooves were made on the base surface of these cylinders for better adhesion of brackets. Brackets were bonded to the cylinders by Araldite Hobby Epoxy glue.

The prescription of bracket torque did not affect our study, since the position of zero torque was used as a baseline to start every test. In order to ensure this, bonding was supported by a mounting device. This device consisted of a calibrator which was adapted and fitted to the walls of the bracket slot, causing it to achieve three-dimensional alignment. It provided bonding to the metallic cylinder that neutralized torque and pre-existing angles of each bracket.

A universal testing machine EMIC DL2000 (Instron Brazil scientific equipament – Paraná – Brazil) was used and adapted to it; a device for torsion tests of wires and brackets was developed to perform the torsion of the wire on both extremities symmetrically. In each test, the machine was reset in the system, and new leveling was performed in order to avoid residual forces and torques of the previous test. After this process, the test was started by adapting the cylinder with bracket to the base of the device, and inserting the wire segment being tested. The system was fixed by screws to prevent dislocations or slides in the set, which could alter the results.

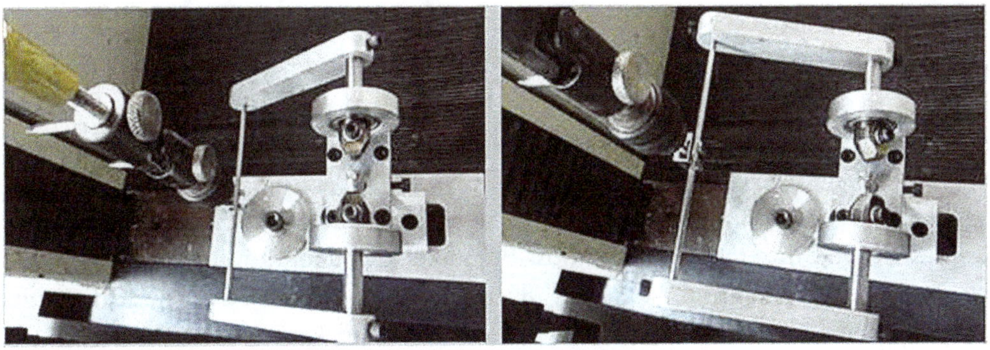

Figure 1 - Torsion device.

The movement (ascent) of the tailstock of the universal testing machine was transmitted to the torsion device by an articulated rod under 0.25 rpm (Fig 1).

A transducer for measurement of force/torque, with strain gauge load cell was used to measure the components of forces and moments (torque) of the bracket/wire combinations tested. The load cell used was "Trd 19" 200 N. There was a sensor that could capture the applied force and torques, as well as the torsion angle, and electronically transfer it in the form of data to a computer, so the results were translated and displayed in graphical form. A data-capture software (version 3.01 Tesc) was used to capture the signal from the transducer and register it to the file.

Each bracket/wire combination was tested ten times, and, for each torsion, a different wire segment was inserted. The combinations were tested in different torsions: 12°, 24°, 36° and 48°, and for every torsion angle in the wire, the moment of force was rated in Nmm.

Statistical analysis

Assessment of data normality was performed through Kolmogorov-Smirnov test, followed by parametric tests. Intergroup comparisons were conducted by one-way ANOVA and Tukey tests.

Regression was performed by the least-squares method in order to assess the trend and the behavior of variables of each brand tested. The coefficient of determination R^2 was employed to assess regression quality and check if the regression found corresponded to the best representative curve of the correlation between the two variables, which explains, in percentage, the relationship between variables ($R^2 \geq 0 \leq 1$). Regression was performed by the least-squares method to generate the mathematical equation of the optimal curve of each bracket brand separately. By the equations, both the angles of initial torque records and the angles regarding torque range that were considered clinically effective were calculated by the Tartaglia-Cardano method.

Statistical analyses were performed with Statistica software (Statistica for Windows 6.0; Statsoft, Tulsa, Oklahoma, USA). Results were considered statistically significant for $p < 0.05$. Regression and equations were obtained in Excel 2007 software.

RESULTS

Intergroup comparisons

At 12°, Bioquick obtained a smaller force x deformation ratio (2.90 Nmm). Shortly thereafter, Portia, with 5.07 Nmm, followed by Roth SLI, with 6.74 Nmm. Roth Max and In-Ovation R brackets came afterwards with statistically similar results (9.97 and 9.14 Nmm, respectively). Damon 3MX showed the greatest force x deformation relationship (12.27 Nmm) (Table 1).

When evaluated at 24°, Bioquick showed the lowest moment (6.19 Nmm), followed by Roth SLI (20.10 Nmm). Shortly after, Roth Max, In-Ovation R and Portia were statistically similar, with values of 26.22, 27.57 and 26.02 Nmm, respectively. Damon 3MX presented the highest moment, 30.42 Nmm (Table 1).

At 36°, Bioquick presented the lowest force x deformation ratio (16.41 Nmm), followed by Roth SLI, 39.45 Nmm. Subsequently, Roth Max presented 45.14 Nmm. In-Ovation R and Portia came afterwards, showing a statistically similar behavior (46.96 and 46.87 Nmm, respectively). Damon 3MX showed the highest value (49.11 Nmm) (Table 1).

At 48°, Bioquick confirmed the lowest force x deformation ratio (40.99 Nmm), followed by Roth SLI (66.63 Nmm) and Roth Max (71.99 Nmm). In-Ovation R, Portia and Damon 3MX brackets had statistically similar results for this angulation (74.49, 73.86 and 75.38 Nmm, respectively) (Table 1).

Regression by the least-squares method

It was observed that torque began to be expressed primarily in Bioquick (1.79°), followed by Roth SLI (3.65°), Roth Max (5.23°), Damon 3MX (5.41°), In-Ovation R (6.91°) and Portia (9.46°). When the values of torque moments were evaluated, it was observed that the effectiveness of torque behaved differently for each bracket type. It was found that, for clinical effects, torque of 5 Nmm first appeared in Damon 3MX, followed by Roth Max, In-Ovation R, Roth SLI, Portia and Bioquick. For a torque of 20 Nmm, the first to be expressed was Damon 3MX, followed by In-Ovation R, Roth Max, Portia, Roth SLI and Bioquick (Tables 2 and 3).

The torsions performed at the orthodontic wire, for most brands tested, should range from approximately 8° to 24°, so that effective clinical results can be achieved. Bioquick presented a very distinct

Table 1 - Intergroup comparison of different brackets used in the trials in the four torsions tested (one-way ANOVA test followed by Tukey test).

Variables	Roth Max (n = 50) Mean (SD)	Roth SLI (n = 50) Mean (SD)	Damon MX (n = 50) Mean (SD)	In-Ovation R (n = 50) Mean (SD)	Bioquick (n = 50) Mean (SD)	Portia (n = 50) Mean (SD)	p-value
12°	9.97 ± 4.10^{A}	6.74 ± 2.05^{B}	12.27 ± 2.56^{C}	9.14 ± 1.21^{A}	2.90 ± 1.00^{D}	5.07 ± 2.41^{E}	0.000*
24°	26.22 ± 4.66^{A}	20.10 ± 2.06^{B}	30.42 ± 2.49^{C}	27.57 ± 1.83^{A}	6.19 ± 2.13^{D}	26.02 ± 2.34^{A}	0.000*
36°	45.14 ± 3.94^{A}	39.45 ± 1.99^{B}	49.11 ± 2.56^{C}	46.96 ± 2.31^{D}	16.41 ± 1.73^{E}	46.87 ± 1.96^{D}	0.000*
48°	71.99 ± 3.89^{A}	66.63 ± 1.97^{B}	75.38 ± 3.02^{C}	73.86 ± 2.62^{C}	40.99 ± 2.48^{D}	74.49 ± 2.01^{C}	0.000*

* Statistically significant for $p < 0.05$. (mean expressed in Nmm). Different letters represent statistically significant differences.

Table 2 - Angle at which the torque expression begins.

Angle at which torque expression begins		Roots of equations of brands (Tartaglia–Cardano's method)		
Bracket tested	Angle	Real root	Complex root	Conjugated root
Bioquick	1.79°	1.79	18.75 + 18.90 i	18.75 - 18.90 i
Roth SLI	3.65°	3.65	21.82 + 53.96 i	21.82 - 53.96 i
Roth Max	5.23°	5.23	24.68 + 52.73 i	24.68 - 52.73 i
Damon 3MX	5.41°	5.41	30.86 + 48.10 i	30.86 - 48.10 i
In-Ovation R	6.91°	6.91	31.71 + 50.83 i	31.71 - 50.83 i
Portia	9.46°	9.46	29.63 + 50.72 i	29.63 - 50.72 i

"i" = Square Root of -1.

Table 3 - Angles for clinically effective torque range.

Torque range clinically effective (Nmm)		Roots of equations of brands for clinically effective torque (Tartaglia–Cardano's Method)					
		Damon 3MX	Roth Max	In-Ovation R	Roth SLI	Portia	Bioquick
Minimum	5.00	7.93°	8.52°	9.62°	10.02°	11.93°	21.4°
		29.61 + 47.48 i	23.24 + 52.20 i	30.36 + 50.22 i	25.01 + 55.71 i	28.39 + 50.28 i	8.94 + 17.70 i
		29.61 - 47.48 i	23.24 - 52.20 i	30.36 - 50.22 i	25.01 - 55.71 i	28.39 - 50.28 i	8.94 - 17.70 i
Maximum	20.00	16.79°	19.48°	19.06°	23.71°	20.19°	39.01°
		25.18 + 46.06 i	17.56 + 51.53 i	25.64 + 48.92 i	31.85 + 61.03 i	24.26 + 49.43 i	0.14 +27.66 i
		25.18 - 46.06 i	17.56 - 51.53 i	25.64 - 48.92 i	31.85 - 61.03 i	24.26 - 49.43i	0.14 - 27.66 i

"i" = Square Root of -1.

behavior from the other brands because even though it began to manifest torque earlier, in order to have moment clinically feasible, it would be necessary to apply greater torsions to the wire used, ranging from 21.4° to 39.01° (Tables 2 and 3).

DISCUSSION

Torque movement is a key element to obtain good results in orthodontic treatments.[14] Great concern about its accuracy is directly related to the desired results of occlusion and esthetics for orthodontic treatment.

In order not to influence the final result, the original torques embedded in the brackets were set to zero through a bonding device that annulled the prescription torque of each bracket. The importance of this procedure has already been reported in the literature seeking distinct forms of parallelism between the wire used in the trials and the accessory slots.[7,15,16]

The analyses of the test results showed that Bioquick presented the lowest torque value in all angles tested. Damon 3MX presented the highest torque value, up to torsion of 36°, equaling subsequently at 48° with In-Ovation R and Portia (Table 1).

Results showed that the behavior of the brackets tested was not dependent on the type of closure. At 12°, the lowest torque expression was Bioquick's which has an active system, followed by Portia, which is considered to be passive, Roth SLI (active), Roth Max (conventional), In-Ovation R (active), and Damon 3MX (passive), all of which presented the highest torque expression (Table 1).

This behavior was repeated in subsequent angles, showing no tendency for active, passive or conventional brackets tested, at higher or lower torque expression (Fig 2) (Table 1).

Regarding active self-ligating brackets, some researches have concluded that they have a higher torque expression than the passive ones.[7,17] This happens due to the fact that the clip constantly presses the wire against the bracket slot, especially as the diameter of the arch increases. They also claim that the active self-ligating ones exert a continuous force on the arch, thereby resulting in better accuracy of orthodontic movement and having the ability to reorient themselves three-dimensionally until the arch is completely inserted into the slot.[18]

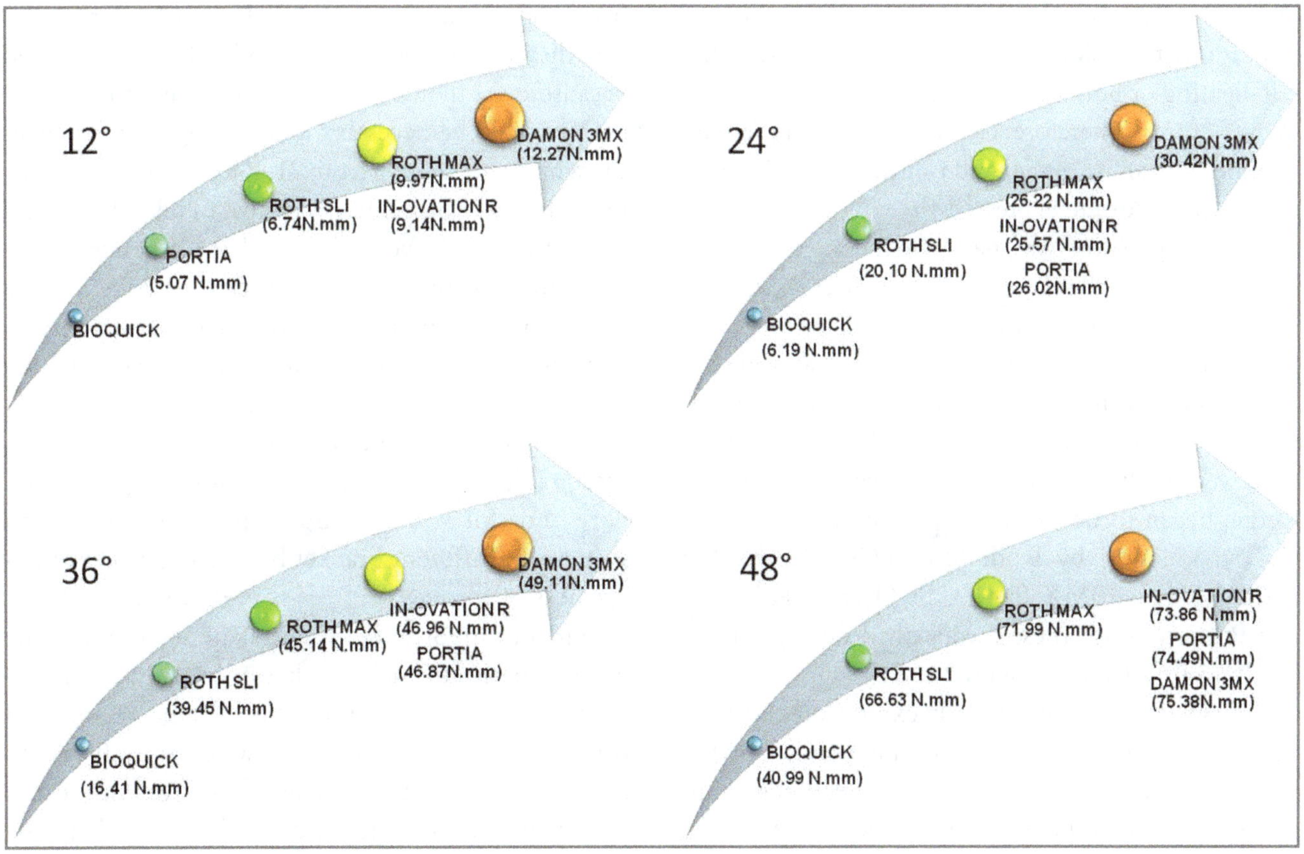

Figure 3 - Intergroup comparison of torque expression.

Some studies, however, corroborated the results found in this research. Morina et al[9] found only minor differences among the various systems of brackets (active, passive self-ligating and conventional brackets), particularly with regards to their effectiveness in relation to expression and correction of torque.[9] Pandis et al[11] and Fansa et al[10] also found that self-ligating brackets are not superior in relation to conventional ones; in terms of biomechanical characteristics, there are no statistically significant differences between them.[10]

It is important to remember that there are many factors that influence torque during orthodontic treatment: torsion magnitude, wire thickness, slot size, bracket positioning, tooth positioning, wire and bracket composition,[17] width and depth of the slot, brackets and wires manufacturing tolerance,[5,20] difference of constituent leagues of the wires, manufacturing process of brackets (injection-molding, casting, or milling).[20,21] All these elements can change the torque expressed in the bracket. Thus, it cannot be said that the active clip, by itself, can effectively increase torque.[16,19]

The conformation and size of the slot appear to be one of the factors that most influence the effectiveness of torque. In several studies, various measurements indicate that the slots of brackets in general, whether self-ligating or not, are above the size reported by the manufacturer. Therefore, clearance between the wire and the slot can be higher and impair mechanics with regard to the torque expressed.[22]

After regression was performed for each brand separately, and the relevant equations were obtained, the torsion angles in which torque began to be expressed (for a torsion angle equal to zero), as well as in which range of the torsion angle each of these brands could reproduce a torque considered clinically effective, were calculated. It was observed that although torque began to be expressed primarily in Bioquick (1.79°), followed by Roth SLI (3.65°), Roth Max (5.23°), Damon 3MX (5.41°), In-Ovation R (6.91°) and Portia (9.46°), these torques had no capacity to be clinically effective (Tables 2 and 3).

It is speculated that this early expression of torque depends on slot depth. This means that when the wire comes into contact with the connection system, a torque begins to be expressed earlier, but the wire has not yet found the cervical and incisal walls of the slot. This early generated torque, however, is not able to perform a third-order effective orthodontic movement yet. To achieve clinic effectiveness, the wire must overcome the slot clearance and touch the cervical and incisal walls of the slot.[3,23]

When the torque moment values of each brand were evaluated over the tests, it was found that the effectiveness of torque behaved differently for each brand. Damon 3MX showed earlier the capacity to express a torque considered clinically effective, i.e., with a 7.93° torsion angle, it could already express 5 Nmm, while Bioquick needs a torsion of 21.4° to achieve the same 5 Nmm.

Based on the literature, the torque range considered clinically effective indicates moments of force ranging from 5 to 20 Nmm.[3,7] It was found that for clinical effects, torque of 5 Nmm first appeared in Damon 3MX, followed by Roth Max, In-Ovation R, Roth SLI, Portia and Bioquick. The first to express a torque of 20 Nmm was Damon 3MX, followed by In-Ovation R, Roth Max, Portia, Roth SLI and Bioquick. This shows that, in order to achieve effective clinical results, the torsions performed on an orthodontic wire, for most brands tested, should range from approximately 8° to 24°. Bioquick presented a very distinct behavior from the other brands evaluated because even though it started to express torque earlier, it would be necessary to apply higher torsions to the wire used, ranging from 21.4° to 39.01°, so that the moment could be clinically feasible (Tables 2 and 3).

As there are several factors that influence brackets manufacture, it would be ideal to have a more rigid control in all manufacturing stages, with constant measurements and a more accurate dimensional control. This is because some distortion may occur during the process. Thus, it seems reasonable to assert that the relationship between wire and slot is more important than the ligation systems of different bracket brands regarding effectiveness of torque.[3,5,9,22,23,24] It is also worth emphasizing the importance of better understanding the particularities of each bracket in relation to the accuracy of their dimensions, as well as to verify what torque should be given to the wire for each case to be treated, so that a clinically effective torque can be performed in conjunction with the bracket chosen by the orthodontist.

CONCLUSIONS

Differences were observed in all torsions studied. Bioquick showed the lowest torque expression in all torsions tested; in contrast, Damon 3MX expressed the highest torque up to 36°. At 48°, In-Ovation R, Portia and Damon 3MX had similar torque moments.

When the torque range considered clinically effective was observed, it was found that Damon 3MX was the first to express clinically effective torque; in contrast, Bioquick was the last to express a clinically effective torque.

The connection system between wire/bracket (active, passive self-ligating or conventional with elastic ligature) seems not to interfere in final torque expression, the latter being dependent on the interaction between the wire and bracket chosen to be used in orthodontic mechanics.

Author contributions

Conceived and designed the study: EMF; Acquisition, analysis or interpretation: EMF, FPV, KMSF Drafting the work: EMF; Data collection: EMF, FPV; Wrote the article: EMF, JBF, RHC, KMSF; Critical revision of the article: FPV, JBF; Final approval of the article: FPV, JBF; Statistical analysis: RHC, KMSF.

REFERENCES

1. Rauch ED. Torque and its application to orthodontics. Am J Orthod. 1959 Nov 45(11):817-30.
2. Kapur R, Sinha PK, Nanda RS. Comparison of load transmission and bracket deformation between titanium and stainless steel brackets. Am J Orthod Dentofacial Orthop. 1999 Sep;116(3):275-8.
3. Meling TR, Odegaard J, Meling EO. On mechanical properties of square and rectangular stainless steel wires tested in torsion. Am J Orthod Dentofacial Orthop. 1997 Mar;111(3):310-20.
4. Odegaard J, Meling T, Meling E. An evaluation of the torsional moments developed in orthodontic applications. An in vitro study. Am J Orthod Dentofacial Orthop. 1994 Apr;105(4):392-400.
5. Sebanc J, Brantley WA, Pincsak JJ, Conover JP. Variability of effective root torque as a function of edge bevel on orthodontic and wires. Am J Orthod. 1984 Jul;86(1):43-51.
6. Balut N, Klapper L, Sandrik J, Bowman D. Variations in bracket placement in the preadjusted orthodontic appliance. Am J Orthod Dentofacial Orthop. 1992 Jul;102(1):62-7.
7. Badawi HM, Toogood RW, Carey JP, Heo G, Major PW. Torque expression of self-ligating brackets. Am J Orthod Dentofacial Orthop. 2008 May;133(5):721-8.
8. Miethke RR. Third order tooth movements with straight wire appliances. Influence of vestibular tooth crown morphology in the vertical plane. J Orofac Orthop. 1997;58(4):186-97.
9. Morina E, Keilig L, Jager A, Bourauel C. [Biomechanical analysis of orthodontic brackets with different closing mechanisms]. Biomed Tech (Berl). 2009 Apr;54(2):89-97.
10. Fansa M, Keilig L, Reimann S, Jager A, Bourauel C. The leveling effectiveness of self-ligating and conventional brackets for complex tooth malalignments. J Orofac Orthop. 2009 Jul;70(4):285-96.
11. Pandis N, Strigou S, Eliades T. Maxillary incisor torque with conventional and self-ligating brackets: a prospective clinical trial. Orthod Craniofac Res. 2006 Nov;9(4):193-8.
12. Rinchuse DJ, Miles PG. Self-ligating brackets: present and future. Am J Orthod Dentofacial Orthop. 2007 Aug;132(2):216-22.
13. Pandis N, Polychronopoulou A, Eliades T. Self-ligating vs conventional brackets in the treatment of mandibular crowding: a prospective clinical trial of treatment duration and dental effects. Am J Orthod Dentofacial Orthop. 2007 Aug;132(2):208-15.
14. Meling TR, Odegaard J. The effect of second-order couple on the application of torque. Am J Orthod Dentofacial Orthop. 1998 Mar;113(3):256-62.
15. Archambault A, Major TW, Carey JP, Heo G, Badawi H, Major PW. A comparison of torque expression between stainless steel, titanium molybdenum alloy, and copper nickel titanium wires in metallic self-ligating brackets. Angle Orthod. 2010 Sep;80(5):884-9.
16. Brauchli LM, Steineck M, Wichelhaus A. Active and passive self-ligation: a myth? Part 1: torque control. Angle Orthod. 2012 Jul;82(4):663-9.
17. Archambault A, Lacoursiere R, Badawi H, Major PW, Carey J, Flores-Mir C. Torque expression in stainless steel orthodontic brackets. A systematic review. Angle Orthod. 2010 Jan;80(1):201-10.
18. Hanson GH. The SPEED system: a report on the development of a new edgewise appliance. Am J Orthod. 1980 Sep;78(3):243-65.
19. Huang Y, Keilig L, Rahimi A, Reimann S, Eliades T, Jäger A, et al. Numeric modeling of torque capabilities of self-ligating and conventional brackets. Am J Orthod Dentofacial Orthop. 2009 Nov;136(5):638-43.
20. Major TW, Carey JP, Nobes DS, Heo G, Major PW. Mechanical effects of third-order movement in self-ligated brackets by the measurement of torque expression. Am J Orthod Dentofacial Orthop. 2011 Jan;139(1):e31-44.
21. Gioka C, Eliades T. Materials-induced variation in the torque expression of preadjusted appliances. Am J Orthod Dentofacial Orthop. 2004 Mar;125(3):323-8.
22. Cash AC, Good SA, Curtis RV, McDonald F. An evaluation of slot size in orthodontic brackets: are standards as expected? Angle Orthod. 2004 Aug;74(4):450-3.
23. Joch A, Pichelmayer M, Weiland F. Bracket slot and archwire dimensions: manufacturing precision and third order clearance. J Orthod. 2010 Dec;37(4):241-9.
24. Kapur-Wadhwa R. Physical and mechanical properties affecting torque control. J Clin Orthod. 2004 Jun;38(6):335-40; quiz 334.

3

Finite element study on modification of bracket base and its effects on bond strength

Tarulatha R. Shyagali[1], Deepak P. Bhayya[2], Chandralekha B. Urs[3], Shashikala Subramaniam[4]

Objective: This article aims to analyze the difference in stresses generated in the bracket-cement-tooth system by means of a peel load in single and double-mesh bracket bases using a three-dimensional finite element computer model. **Material and Methods:** A three-dimensional finite element model of the bracket-cement-tooth system was constructed and consisted of 40,536 bonds and 49,201 finite elements using a commercial mesh generating programmer (ANSYS 7.0). Both single and double-mesh bracket bases were modified by varying the diameter from 100-400 μm progressively, and the spacing between the mesh wires was kept at 300 μm for each diameter of wire. A peel load was applied on the model to study the stresses generated in different layers. **Results:** In case of double-mesh bracket base, there was reduction in stress generation at the enamel in comparison to single-mesh bracket base. There was no difference in stress generated at the bracket layer between single and double-mesh bracket bases. At the impregnated wire mesh (IWM), layer stresses increased as the wire diameter of the mesh increased. **Conclusion:** Results show that bracket design modification can improve bonding abilities and simultaneously reduce enamel damage while debonding. These facts may be used in bringing about the new innovative bracket designs for clinical use.

Keywords: Finite element analysis. Orthodontic brackets. Mechanical stress.

[1] Professor, Darshan Dental College and Hospital, Department of Orthodontics and Dentofacial Orthopedics, Udaipur, India.
[2] Professor, Darshan Dental College and Hospital, Loyara, Department of Pediatric and Preventive Dentistry, Udaipur, India.
[3] Former professor and head, Vaidehi Dental College and Hospital, Department of Orthodontics and Dentofacial Orthopedics, Bangalore, India.
[4] Professor, KGM Dental College and Hospital, Department of Orthodontics and Dentofacial Orthopedics, Kolar, India.

» The authors report no commercial, proprietary or financial interest in the products or companies described in this article.

Tarulatha R Shyagali
Quarter No 6, Darshan Dental College and Hospital Campus,
Loyara, Udaipur, Rajasthan, India. E -mail ID : drtarulatha@gmail.com

INTRODUCTION

The key to successful malocclusion correction is the application of sustained force. Force is applied to teeth via brackets, thus, brackets play a major role in the system of correction of malocclusion.

Bonding has been a boon granted to the branch of Orthodontics since its introduction by Buonocore.[1] It has solved the major problem of attaching brackets to teeth. Newman was the first to directly bond brackets to the enamel surface;[2,3] however, problems were persistent. As more and more adults started enjoying the benefits of Orthodontics, the problem of visibility of metal brackets surfaced.

An obvious choice to overcome this was the use of esthetic brackets (ceramic, plastic, etc.) and lingual Orthodontics, both of which had their own set of disadvantages and advantages. Ceramic brackets, having a chemical bond with teeth, posed the problem of enamel damage during debonding as well as increased brittleness leading to wing fracture.[4-8] In addition, there is the issue of frictional resistance and iatrogenic enamel damage.[9] Lingual Orthodontics can be performed in selected cases. Overtime, most disadvantages related to ceramic brackets were quite effectively addressed. Nevertheless, the technique never met the gold standard of metal brackets, as it clearly lacked their ductility. In order to overcome the issue of enamel damage caused by ceramic brackets debonding, many adhesive material[10] and debonding techniques[11] (laser operate debonding) have surfaced. Nevertheless, that again is an addition to the inventory, which can be an economical burden to orthodontists as well as patients. Thus, metal brackets still dominate the scene with their intact gold standard. With a view to rendering metal brackets more patient–friendly, their bulk was significantly reduced and mini brackets made their way into the field.

Logically speaking, reducing the bulk resulted in decreased surface area for bracket bonding, which significantly affects bond strength.[12] This has paved the way for researchers to study different bracket modifications so as to improve bond strength. Gradual evolution in the context of bracket material and mesh design is an inevitable change. Considering that the ideal bracket requirement does not change much, it should have the adequate bond strength to withstand the forces of the wire, in addition to causing minimal damage to the enamel while debonding. Meanwhile, it should not be bulky enough so as to compromise patient's esthetics.[13] Production of such a bracket is the requirement of the day.

Studying such complex designs *in vivo* is a time-consuming and tedious work. Virtual models are ideal to deal with complex set ups within time constraints and without much economic burden. To date, the most popular virtual modelling system prevalent in the field of Orthodontics is the finite element method (FEM).[14-18] FEM analyzes the stress distribution factor of different components, thus enabling researchers to understand the practicality of using certain models.

Studying stress distribution in different layers of bracket bonding systems, i.e bracket-cement-tooth system, may give us the insight into the potential possibility of producing an ideal bracket system. In this context, many studies explored the possibilities of bracket modification, including the double-mesh bracket base.[18-24] Double-mesh bracket studies have divided the double-mesh layers as coarse and fine mesh. These studies report that in the superficial layer of the double-mesh bracket, stress was reduced.[18] This fact did not put much light on the stress produced on the other layers of the bracket-cement-tooth interface. Presently, there is a need for a technological revolution aiming at achieving favorable clinical outcomes in the field of bracket mesh base design. The present article enjoys the benefits of the finite element method to construct a computerized three-dimensional virtual model of bracket-cement-tooth interface with a view to assessing and analyzing stress distribution produced by modifying the bracket base geometry in single-mesh bracket base, and to compare it with the double-mesh bracket base design using peel load, all of which to bring about the favorable bracket mesh base design.

MATERIAL AND METHODS

The geometric image of a maxillary first premolar was determined by taking 0.5-mm longitudinal sections of a representative tooth by means of computer tomography (General Electronics, USA). These sections were then transferred to AutoCAD software (Autodesk Inc., USA) to get the geometric model of the maxillary first premolar. The model generated was transferred to a finite element package in

IGES (initial graphics exchange specification) format. IGES files are neutral files that can support almost all CAD software and are also amenable for analysis.

Using digital measurements of these sections, the three-dimensional coordinates of the tooth were recorded and a finite element mesh was generated using a commercial mesh generating programmer (ANSYS 7.0). Only the area of the tooth required for bracket placement was generated and secured by appropriate boundary conditions. This helped to reduce the size of the overall model.

A maxillary first premolar bracket (MBT bracket system, Ortho Organizer) was modeled using the geometric measurements obtained by the digital vernier caliper. Apart from the tooth and bracket, an impregnated wire mesh (IWM) layer was constructed using previous data from the literature (Figs 1, 2, 3).[18,24,25] IWM is a layer where cement and metal mesh are joined or intermingled. All layers of the tooth-IWM-bracket system were kept linear, elastic, isotropic and homogeneous. Theory of composite material was applied to generate the properties of IWM layer as per the recommendation of earlier studies of similar nature (Table 1).[18,24,25]

The material parameters used in the computations are similar to those used in previous studies.[24,25] However, Poisson's ratio for IWM for each modification was calculated separately for single and double-mesh bracket base models, as depicted in Tables 2 and 3, respectively. The complete three-dimensional finite element model of the bracket-cement-tooth system consisted of 40,536 bonds and 49,201 finite elements (Fig 4). The mesh base is the crisscross of stainless steel wire with a gap between the wire for cement retention. The geometry of the mesh base was altered by increasing the mesh wire diameter sequentially from 100 μm to 400 μm consecutively, while spacing was kept constant at 300 μm.

The guidelines from a previous study were taken into consideration to prepare the double-mesh base geometry.[18] Each layer was homogenized separately before introducing them into the overall FE model.

To assess the stress generated by altering the geometry of the bracket mesh base, peel load of 1 N was used (Fig 4). The obtained results were tabulated and subjected to percentile calculation for comparison of single and double-mesh bracket bases for different layers of tooth-cement-bracket continuum.

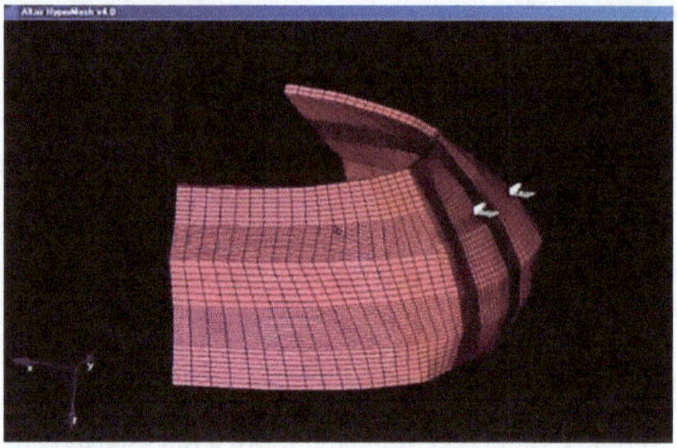

Figure 1 - Finite element model of enamel.

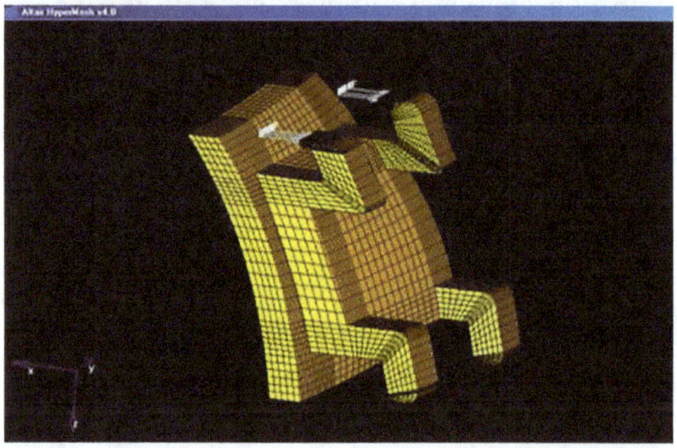

Figure 2 - Finite element model of bracket.

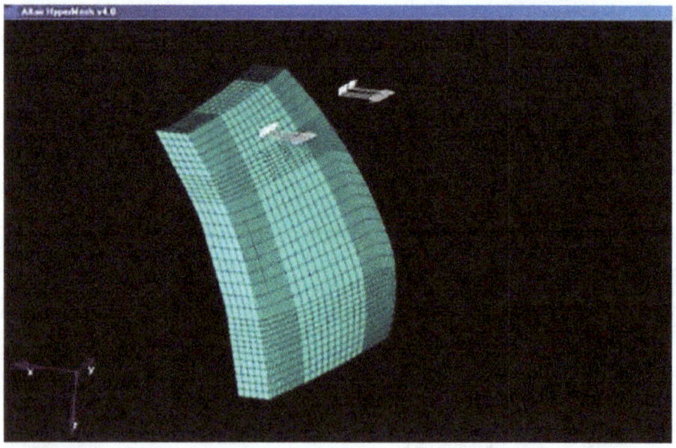

Figure 3 - Finite element model of IWM.

Table 1 - Material properties employed.

Material	Young's modulus (MPa)	Poisson's ratio
Enamel	46.890	0.30
Cement	11.721	0.21
Stainless steel	210.00	0.30

Table 2 - Material properties of IWM layer in single-mesh bracket base for different diameters and spacing.

Diameter (µm)	Spacing (µm)	Length (µm)	Width (µm)	Area (µm²)	Long. deflection	Lat. deflection	E	Long. strain	Lat. strain	Poisson's ratio
100	300	200	400	160000	1.18E-15	3.10E-16	1.059E+08	5.900E-18	7.750E-19	0.131
200	300	400	500	250000	1.32E-15	3.46E-16	1.212E+08	3.300E-18	6.920E-19	0.210
300	300	600	600	360000	1.22E-15	3.23E-16	1.366E+08	2.033E-18	5.383E-19	0.265
400	300	800	700	490000	1.07E-15	2.84E-16	1.526E+08	1.338E-18	4.057E-19	0.303

Table 3 - Material properties of IWM layer in double-mesh bracket base for different diameters and spacing.

Diameter (µm)	Spacing (µm)	Length (µm)	Width (µm)	Area (µm²)	Long. deflection	Lat. deflection	E	Long. strain	Lat. strain	Poisson's ratio
100	300	400	400	160000	2.04E-15	3.86E-16	1.225E+08	5.100E-18	9.650E-19	0.189
200	300	800	500	250000	2.09E-15	3.59E-16	1.531E+08	2.613E-18	7.180E-19	0.275
300	300	1200	600	360000	1.86E-15	3.21E-16	1.792E+08	1.550E-18	5.350E-19	0.345
400	300	1600	700	490000	1.61E-15	2.80E-16	2.028E+08	1.006E-18	4.000E-19	0.398

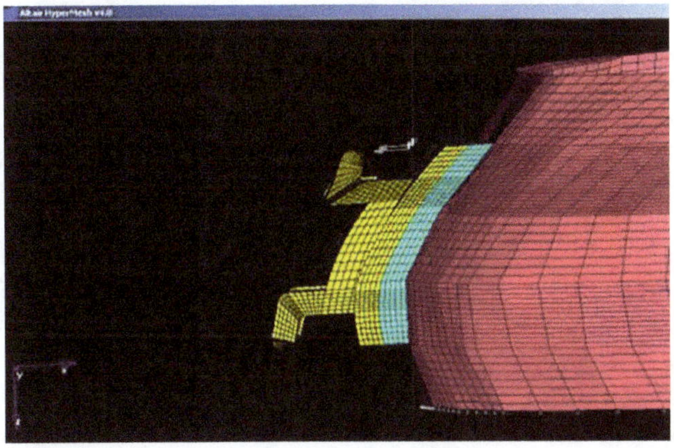

Figure 4 - Finite element model of the tooth-cement-bracket continuum.

RESULTS

The results are represented in the form of charts. Figure 5 represents the difference in the stresses generated at the enamel layer for single and double-mesh bracket bases. Stress was higher on enamel as the wire diameter decreased. The single mesh produced more stress on the enamel than the double-mesh bracket base.

The range of stresses for the IWM layer in single and double-mesh bracket bases is depicted in Figure 6. Stresses nearly remained the same for single and double-mesh bracket bases, but were high on IWM when wire diameter increased.

For the bracket layer of the single and double-mesh base model, stress remained constant, as presented in Figure 7. Stress ranged from 9.4 to 9.7 MPa and remained the same for both single and double-mesh bracket systems.

DISCUSSION

The study used a three-dimensional finite element model of the tooth-bracket-cement system to assess the stress generated by altering the mesh base design. A peel force of 1 N was applied and the stresses generated were registered.

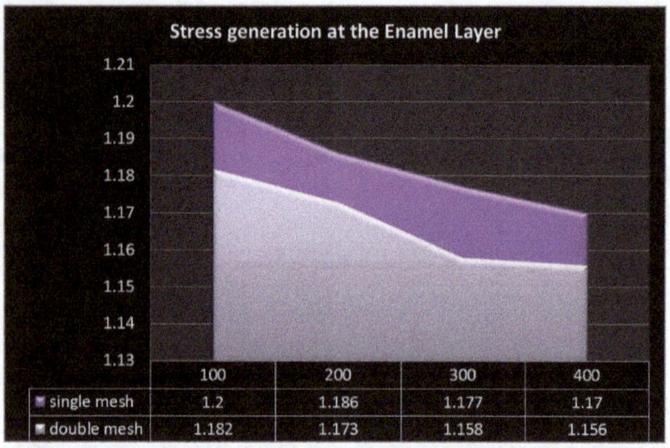

Figure 5 - Comparison of stress generated at the enamel layer for single- and double-mesh bracket bases.

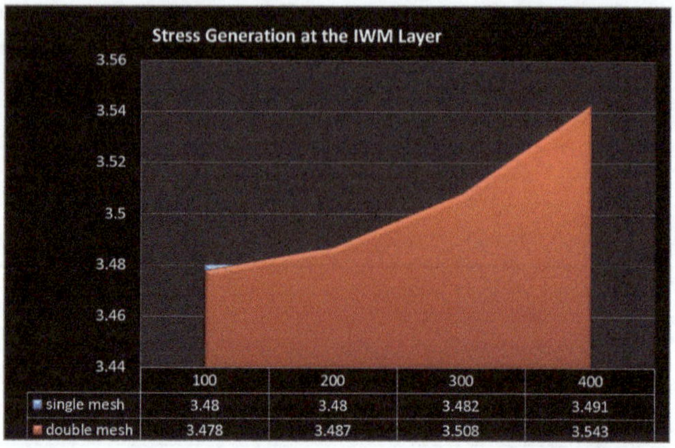

Figure 6 - Comparison of stress generated at the IWM layer for single and double-mesh bracket bases.

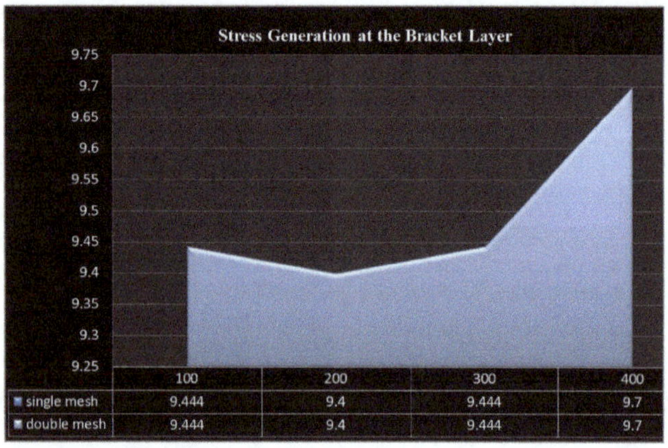

Figure 7 - Comparison of stress generated at the bracket layer for single- and double-mesh bracket bases.

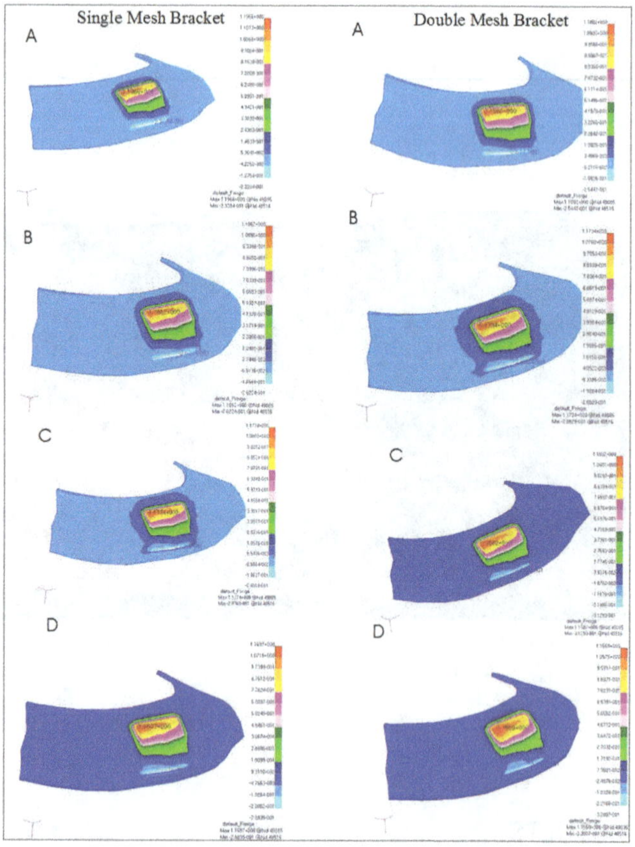

Figure 8 - Stress on enamel at different wire diameters of the mesh for single and double-mesh bracket bases.

The stress generated in the enamel layer of the single-mesh bracket base model decreased progressively as the diameter of the mesh wire increased (Fig 8). As the wire diameter of the mesh base increased, the surface area also increased, thus, inuring the distribution of force evenly over the large surface. This is probably the reason behind the decrease in stress on enamel, as the wire diameter of the bracket mesh base increases.

A similar phenomenon was noticed in the double-mesh bracket base at the enamel layer (Fig 8). However, when single and double-mesh bracket bases were compared, the stress in the double-mesh bracket base at the enamel remained low in comparison to the single-mesh bracket modification. This assures less damage to the enamel layer while orthodontic bracket debonding procedure is carried out. Double-mesh bracket design has greater surface area in comparison to the single-mesh bracket base, thus, stress distribution on the mesh is generous, which ensures less stress concentration on the enamel.

Nevertheless, a previous study checking the efficiency of different bracket designs showed that double-mesh bracket produced greater bond strength in comparison to other bracket designs.[26]

Of all the different layers of the FEM model applied to the bracket-cement-tooth continuum, the stress generated at the bracket remained high for both single and double-mesh bracket bases. The point of force application is on the bracket and, owing to this factor, the stress generated at the bracket was greater.

In case of an IWM layer, stress increased progressively with the increase in wire diameter for both models. As wire diameter increased, the part of the impregnated wire mesh constituted by the cement decreased and there was a smaller area of cement impregnating the wire mesh, which can take up the stress. This criterion led to the increase in stress at the IWM layer as the wire mesh diameter increased.

Further, previous researchers have shown that the success of bracket base design in increasing bonding strength is not only dependent on the bracket base, but also on the type of bonding agent selected. Additionally, certain brackets performed well with a particular brand of bonding agent.[27]

When one has the bird view of the stress generated in both models, it is evident that maximum stresses were noticed at the bracket, followed by the IWM layer of the tooth-cement-bracket continuum. This indicates the possible fracture site of the continuum when the debonding procedure is performed. Nevertheless, the above point is advantageous for the orthodontist, as one can safeguard the enamel wear and tear, which ultimately is the concern of every orthodontist.

As the wire diameter increased, the possible retentive unit area for the cement decreased and the load was taken up by the increased surface area of the wire, which in turn produced less impact on the enamel. With all due respect to the above finding, one has to ponder around the fact that the profile of the bracket might increase significantly with double-mesh design.

The results of the present study indicate that altering the mesh geometry affects the bonding strength of the bracket. Both contrasting and accordance evidence was found in earlier studies of similar nature.[21,23] Nevertheless, for better bonding, with smaller chances of enamel damage during the debonding procedure, double-mesh bracket base can be an ideal choice.

A previous study reports that single and double-mesh bracket bases had comparable bonding strength and bracket failure modes.[19] This study is quite contrasting to the findings of the present study, as there existed a difference in stress noted in different layers of the tooth-cement-bracket system.

Other than wire diameter and wire spacing, the researchers have identified a number of variables in the bracket mesh which might exert some influence on the bonding strength of the bracket, namely: weld spots, weld spurs, location of weld spots and air entrapment.[20] While the present study mainly emphasized the difference in the behavior of single and double-mesh bracket bases, the above mentioned variables should be taken into consideration and a study of more extensive nature should be conducted.

CONCLUSION

Modifying the bracket mesh base by varying the diameter of the wire mesh significantly influences the amount of stress generated in the bracket-cement-tooth continuum.

The double-mesh bracket base can be an answer for the potential reduction of enamel wear and tear during debonding.

Further in-depth investigations are needed on other bracket base mesh designs and related variables influencing them, as there are relatively few studies in this regard. This study can be used as reference for future investigation.

In today's world of inventory abundance, the orthodontist should be well equipped with evidence-based material to be for individual cases. The present article tried to address past unsolved issues of bonding strength and found the solution which will guide the clinician to choose the best bracket mesh base for efficient bonding with least enamel damage possible during debonding processes.

REFERENCES

1. Buonocore MG. A simple method of increasing the adhesion of acrylic filling materials to enamel surfaces. J Dent Res. 1955;34(6):849-53.
2. Newman GV. Epoxy adhesives for orthodontic attachments: progress report. Am J Orthod.1965;12:90-1.
3. Newman GV. The effects of adhesive systems on tooth surfaces. Am J Orthod. 1971;59(1):67-75.
4. Bishara SE, Olsen ME, Von Wald L. Evaluation of debonding characteristics of a new collapsible ceramic bracket. Am J Orthod Dentofacial Orthop. 1997;112(5):552-9.
5. Sinha PK, Nanda RS. The effect of different bonding and debonding techniques on debonding ceramic orthodontic brackets. Am J Orthod Dentofacial Orthop. 1997;112(2):132-7.
6. Theodorakopoulou LP, Sadowsky PL, Jacobson A, Lacefield W Jr. Evaluation of the debonding characteristics of 2 ceramic brackets: an in vitro study. Am J Orthod Dentofacial Orthop. 2004;125(3):329-36.
7. Flores DA, Caruso JM, Scott GE, Jeiroudi MT. The fracture strength of ceramic brackets: a comparative study. Angle Orthod. 1990 Winter;60(4):269-76.
8. Holt MH, Nanda RS, Duncanson MG. Fracture resistance of ceramic brackets during arch-wire torsion. Am J Orthod Dentofacial Orthop. 1991;99(4):287-93.
9. Russell JS. Current products and practice aesthetic orthodontic brackets. J Orthod. 2005;32:146-63.
10. Ryu C, Namura Y, Tsuruoka T, Hama T, Kaji K, Shimizu N. The use of easily debondable orthodontic adhesives with ceramic brackets. Dent Mater J. 2011;30(5):642-7.
11. Ahrari F, Heravi F, Fekrazad R, Farzanegan F, Nakhaei S. Does ultra-pulse CO2 laser reduces the risk of enamel damage during debonding of ceramic brackets? Lasers Med Sci. 2012;27(3):567-74.
12. Sharma-Sayal SK, Rossouw PE, Kulkarni GV, Titley KC. The influence of orthodontic bracket base design on shear bond strength. Am J Orthod Dentofacial Orthop. 2003;124(1):74-82.
13. Oesterle LJ, Shellhart CW, Fisher A. Effect of primer precuring on the shear bond strength of orthodontic brackets. Am J Orthod Dentofacial Orthop. 2004;126(6):699-702.
14. McGuiness NJP, Wilson A, Jones ML, Middleton J, Robertson NR. Stresses induced by edgewise appliances in the periodontal ligament: a finite element study. Angle Orthod. 1992;62(1):15-22.
15. Calao E, Becerra F, Ossa J, Enríquez C, Fresneda E. Initial stress differences between sliding and sectional mechanics with an endosseous implant as anchorage: a 3-dimensional finite element analysis. Angle Orthod. 2001;71(4):247-56.
16. Geramy A. Initial stress produced in the periodontal membrane by orthodontic loads in the presence of varying loss of alveolar bone: a three-dimensional finite element analysis. Eur J Orthod. 2002;24(1):21-33.
17. Jafari A, Shetty KS, Kumar M. Study of stress distribution and displacement of various craniofacial structures following application of orthopedic forces: a three-dimensional fem study. Angle Orthod. 2003;73(1):12-20.
18. Knox J, Kralj B, Hubsch P, Middleton J, Jones ML. An evaluation of the quality of orthodontic attachment offered by single- and double-mesh bracket bases using the finite element method of stresses analysis. Angle Orthod. 2001;71(2):149-55.
19. Bishara SE, Manal MA. Soliman, Oonsombat C, Laffoon JF, Ajlouni R. The effect of variation in Mesh-Base Design on the shear bond strength of orthodontic brackets. Angle Orthod. 2004;74(3):400-4.
20. Maijer R, Smith DC. Variables influencing the bond strength of metal orthodontic bracket bases. Am J Orthod. 1981;79(1):20-34.
21. Cucu M, Driessen CH, Ferreira PD. The influence of orthodontic bracket base diameter and mesh size on bond strength. SADJ. 2002;57(1):16-20.
22. Fox NA, McCabe JF, Buckley JG. A critique of bond strength testing in orthodontics. Br J Orthod. 1994;21(1):33-43.
23. Smith NR, Reynolds IR. A comparison of three bracket bases: an in vitro study. Br J Orthod. 1991;18(1):29-35.
24. Millett DT, McCabe JF. Orthodontic bonding with Glass Ionomer cement: a review. Eur J Orthod.1996;18:385-99.
25. Yettram AL, Wright KW, Pickard HM. Finite element stress analysis of the crown of normal and restored teeth. J Dent Res. 1976;55(6):1004-11.
26. Wang WN, Li CH, Chou TH, Wang DDH, Lin LH, Lin CT. Bond strength of various bracket base designs. Am J Orthod Dentofacial Orthop. 2004;125(1):65-70.
27. Knox J, Hubsch P, Middleton J. The Influence of Bracket Base Design on the Strength of the Bracket–Cement Interface. J Orthod. 2000;27(3):249-54.

4

In vitro study of color stability of polycrystalline and monocrystalline ceramic brackets

Cibele Braga de Oliveira[1], Luiz Guilherme Martins Maia[2], Ary Santos-Pinto[3], Luiz Gonzaga Gandini Júnior[3]

Objective: The aim of this *in vitro* study was to analyze color stability of monocrystalline and polycrystalline ceramic brackets after immersion in dye solutions. **Methods:** Seven ceramic brackets of four commercial brands were tested: Two monocrystalline and two polycrystalline. The brackets were immersed in four dye solutions (coffee, red wine, Coke and black tea) and in artificial saliva for the following times: 24 hours, 7, 14 and 21 days, respectively. Color changes were measured by a spectrophotometer. Data were assessed by Multivariate Profile Analysis, Analysis of Variance (ANOVA) and Multiple Comparison Tests of means. **Results:** There was a perceptible change of color in all ceramic brackets immersed in coffee (ΔE^* Allure = 7.61, Inspire Ice = 6.09, Radiance = 6.69, Transcend = 7.44), black tea (ΔE^* Allure = 6.24, Inspire Ice = 5.21, Radiance = 6.51, Transcend = 6.14) and red wine (ΔE^* Allure = 6.49, Inspire Ice = 4.76, Radiance = 5.19, Transcend = 5.64), but no change was noticed in Coke and artificial saliva ($\Delta E < 3.7$). **Conclusion:** Ceramic brackets undergo color change when exposed to solutions of coffee, black tea and red wine. However, the same crystalline structure, either monocrystalline or polycrystalline, do not follow the same or a similar pattern in color change, varying according to the bracket fabrication, which shows a lack of standardization in the manufacturing process. Coffee dye produced the most marked color changes after 21 days of immersion for most ceramic brackets evaluated.

Keywords: Color. Ceramics. Orthodontic brackets.

[1] MSc in Orthodontics, State University of São Paulo (UNESP).
[2] Professor, Department of Orthodontics, UNIT/SE.
[3] Full professor, Department of Orthodontics, State University of São Paulo (UNESP).

Cibele Braga de Oliveira
Universidade Estadual Paulista, UNESP, Departamento de Ortodontia
Rua Humaitá, 1680 – Araraquara/SP — Brazil
CEP: 14.801-385 – E-mail: cibeleodonto@yahoo.com.br

» The authors report no commercial, proprietary or financial interest in the products or companies described in this article.

INTRODUCTION

The first esthetic brackets appeared in the 70's and were made from polycarbonate, a plastic material. Although these brackets were reasonably esthetic, this material did not present suitable properties for clinical use. Several studies showed clinical problems such as deformation and structural weakness, poor adhesion and poor stain resistance during treatment.[1,2,3]

In the mid-1980s, other types of material were tested to meet the esthetic needs of the orthodontic market, and that was when esthetic ceramic brackets appeared. These brackets are mainly made from aluminum oxide and are available in two forms according to the manufacturing process: polycrystalline or monocrystalline.[4,5]

Polycrystalline or alumina polycrystalline brackets are made of aluminum oxide crystals fused at high temperatures (near 1950°C).[6] Monocrystalline brackets are made of a single crystal produced from the combination of particles of aluminum oxide fused at a higher temperature (2100°C) and cooled slowly, thus enabling thorough control of crystallization.[4,7]

Thus, the manufacturing process produces translucent and nontranslucent ceramic brackets. Monocrystalline brackets are included in the translucent brackets group while polycrystalline brackets are nontranslucent.[8] The translucency of monocrystalline brackets is due to the structure of a single crystal that provides passage of light. Polycrystalline brackets are not translucent because their structure presents lack of boundaries between the crystals and impurities incorporated during the manufacturing process, thereby hindering passage of light.[9]

To have a good esthetic appearance, nontranslucent brackets need to be similar in color and fluorescence to the underlying tooth, whereas translucent brackets need to have sufficient translucency so as to allow the color and fluorescence of the tooth to pass through them. However, it is essential that both have good color stability.[8]

Even if esthetics is the only advantage of ceramic brackets in relation to metal brackets, they are not color stable in the long term. As reported by some authors, the color of these accessories changes in the oral environment due to staining from substances containing pigments commonly found in food and drinks.[3,6,10,11,12]

Nevertheless, only a few studies have been conducted to investigate the color changes and the factors that lead to such changes. Therefore, this study aims to analyze *in vitro* the color stability of monocrystalline and polycrystalline esthetic ceramic brackets after immersion in dye solutions commonly present in food and drinks in order to know if the crystal structure of these brackets follow a similar pattern of color change.

MATERIAL AND METHODS

The sample comprised maxillary right central incisors ceramic brackets, slot size 0.022 x 0.028-in in Roth prescription. Four commercial brands were selected: Two brands were monocrystalline brackets — Inspire Ice from Ormco® (Orange, California) and Radiance from American Orthodontics® (Sheboygan, Wisconsin); and two were polycrystalline brackets — Allure MB from GAC® (Bohemia, New York) and Transcend from 3M Unitek® (Monrovia, California). To prevent the glue surfaces of different brands from interfering in the staining process, all surfaces were worn with a diamond drill bit. Seven brackets of each brand were tested.

The brackets were immersed in solutions of coffee, dry red wine, Coke, black tea and artificial saliva (control group) (Table 1). Each one of these solutions was distributed into glass chambers with partitions to separate the different brands of brackets. These containers were placed in an incubator at a temperature of 37°C wrapped in black plastic bags to eliminate the interference of light. The solutions were changed every 24 hours and their pH was measured with a pH meter (Model 8010, Qualxtron) at each change to check whether it remained the same.

The color parameters of brackets were measured at the following times: T_0 (initial measurement), T_1, T_2, T_3 and T_4 (brackets immersed in dye solution for 24 hours, 7, 14 and 21 days, respectively). Before each color reading, brackets were washed with distilled water and blotted dried to remove any residual waste from the dyes on the brackets.

Color measurements of each group of brackets were obtained using a portable reflectance spectrophotometer Spectro-guide (Byk Gardner®, Columbia, USA). Spectro-guide measures the intensity of each wavelength of light reflected by the sample when illuminated by a polychromatic light (illuminant D65) emitted from the device at an angle of 45°. Light reflected from the sample is captured by a viewing angle of 0°. The measuring aperture diameter size was 3 mm. Tristimulus values (L★, a★ and b★) were supplied by the device from the captured light.

Table 1 - Solutions, brands, pH values and preparation methods.

Solution	pH	Brand	Preparation
Coffee	5	Nescafé (Nestlé, Brazil Ltda, Brazil)	Solution prepared with 50 g of instant coffee added to 200 ml of boiling distilled water.
Red wine	3.3	Dry red wine (Canção - Serra Gaúcha, Rio Grande do Sul, Brazil)	Solution ready for consumption
Black tea	5.2	Black tea sachet (Leão Junior S.A., Brazil)	Solution prepared with one black tea sachet immersed in 200 ml of boiling distilled water
Coke	2.4	Coke (Coca-Cola Co.)	Solution ready for consumption
Artificial saliva	7	Artificial saliva (Farmácia Santa Paula – Araraquara, São Paulo, Brazil).	Prepared solution (neutral pH, tasteless and odorless)

* All solutions were distributed into containers at ambient temperature.

Potential color changes of brackets were measured in accordance with the Commission Internationale de l'Eclairage (CIE) L★, a★, b★ (LAB) color scale.[13] This color measurement system[14] quantitatively determines color by using three parameters (L★, a★ and b★). On the CIELAB color scale, L★ is a measure of brightness of an object. It is quantified on a scale in which black has a L★ value of zero; and light, which is totally reflected, has a L★ value of 100. On the same scale, a★ accounts for the amount of red (+ a★) and green (-a★), whereas b★ accounts for the amount of yellow (+ b★) and blue (- b★). Color change (ΔE★) was calculated using the equation: $\Delta E^\star = [(\Delta L^\star)^2 + (\Delta a^\star)^2 + (\Delta b^\star)^2]^{1/2}$. Changes in color parameters ΔL★, Δa★ and Δb★ were obtained by subtracting the final values from the baseline (T_0).

For color measurements, brackets were positioned in a matrix of white silicone rubber from Redelease® (4 matrices were made for the four brands of brackets) coupled to a positioner where the spectrophotometer was embedded. Thus, the brackets and the spectrophotometer were always in the same position for all measurements.

Statistical analysis

To evaluate the error of the method, two measurements were made for each variable. Reproducibility was assessed by means of the Intraclass Correlation Coefficient (ICC).

Multivariate Profile Analysis, carried out by means of the Pillai Trace test, was used to evaluate the effect of time.

Analysis of Variance (ANOVA) with one classification criterion and Bonferroni Test of Multiple Comparison of means were used to define any statistical difference of color change between brands and between solutions. These analyses were preceded by a test of homogeneity of variances. Should homogeneity of variances be rejected, ANOVA was replaced by Brown-Forshyte test and the Multiple Comparison Tests of means was conducted with the Tamhane test.

The statistical software SPSS version 16.0 (Statistical Package for Social Sciences, SPSS Inc., Chicago, IL, USA) was used to tabulate and analyze data. Statistical significance was adopted at 95% confidence interval.

RESULTS

Results of intraclass correlation coefficients (ICC) revealed that the method for measuring the color of ceramic brackets was effective. A high degree of reproducibility as obtained for all parameters of color (L★, a★, b★), thus indicating a negligible method error (range limit top and bottom of the ICC: 0.8 to 1.00).

Table 2 presents the results of the multivariate tests for assessing color change over time. Results show that color of ceramic brackets changes over time. Furthermore, there is no similarity of color change over time among all brackets. A significant difference in bracket staining between solutions was also observed over immersion time. Thus, color change over time depends on a brand-solution combination.

Comparative study of ceramic brackets staining by solution and immersion time

Bracket brands (two monocrystalline and two polycrystalline) were assessed for color change produced by each solution within each time period. Results are shown in Table 3 and Figure 1.

Table 2 - Pillai trace multivariate test for significance of color change. Intra individual factor = time.

Effect	Pillai trace	F test				Power
		F	df1	df2	p	
Time	0.945	1419.643	3	250	<0.001	> 0.999
Time * brand	0.776	29.296	9	756	<0.001	> 0.999
Time * solution	1.441	58.208	12	756	<0.001	> 0.999
Time * brand * solution	0.56	4.816	36	756	<0.001	> 0.999

Note: df1 = numerator degrees of freedom; df2 = denominator degrees of freedom.

Table 3 - Mean and standard deviation of color change (ΔE*) dof ceramic brackets in each solution and time, result of the Variance Analysis and multiple comparison of means.

Time of immersion	ALLURE ΔE* Mean ± SD	INSPIRE ICE ΔE* Mean ± SD	RADIANCE ΔE* Mean ± SD	TRANSCEND ΔE* Mean ± SD	ANOVA F	ANOVA P
			ARTIFICIAL SALIVA			
24 hours	$1.26^{A} \pm 0.20$	$1.07^{AB} \pm 0.13$	$0.81^{B} \pm 0.47$	$0.29^{C} \pm 0.14$	16.79	0.000
7 days	$1.27A^{B} \pm 0.27$	$1.10^{A} \pm 0.32$	$1.68^{B} \pm 0.48$	$0.41^{C} \pm 0.09$	19.35	0.000
14 days	$1.43^{A} \pm 0.29$	$1.06^{A} \pm 0.12$	$1.37^{A} \pm 0.40$	$0.44^{B} \pm 0.17$	20.09	0.000
21 days	$1.45^{A} \pm 0.30$	$0.46^{B} \pm 0.10$	$1.82^{C} \pm 0.30$	$0.64^{B} \pm 0.17$	53.58	0.000
			COKE			
24 hours*	$1.40^{A} \pm 0.21$	$2.22^{B} \pm 0.10$	$1.29^{A} \pm 0.14$	$1.65^{AB} \pm 0.78$	7.01	0.014
7 days	$2.43^{A} \pm 0.20$	$2.02^{B} \pm 0.21$	$2.29^{AB} \pm 0.13$	$1.53^{C} \pm 0.30$	23.03	0.000
14 days	$2.50^{A} \pm 0.33$	$2.13^{BC} \pm 0.19$	$2.43^{AC} \pm 0.18$	$1.89^{B} \pm 0.13$	11.11	0.000
21 days	$2.63^{A} \pm 0.21$	$2.02^{B} \pm 0.25$	$2.48^{A} \pm 0.18$	$1.89^{B} \pm 0.18$	20.61	0.000
			COFFEE			
24 hours	2.28 ± 0.27	2.44 ± 0.18	2.16 ± 0.34	2.47 ± 0.24	2.14	0.126
7 days	$5.16^{A} \pm 0.48$	$3.57^{B} \pm 0.34$	$5.33^{A} \pm 0.30$	$5.05^{A} \pm 0.23$	37.75	0.000
14 days	$5.47^{A} \pm 0.32$	$4.97^{B} \pm 0.37$	$5.91^{A} \pm 0.34$	$5.94^{A} \pm 0.22$	14.44	0.000
21 days	$7.61^{A} \pm 0.44$	$6.09^{B} \pm 0.38$	$6.69^{C} \pm 0.42$	$7.44^{A} \pm 0.31$	22.59	0.000
			BLACK TEA			
24 hours	$0.99^{A} \pm 0.24$	$1.74^{B} \pm 0.22$	$1.27^{A} \pm 0.25$	$1.19^{A} \pm 0.15$	14.84	0.000
7 days	$3.23^{A} \pm 0.34$	$2.17^{B} \pm 0.20$	$3.51^{A} \pm 0.24$	$3.15^{A} \pm 0.13$	41.09	0.000
14 days	$4.77^{A} \pm 0.23$	$4.29^{B} \pm 0.28$	$5.44^{C} \pm 0.24$	$4.73^{A} \pm 0.30$	22.72	0.000
21 days	$6.24^{A} \pm 0.39$	$5.21^{B} \pm 0.38$	$6.51^{A} \pm 0.20$	$6.14^{A} \pm 0.39$	18.42	0.000
			RED WINE			
24 hours*	$3.07^{A} \pm 0.51$	$3.62^{A} \pm 0.27$	$1.83^{B} \pm 0.27$	$2.04^{B} \pm 0.14$	47.30	0.000
7 days	$5.21^{A} \pm 0.44$	$3.63^{B} \pm 0.39$	$4.24^{C} \pm 0.43$	$3.50^{B} \pm 0.24$	28.84	0.000
14 days	$5.76^{A} \pm 0.33$	$4.53^{B} \pm 0.57$	$5.26^{AC} \pm 0.21$	$4.91^{BC} \pm 0.29$	13.67	0.000
21 days	$6.49^{A} \pm 0.47$	$4.76^{B} \pm 0.69$	$5.19^{BC} \pm 0.31$	$5.64^{C} \pm 0.33$	16.94	0.000

Notes: 1) In times marked with a *, brands are not equal. In this case, ANOVA was replaced by Brown-Forsythe test. 2) Same letters account for statistically similar means. Letters are not displayed when the result of ANOVA was not significant or when multiple comparison of means was not able to detect different means.

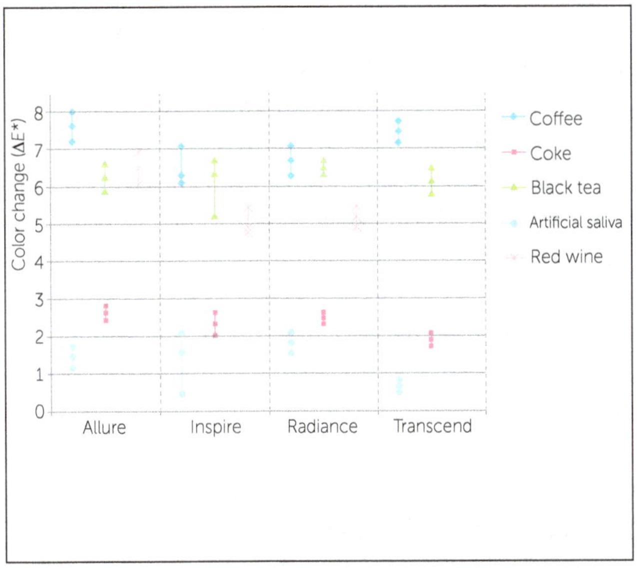

Figure 1 - Mean values and 95% confidence intervals of color change by brand in coffee, black tea, red wine, Coke and artificial saliva solutions.

There was an overall pattern of increasing color change for all brands. However, brackets with the same crystal formation do not follow the same or similar patterns in terms of color change. In other words, monocrystalline or polycrystalline structures do not interfere in how brackets are stained. Furthermore, Inspire Ice bracket had the lowest color change mean after 21 days.

Comparative study of dye solutions for color change produced on brackets within each immersion time.

In this analysis, solutions were compared for color changes produced on brackets of each brand tested within each time period, as shown in Table 4.

Color change was considered clinically significant only for values of $\Delta E^{\star} > 3.7$.[15,16,17] Thus, artificial saliva and Coke solutions did not produce major changes

Table 4 - Mean and standard deviation of color change (ΔE*) produced by solutions on ceramic brackets over time; result of Variance Analysis and multiple comparison of means.

Time of immersion	ARTIFICIAL SALIVA ΔE* Mean ± SD	COKE ΔE* Mean ± SD	COFFEE ΔE* Mean ± SD	BLACK TEA ΔE* Mean ± SD	RED WINE ΔE* Mean ±SD	ANOVA F	ANOVA P
			ALLURE				
24 hours	$1.26^{A} \pm 0.2$	$1.4^{A} \pm 0.21$	$2.28^{B} \pm 0.27$	$0.99^{A} \pm 0.24$	$3.07^{B} \pm 0.51$	53.53	0.000
7 days	$1.27^{A} \pm 0.27$	$2.43^{B} \pm 0.2$	$5.16^{C} \pm 0.48$	$3.23^{D} \pm 0.34$	$5.21^{C} \pm 0.44$	158.86	0.000
14 days*	$1.43^{A} \pm 0.29$	$2.5^{B} \pm 0.33$	$5.47^{C} \pm 0.32$	$4.77^{D} \pm 0.23$	$5.76^{C} \pm 0.33$	280.48	0.000
21 days	$1.45^{A} \pm 0.3$	$2.63^{B} \pm 0.21$	$7.61^{C} \pm 0.44$	$6.24^{D} \pm 0.39$	$6.49^{D} \pm 0.47$	359.29	0.000
			INSPIRE ICE				
24 hours	$1.07^{A} \pm 0.13$	$2.22^{B} \pm 0.1$	$2.44^{B} \pm 0.18$	$1.74^{C} \pm 0.22$	$3.62^{D} \pm 0.27$	173.66	0.000
7 days*	$1.1^{A} \pm 0.32$	$2.02^{B} \pm 0.21$	$3.57^{C} \pm 0.34$	$2.17^{B} \pm 0.2$	$3.63^{C} \pm 0.39$	90.93	0.000
14 days*	$1.06^{A} \pm 0.12$	$2.13^{B} \pm 0.19$	$4.97^{C} \pm 0.37$	$4.29^{D} \pm 0.28$	$4.53^{CD} \pm 0.57$	173.26	0.000
21 days	$0.46^{A} \pm 0.1$	2.02B ± 0.25	$6.09^{C} \pm 0.38$	$5.21^{D} \pm 0.38$	$4.76^{D} \pm 0.69$	233.33	0.000
			RADIANCE				
24 hours	$0.81^{A} \pm 0.47$	$1.29^{BCD} \pm 0.14$	$2.16^{B} \pm 0.34$	$1.27^{C} \pm 0.25$	$1.83^{D} \pm 0.27$	33.9	0.000
7 days	$1.68^{A} \pm 0.48$	$2.29^{B} \pm 0.13$	$5.33^{C} \pm 0.3$	$3.51^{D} \pm 0.24$	$4.24^{E} \pm 0.43$	497.23	0.000
14 days	$1.37^{A} \pm 0.4$	$2.43^{B} \pm 0.18$	$5.91^{C} \pm 0.34$	$5.44^{D} \pm 0.24$	$5.26^{D} \pm 0.21$	706.24	0.000
21 days*	$1.82^{A} \pm 0.3$	$2.48^{B} \pm 0.18$	$6.69^{C} \pm 0.42$	$6.51^{D} \pm 0.2$	$5.19^{E} \pm 0.31$	713.58	0.000
			TRANSCEND				
24 hours	$0.29^{A} \pm 0.14$	$1.65^{A} \pm 0.78$	$2.47^{B} \pm 0.24$	$1.19^{A} \pm 0.15$	$2.04^{B} \pm 0.14$	19.64	0.000
7 days*	$0.41^{A} \pm 0.09$	$1.53^{B} \pm 0.3$	$5.05^{C} \pm 0.23$	$3.15^{D} \pm 0.13$	$3.5^{E} \pm 0.24$	131.54	0.000
14 days	$0.44^{A} \pm 0.17$	$1.89^{B} \pm 0.13$	$5.94^{C} \pm 0.22$	$4.73^{D} \pm 0.3$	$4.91^{D} \pm 0.29$	358.04	0.000
21 days	$0.64^{A} \pm 0.17$	$1.89^{B} \pm 0.18$	$7.44^{C} \pm 0.31$	$6.14^{C} \pm 0.39$	$5.64^{D} \pm 0.33$	415.68	0.000

Note: 1) In times marked with a *, brands are not equal. In this case ANOVA was replaced by Brown-Forsythe test. 2) Same letters account for statistically similar means. Letters are not displayed when the result of ANOVA was not significant or when multiple comparison of means was not able to detect different means.

distinguished by the naked eye. Conversely, coffee, black tea and red wine promoted visible changes, in general, from the 14th day of immersion on.

Coffee dye solution produced the most marked color changes after 21 days of immersion for most brackets, except for Transcend brackets that, despite having the highest average, were statistically similar to black tea.

DISCUSSION

The results of this study led to the conclusion that all ceramic brackets change in color. However, brackets with the same crystal formation did not follow the same or similar patterns of color change when exposed to the same dye solutions under the same conditions. Thus, the degree of staining was different in several brands, and monocrystalline or polycrystalline structure did not affect staining, thereby showing that esthetic behavior depends on the bracket manufacturer.

In the literature, there are few studies about color changes of different esthetic ceramic brackets after immersion in dye solutions. According to them,[16-19] the color of ceramic brackets changes over time when exposed to potentially dye solutions commonly present in people's diet. In addition, staining is cumulative, it increases as the time of exposure to the coloring elements increases. Nevertheless, only a few studies were comparable with the results of this study, given that most of them compare ceramic and plastic brackets.

Among them, a recent work[19] obtained similar findings to our study. The authors confirmed that the crystal structure of ceramic brackets has no effect on staining. This conclusion was obtained after confirming that Inspire Ice and Radiance, two monocrystalline brackets, had the lowest and highest values of color change, respectively.

Other authors[20] are in agreement with these findings. They report that brackets with the same composition made by different manufacturers had different behaviors in color change. This shows a discrepancy in the manufacturing process of brackets and its influence on their esthetic performance.

Only one research[16] yielded opposite results. According to the authors, color stability of monocrystalline and polycrystalline ceramic brackets remained statistically equal after 14 days. Nevertheless, color was measured at the base brackets worn by drill, thereby not corresponding to the actual surface area exposed to the oral environment or to the entire surface conditions produced by the manufacturer.

According to Yu and Lee,[20] variation in staining between brackets with the same crystalline formation can be explained by lack of evidence proving that brackets classified within the same composition category, but made by different manufacturers, are actually made of the same material. Moreover, they also raised the possibility that size, shape and roughness could be the cause of this divergence in the optical properties of ceramic brackets. Lee[15] corroborates the aforementioned work by asserting that bracket surface, size and type of accessories may influence color stability . He also suggests that further studies on the influence of surface on color stability be conducted in order to yield results that can be used to develop esthetic brackets with improved color stability. However, there is no scientific evidence supporting these theories.

For the present study, Inspire Ice bracket had the lowest mean value of color change in most solutions. However, there was a variation in staining, depending on the interaction between the bracket brand and solution. For this reason, we cannot determine which bracket has the best or worst color stability. These results confirm previous studies[16,19,20] that assessed staining of ceramic brackets and also found many levels of staining, depending on the solution assessed.

The clinical relevance of color changes in the ceramic brackets should also be addressed in terms of dye potential. For Cosmetic Dentistry, color change greater than 2 is already visible for all observers.[21] Nevertheless, we adopted a parameter of 3.7. This value is based on the limits of color change that are clinically visible and used in studies with ceramic facets [22] and esthetic brackets.[15,16]

Considering the value of $\Delta E^\star > 3.7$ as clinically significant staining, artificial saliva and Coke did not produce color changes that were perceptible to the naked eye. Conversely, coffee, black tea and red wine produced visible changes ($\Delta E^\star > 3.7$) from the 14th day of immersion on. Coffee solution produced the most marked color changes for all brackets after 21 days of immersion, except for Transcend brackets that, despite having the highest mean value, were statistically similar to black tea.

Our results are in agreement with a previous study[17] that showed that mean values above 3.7 were obtained for Transcend and INVU ceramic brackets immersed in coffee solution after 14 days. Artificial saliva did not visibly alter the color of these brackets.

Different values of perceptible color changes were used in a different study[18] which assert that the range of $5 < \Delta E^{\star} < 10$ is noticeable. The authors also claim that mean values greater than 10 account for indisputable discoloration of brackets. Thus, they concluded that all brackets immersed in black tea, coffee or red wine showed similar reactions with a marked increase in discoloration after 5 days. This study corroborates our results; however, with a staining power achieved within a shorter period of time, since, after 24 hours, color change was observed with $\Delta E^{\star} > 3.7$ for all brackets.

Divergent results were found in another study[16] in which color change values were below clinically significant values ($\Delta E^{\star} > 3.7$) for all brackets in all solutions. However, these values cannot be compared to other studies, since their spectrophotometric evaluation was performed on the base of worn brackets, unlike most studies that measured color on the vestibular surface of these accessories.

It has been shown that even though Coke has a lower pH value that can damage surface integrity of material, it does not promote clinically significant color changes like coffee and black tea do, possibly due to lack of yellow dye in its constitution.[23] Coffee and tea have yellow dye, but with different polarities, which differs in their interaction with material surface. Park et al[24] also showed that pH was not the main element responsible for color changes. According to the authors, the amount and type of pigment was the main reason, thereby confirming the previous study. Studies on color change and ceramic brackets do not usually investigate the physical and chemical interaction between dye solutions and material components. Fort his reason, additional studies are warranted to further investigate this topic.

By comparing the *in vitro* results of this study with the clinical practice, some limitations are encountered, namely: Complex flora of the oral cavity and its by-products, as well as the buildup of biofilm on tested material.[25] Therefore, the present study as well as other *in vitro* studies showed overestimated values of color change. Since no *in vivo* studies have been conducted to demonstrate the real-time parameters for visible color changes, additional studies are warranted to further investigate this topic.

Nevertheless, *in vitro* studies may provide an initial estimate. This estimate was calculated on the basis of a research[26] in which, according to coffee producers, the average time spent to consume a cup of coffee is 15 minutes and the average number of cups of coffee consumed per day is 3.2 cups. Therefore, 24 hours of immersion in coffee represents a monthly consumption of coffee. Thus, 21 days of immersion *in vitro*, as used in this study, simulates the susceptibility of ceramic brackets to coffee staining within 1 year and 9 months of orthodontic treatment.

This calculation can be individualized for each person, thereby allowing the risk of color change to be estimated according to orthodontic treatment time expected by the orthodontist and information on average color change provided by *in vitro* studies.

Akyalcin et al[19] conducted an *in vitro* study to reproduce the exposure time necessary for a dye drink to act on brackets inside the mouth. The total time of the experiment was 26 weeks (equivalent to 6 months), with daily exposures of 10 minutes alternated by baths of water at 37°C. The amount of bracket exposure to dye solution differed according to the frequency of use of each drink, as limited by the authors. A total time ranging from 13 to 60 hours of exposure was used for the entire study period.

In any *in vitro* study, the biggest challenge is to reproduce the real conditions of the oral cavity. Under the conditions of our study, we are not able to provide the real time of bracket staining. Nevertheless, bracket structures should be improved by manufacturers in order to increase color stability and standardize the production process of these accessories. To this end, additional research about the possible factors that might promote color change of esthetic brackets is necessary, since the mechanism of staining is not clear in the literature.

CONCLUSION

The methodology of this study let us to conclude that ceramic brackets undergo color change when exposed to solutions of coffee, black tea and red wine, drinks commonly present in people's diet. However, the same crystalline structure, either monocrystalline or polycrystalline, do not follow the same or a similar pattern in color change, but vary from manufacturer to manufacturer;

thereby showing lack of standardization in the manufacturing process of these brackets. Coffee dye produced the most marked color changes after 21 days of immersion for most ceramic brackets assessed.

ACKNOWLEDGMENTS

This study was supported by FAPESP (Process #2010/03491-7, (Research Support Foundation of the State of São Paulo).

REFERENCES

1. Newman GV. Adhesive and orthodontic plastic attachments. Am J Orthod. 1969;56(6):573-88.
2. Olsen ME, Bishara SE, Jakobsen JR. Evaluation of the shear bond strength of different ceramic bracket base designs. Angle Orthod. 1997;67(3):179-82.
3. Fernandez L, Canut JA. In vitro comparison of the retention capacity of new aesthetic brackets. Eur J Orthod. 1999;21(1):71-7.
4. Maltagliati LA, Feres R, Figueiredo MA, Siqueira DF. Braquetes estéticos: considerações clínicas. Rev Clín Ortod Dental Press. 2006;5(3):89-95.
5. Liu JK, Chung CH, Chang CY, Shieh DB. Bond strength and debonding characteristics of a new ceramic bracket. Am J Orthod Dentofacial Orthop. 2005;128(6):761-5; quiz 802.
6. Ghafari J. Problems associated with ceramic brackets suggest limiting use to selected teeth. Angle Orthod. 1992;62(2):145-52.
7. Omana HM, Moore RN, Bagby MD. Frictional properties of metal and ceramic brackets. J Clin Orthod. 1992;26(7):425-32.
8. Lopes Filho H, Maia LEG, Araujo MVA, Ruellas ACO. Influence of optical properties of esthetic brackets (color, translucence, and fluorescence) on visual perception. Am J Orthod Dentofacial Orthop. 2012;141(4):460-7.
9. Jena AK, Duggal R, Mehrotra AK. Physical properties and clinical characteristics of ceramic brackets: a comprehensive review. Trends Biomater Artif Organs. 2007;20(2):101-15.
10. Bishara SE, Fehr DE. Ceramic brackets: something old, something new, a review. Semin Orthod. 1997;3(3):178-88.
11. Karamouzos A, Athanasiou AE, Papadopoulos MA. Clinical characteristics and properties of ceramic brackets: a comprehensive review. Am J Orthod Dentofacial Orthop. 1997;112(1):34-40.
12. Bishara SE. Ceramic brackets: a clinical perspective. World J Orthod. 2003;4(1):61-6.
13. O`Brien WJ. Dental Materials and their selection. 3ª ed. São Paulo: Quintessence Books; 2002.
14. Commission Internationale de l'Eclairage. Colorimetry technical report. CIE publication no 15. 3rd ed. Vienna: Bureau Central de la CIE; 2004.
15. Lee Y. Changes in the reflected and transmitted color of esthetic brackets after thermal cycling. Am J Orthod Dentofacial Orthop. 2008;133(5):641e1-6.
16. Guignone BC. Avaliação in vitro da estabilidade de cor de braquetes cerâmicos imersos em soluções potencialmente corantes [dissertação]. Belo Horizonte (MG): Pontifícia Universidade Católica de Minas Gerais; 2008.
17. Mendonça MR, Fabre AF, Goiatto MC, Cuoghi OA, Martins LP, Verri ACG. Spectrophotometric evaluation of color changes of esthetic brackets stored in potentially staining solutions. RPG Rev Pós Grad. 2011;18(1):20-7.
18. Wriedt S, Schepke U, Wehrbein H. The Discoloring effects of food on the color stability of esthetic brackets: an in-vitro study. J Orofac Orthop. 2007;68(4):308-20.
19. Akyalcin S, Rykiss J, Rody WJ, Wiltshire WA. Digital analysis of staining properties of clear aesthetic brackets. J Orthod. 2012;39(3):170-5.
20. Yu B, Lee YK. Aesthetic color performance of plastic and ceramic brackets: an in vitro study. J Orthod. 2011;38(3):167-74.
21. Seghi RR, Hewlett ER, Kim J. Visual and colorimetric assessments of small color differences on translucent dental porcelain. J Dent Res. 1989;68(12):1760-4.
22. Johnston WM, Kao EC. Assessment of appearance match by visual observation and clinical colorimetry. J Dent Res. 1989;68(5):819-22.
23. Um CM, Ruyter IE. Staining of resin-based veneering materials with coffee and tea. Quintessence Int. 1991;22(5):377-86.
24. Park K, Yoon H, Kim S, Lee G, Park H, Park Y. Surface roughness analysis of ceramic bracket slots using atomic force microscope. Korean J Orthod. 2010;40(5):294-303.
25. Eliades T, Bourauel C. Intraoral aging of orthodontic materials: the picture we miss and its clinical relevance. Am J Orthod Dentofacial Orthop. 2005;127(4):403-12.
26. Erta E, Güler AU, Yücel AAN, Köprülü H, Güler E. Color stability of resin composites after immersion in different drinks. Dent Mater. 2006;2(52):371-6.

5

Influence of bleaching and desensitizing gel on bond strength of orthodontic brackets

Fernanda Alves Rodrigues Britto[1], Adriana Simoni Lucato[2], Heloisa Cristina Valdrighi[2], Sílvia Amélia Scudeler Vedovello[2]

Objective: The objective of this study was to assess, *in vitro,* the influence of bleaching gel and the use of desensitizing agent over bond strength of ceramic brackets bonded to bovine enamel. **Methods:** One hundred bovine incisors were selected and randomly divided into five groups (n = 20): Group 1, control group (without bleaching); Group 2, bleached with 35% hydrogen peroxide; Group 3, bleached with 35% hydrogen peroxide (three applications, 15 minutes each) and desensitizing agent applied for 10 minutes; Group 4, bleached with 35% hydrogen peroxide for 40 minutes; Group 5, bleached with 35% hydrogen peroxide for 40 minutes with desensitizing agent applied for 10 minutes. Brackets were bonded 7 days after bleaching and submitted to shear bond strength test after 24 hours at a compression rate of 1 mm/minute. After fracture, the adhesive remnant index (ARI) was assessed under stereoscopic at 40 x magnification. Shear strength data (MPa) were submitted to one-way ANOVA and Tukey's test with significance level set at 5%. **Results:** Group 5 (29.33 MPa) showed significantly higher bond strength than Group 1 (19.19 MPa), Group 2 (20.59 MPa) and Group 4 (23.25 MPa), but with no difference in comparison to Group 3. There was no significant difference among the other groups. The adhesive remnant index showed predominance of score 3, that is, all resin remained adhered to enamel for all groups. **Conclusion:** Bleaching with 35% hydrogen peroxide with calcium associated with desensitizing agent application produced higher bond strength values of brackets bonded to bovine enamel.

Keywords: Tooth bleaching. Hydrogen peroxide. Shear strength.

[1] Master's student in Orthodontics, Centro Universitário Hermínio Ometto (UNIARARAS), Araras, São Paulo, Brazil.

[2] Professor, Centro Universitário Hermínio Ometto (UNIARARAS), Postgraduate program, Department of Orthodontics, Araras, São Paulo, Brazil.

» The authors report no commercial, proprietary or financial interest in the products or companies described in this article.

Fernanda Alves Rodrigues Brito
Av. Dr. Maximiliano Baruto, 500 - Jd. Universitário
Araras - SP - Brazil — CEP: 13607-339 - E-mail: amerbc@yahoo.com.br

INTRODUCTION

Esthetics is one of patients' demands when seeking dental offices to change the angle, position and color of their teeth.[1] One of the most common esthetic complaints involves changes in the color of teeth, in addition to disproportionate shape and misalignment. Tooth bleaching is indicated to improve the esthetics of the smile, and must be performed before restorative and rehabilitative procedures.[2]

The most frequently used bleaching agents are hydrogen peroxide and carbamide peroxide in various concentrations, and bleaching may be performed by means of two techniques: at-home or in-office bleaching.[3] In procedures performed at the dentist's office, 35% hydrogen peroxide is usually used, and should be applied and supervised by duly qualified professionals.[4] Both techniques are equally effective.[5]

Tooth bleaching promotes rupture of the pigmented molecules impregnated in the dental structures, making them smaller, with significant reduction in the tonalities of their color, so that the tooth becomes whiter.[6,7,8] Bleaching may be redone after 14 months.[8]

Various studies have demonstrated that changes occur in the morphology, microhardness and permeability of bleached enamel.[10,11] This is believed to occur due to the demineralizing potential of bleaching agents.[11] Thus, some undesirable effects may be generated.

One of the undesirable effects reported by patients is tooth sensitivity which occurs due to an increase in enamel and dentin permeability by the bleaching agents.[11] This allows penetration of fluids into the dentinal tubules, stimulating nerve fibers and consequently leading to sensitivity. This may be reverted by the use of desensitizing agents, with emphasis on the use of potassium nitrate, which reduces sensitivity by means of diminishing the ability of nerve fibers in dental pulp to transmit pain;[12] and fluorides that obstruct dentinal tubules and, thereby, also promote the inhibition of pain.[13,14]

Adding calcium to the composition of bleaching agents is another alternative to reduce the adverse effects caused by bleaching. The presence of calcium in the composition of bleaching agents probably contributes, directly and indirectly, to reduce sensitivity.[15] The goal of this addition is to increase the saturation of gels with ions, thereby reducing mineral losses and increasing enamel resistance to demineralization caused by peroxides.[16] Studies have evinced that the presence of calcium in 35% hydrogen peroxide-based bleaching agents increased microhardness of bleached enamel, thus resulting in remineralization of this substrate.[17] Therefore, the addition of calcium and fluoride helps to control mineral loss in enamel submitted to different bleaching treatments.[18]

Studies have reported increase in resin bond strength to enamel submitted to bleaching.[19,20] The application of bleaching agents may also cause surface porosities that change enamel permeability and interfere in bond strength in bracket bonding.[21] There is some discrepancy in the results found in the literature with respect to the reduction in bond strength of brackets bonded to bleached teeth. However, changes caused by bleaching are undeniable, making it necessary to wait for a period of at least seven days in order to perform orthodontic bracket bonding more safely.[22]

Patients who need orthodontic treatment and choose esthetic brackets give much importance to the smile. Some of them have stained teeth and request that bleaching treatment be performed prior to orthodontic treatment. This is because they do not want to remain with stained teeth throughout all orthodontic treatment, which can last more than three years. Therefore, it is important to assess the influence of bleaching treatment associated with desensitizing agents on the bond strength of brackets to enamel.

Therefore, the aim of this study was to assess the influence of bleaching agents, with and without calcium, and desensitizing agents on the bond strength of ceramic brackets bonded to bovine enamel, in addition to assessing the adhesive remnant index (ARI) after the bond strength test.

MATERIAL AND METHODS

This study began after being approved by UNIARARAS Institutional Review Board under protocol #560/2011.

One hundred recently extracted bovine teeth were selected, based on the following inclusion criteria: teeth with intact crowns, absence of white spot lesions, cracks and fractures, and teeth originating from the same lot. These teeth were included in PVC tubes with polystyrene (Resina Cristal, Piraglass, Piracicaba, SP, Brazil), with the buccal surface exposed, and submitted to prophylaxis with pumice stone and water, using a Robson brush. Teeth were divided into five groups (n = 20), according to the bleaching and desensitizing agent.

» Group 1: control group in which specimens received no bleaching before bracket bonding.

» Group 2: bleached with 35% hydrogen peroxide (Whiteness HP Maxx 35%, FGM, Joinville, Santa Catarina, Brazil), with three applications for 15 minutes each, as recommended by the manufacturer, using the light polymerizing appliance Radii (SDI, Australia). At the end of treatment, the samples were washed with water and polished with a felt disc.

» Group 3: bleached with 35% hydrogen peroxide (Whiteness HP Maxx 35%, FGM, Joinville, Santa Catarina, Brazil) according to the protocol described for Group 2. After bleaching, teeth were washed and dried, and the desensitizing agent was applied (KF 2%, FGM, Joinville, Santa Catarina, Brazil) for 10 minutes, followed by washing and polishing with a felt disc.

» Group 4: bleached with 35% hydrogen peroxide (Whiteness Blue 35% Calcium, FGM, Joinville, Santa Catarina, Brazil) for 40 minutes, as recommended by the manufacturer, and subsequently washed, dried and polished with a felt disc.

» Group 5: bleached with 35% hydrogen peroxide (Whiteness Blue 35% Calcium, FGM, Joinville, Santa Catarina, Brazil) for 40 minutes. After bleaching, teeth were washed and dried, and the desensitizing agent was applied (KF 2%, FGM, Joinville, Santa Catarina, Brazil) for 10 minutes, followed by washing and polishing with a felt disc.

After the bleaching procedure, all samples were stored in distilled water for seven days after which the brackets were bonded. Prophylaxis of the bonding area was performed with pumice stone and a Robson brush. The enamel was etched with 37% phosphoric acid for 15 seconds and subsequently washed and dried. Afterwards, Transbond XT Primer (3M Unitek, Monrovia, USA) adhesive was applied and light activated for 10 seconds with the Radii (SDI, Australia) light curing appliance. Transbond XT (3M Unitek, Monrovia, USA) resin was applied at the base of the Edgewise prescription ceramic brackets for maxillary central incisors (Morelli, Sorocaba, SP, Brazil). Brackets were manually positioned on the tooth surface until the material flowed, and were then polymerized for 40 seconds, 10 seconds on each surface (distal, mesial, gingival and occlusal).

Table 1 - Study groups divided according to the bleaching agent and desensitizing gel.

Group	Bleaching agent	Desensitizing
Group 1 (control)	---	---
Group 2	35% hydrogen peroxide (Whiteness HP Maxx, FGM)	---
Group 3	35% hydrogen peroxide (Whiteness HP Maxx, FGM)	Desensitizing (KF 2%, FGM)
Group 4	35% hydrogen peroxide (Whiteness Blue Calcium, FGM)	---
Group 5	35% hydrogen peroxide (Whiteness Blue Calcium, FGM)	Desensitizing (KF 2%, FGM)

Specimens were stored in distilled water at 37 °C for 24 hours[23,24] and submitted to shear bond strength test in an Instron 4411 universal testing machine (Instron Corp, USA) at a compression speed rate of 1 mm/minute. Shear bond strength was tested for normal distribution by means of Kolmogorov-Smirnov test. One-way ANOVA and Tukey's multiple comparison tests were used to assess the influence of bleaching on shear bond strength results at a significance level of 5%.

After the shear bond strength test, the adhesive remnant index (ARI) was assessed in accordance with the method proposed by Artun and Bergland,[25] and determined by scores that ranged from 0 to 3:

» Score 0 — absence of any residue of adhesive layer on enamel;

» Score 1 — presence of less than half resin remnant on enamel;

» Score 2 — presence of more than half resin remnant on enamel;

» Score 3 — presence of all resin remnant on enamel, together with impression of the bracket base design.

Adhesive remnant was evaluated under a stereoscopic microscope (Carl Zeiss, MC 63A, Germany) under 40 x magnification.

RESULTS

Analysis of variance showed significant difference among the different types of material ($P < 0.001$). Tukey's test (Table 2) showed that the samples submitted to bleaching with HP Blue and later application of 2% KF desensitizing agent presented significantly higher bond strength in comparison to control and the samples submitted to bleaching with HP Blue and HP

Table 2 - Shear strength (MPa) of brackets bonded to enamel and subjected to different bleaching protocols.

Material	Shear strength (MPa)
Group 5: HP Blue + KF a 2%	29.33 (6.03) A
Group 4: HP Blue	23.25 (6.85) B
Group 3: HP Maxx + KF a 2%	24.22 (5.45) AB
Group 2: HP Maxx	20.59 (7.17) B
Group 1: Control	19.19 (6.12) B

Different letters stand for significant difference ($P < 0.05$).

Table 3 - Frequency (%) of ARI distribution after applying different bleaching agents.

Scores	HP Blue + 2% KF	HP Blue	HP Maxx + 2% KF	HP Maxx	Control
Score 0	1 (5%)	1 (5%)	1 (5%)	2 (10%)	1 (5%)
Score 1	0 (0%)	0 (0%)	0 (0%)	0 (0%)	2 (10%)
Score 2	1 (5%)	2 (10%)	0 (0%)	2 (10%)	4 (20%)
Score 3	18 (90%)	17 (85%)	19 (95%)	16 (80%)	13 (65%)

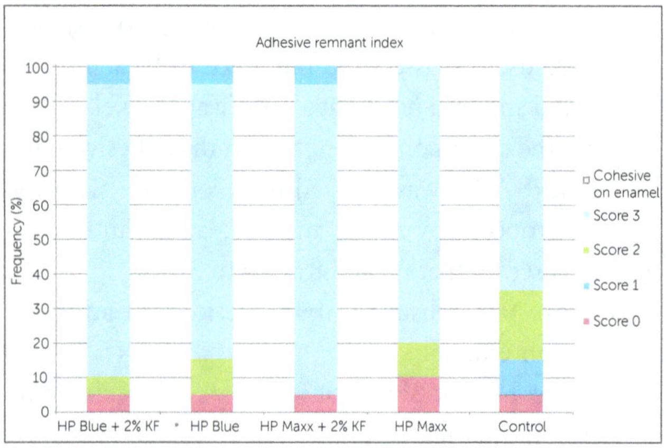

Figure 1 - Frequency (%) of adhesive remnant index after application of different bleaching agents.

Maxx; however, no differences were found in comparison to those bleached with HP Maxx and later application of 2% KF desensitizing agent. There was no significant difference between the bond strength values of other groups.

Assessment of the adhesive remnant index (ARI) showed predominance of score 3; that is, all resin remained adhered to the enamel for all groups. For the control group, there was a trend towards scores 1 and 2 (Fig 1). The groups bleached with HP Blue, with and without desensitizing agent, and the HP Maxx group with desensitizing agent presented cohesive fracture in enamel.

DISCUSSION

Many patients have some trouble using orthodontic appliances, even ceramic ones. In order to reduce the color contrast between teeth and ceramic brackets, patients are subjected to bleaching procedures before bracket bonding, which leads orthodontists to question the influence of bleaching agent on the bonding procedure.

One of the most common effects resulting of hydrogen peroxide or carbamide peroxide on bleaching treatment in Dentistry is the change in bond strength to enamel and dentin. The reduction in bond strength of resin to enamel and dentin may be related to the presence of free radicals of oxygen that interfere in the polymerization of resin material.[26,27] Therefore, the most used clinical approach to eliminate or reduce the effects of residual oxygen is to wait a few days after the end of bleaching treatment before bonding brackets.[28,29]

This study demonstrated that the samples submitted to bleaching with HP Blue Calcium and subsequent application of 2% KF desensitizing agent presented a significantly higher bond strength compared with non-bleached teeth and teeth bleached without later desensitizing application. Assessment of adhesive remnant index (ARI) showed predominance of score 3, failures between bracket and resin, thereby confirming that bleaching did not negatively influence the bond strength of brackets to enamel.

The high bond strength values shown in this study are possibly due to the time interval of seven days between the end of bleaching and orthodontic bracket bonding. Within this period, residual oxygen must have been neutralized, thus not interfering in polymerization of resin composite for bonding. This may be proved by the absence of significant differences between the bleached groups and the control group (without bleaching). Some authors[30,31] suggest that orthodontic bonding should be delayed for one week after bleaching so as to ensure adequate bond strength. Other authors[32,33] also recommend postponing bonding after bleaching for periods ranging from 24 hours to four weeks. Thus, according to these authors,[22,34] a period of at least seven days of waiting time is necessary so that orthodontic bracket bonding can be performed more safely. This is in agreement with the results obtained in the present study in which the waiting time was of seven days before bonding orthodontic brackets to bovine enamel after bleaching.

The release of oxygen may cause morphological alterations in mineralized tissues.[4,8,33] The reduction in bond strength of dentin to bleached teeth has been related to changes in the mineral and protein content of enamel, and not to the effect of residual oxygen.[35] Soares et al[36] demonstrated that the addition of calcium and fluoride ions to the gel reduced mineral loss, thereby increasing resistance to demineralization.

Giannini et al[16] reported that if mineral ions were added to the gel during bleaching and ionic exchange, they could perhaps be taken up and increase enamel resistance to demineralization. Since fluoride and calcium ions increase the saturation of the bleaching gel, lower mineral loss could occur during bleaching; therefore, gels with the addition of fluoride or calcium could reduce or overcome the adverse effects of bleaching treatment. This result was obtained in the present study, in which the presence of calcium in the bleaching gel and application of a desensitizing agent must have remineralized this substrate, showing an increase in bond strength in teeth bleached with a bleaching agent containing calcium, and application of the desensitizer.

Another result found in this study was that the association of bleaching agent with calcium and desensitizing agent produced the highest shear bond strength. Nevertheless, a previous study found that bleaching with the application of desensitizing agent significantly reduced the bond strength of orthodontic brackets bonded to human enamel.[37] Reduction in bond strength in that study was probably due to a post-bleaching bonding time of two days, in disagreement with studies that indicate that the ideal should be waiting for at least seven days, as it was done in the present experiment. This waiting time would be necessary for complete release of residual oxygen.[29] Moreover, the calcium present in the bleaching agent could reduce demineralization during tooth bleaching, and the fluoride ions released from desensitizing agent could promote ions change with enamel and form fluoridated apatite on tooth surface that could be related to the highest shear bond strength for Group 5.

Another study reported that in order to reduce the effects of residual oxygen on bonding procedures performed right after bleaching, fluoride in gel could be applied to the enamel.[27] The presence of sodium fluoride in the desensitizing agent may act as a remineralizing agent, thereby forming a layer of calcium fluoride on the enamel surface.[38] Thus, the application of the desensitizing agent may have removed the layer of residual oxygen, which did not interfere negatively in orthodontic bracket bonding to bleached enamel.

Although the ideal substrate for this type of study is the human tooth, bovine teeth were used as a substitute because extracted human teeth are becoming difficult to obtain due to progress in conservative dental treatment.[38] Bovine teeth are easily obtainable and are reported to be a reliable substitute for human teeth in enamel bonding.[39]

Clinically, the application of desensitizing agent after bleaching with hydrogen peroxide can be a good option to reduce the negative effects of residual oxygen on bond strength of brackets bonded to bleached enamel. However, further studies must be conducted to investigate the effect of associating bleaching gel with calcium and desensitizing agent applied to the dental structure.

CONCLUSION

Bleaching agent with calcium associated with desensitizing gel increased the shear bond strength of ceramic brackets bonded to the enamel. Bleaching did not reduce shear strength between bracket and teeth.

The adhesive remnant index (ARI) revealed that score 3 was predominant, that is, all resin remained adhered to the enamel.

REFERENCES

1. Baratieri LN, Monteiro Junior S, Andrada MAC, Vieira LCC. Clareamento dental. 2a ed. São Paulo: Ed. Santos; 1993.
2. Zanin F, Brugnera Júnior A, Zanin S, Campos DHS, Zanin VOZ. Clareamento dental com laser e led. Rev Gauch Odontol. 2003;51(3):143-6.
3. Soares CJ, Santos Filho PCF, Barreto BCF, Mota AS. Effect of previous desensitizer and rewetting agent application on shear bond strength of bonding systems to dentin. Cienc Odontol Bras. 2006;9(4):6-11.
4. Pinto C, Oliveira R, Cavalli V, Giannini M. Peroxide bleaching agent effects on enamel surface microhardness, roughness and morphology. Braz Oral Res. 2004;18(4):306-11.
5. Almeida LC, Riehl H, Santos PH, Sundfeld ML, Briso AL. Clinical evaluation of the effectiveness of different bleaching terapies in vital teeth. Int J Periodontics Restorative Dent. 2012;32(3):303-9.
6. Pécora JD, Cruzfilho AM, Sousaneto MD, Silva RG. In vitro action of various bleaching agents on the microhardnesse of human dentin. Braz Dental J. 1994;5(2):129-34.
7. Baratieri LN. Clareamento dental. São Paulo: Ed. Santos; 1995.
8. Novais RCP, Toledo OA. Estudo in vitro das alterações do esmalte dentário submetido à ação de um agente clareador. J Bras Clín Estét Odontol. 2000;4(20):48-51.

9. Grobler SR, Mjeed A, Moola MH, Rossouw RJ, Van wyk kotze T. In vivo Spectrophotometric assessment of the tooth whitening effectiveness of nite White 10% with amorphous calcium phosphate, potassium nitrate and fluoride, over a 6 month. Period Open Dent J. 2011;2(5):18-23.
10. Basting RT, Rodrigues Jr AL, Serra MC. The effects of seven carbamide peroxide bleaching agents on enamel microhardness over time. J Am Dent Assoc. 2003;134(10):335-42.
11. Lewinstein I, Fuhrer N, Churaru N, Cardash H. Effect of different peroxide bleaching regiments and subsequent fluoridation on the hardness of human enamel and dentin. J Prosth Dent. 2004;92(4):337-42.
12. Ajcharanukul O, Kraivaphan P, Wanachantararak S, Vongsavan N, Matthews B. Effects of potassium íons on dentine sensitivity in man. Arch Oral Biol. 2007;52(7):632-9.
13. Addy M, Mostafa P. Dentine hypersensitivity. Effects produced by the uptake in vitro of metal ions, fluoride and formaldehyde onto dentine. J Oral Rehabil. 1988;15(6):575-85.
14. Paes-Leme AF, Santos JCRG, Giannini M, Wada RS. Occlusion of dentin tubules by desensitizing agents. Am J Dent. 2004;17:368-72.
15. Matins GC, Izidora ACSA, Meister LMB, Kossatz S, Gomes OMM, Loguercio DA, et al. Avaliação clínica do uso de um dessensibilizante antes do clareamento de consultório. Rev Assoc Paul Cir Dent. 2011;65(2):119-23.
16. Giannini M, Silva AP, Cavalli V, Paes Leme AF. Effect of carbamide peroxide-based bleaching agents containing fluoride or calcium on tensile strength of human enamel. J Appl Oral Sci. 2006;14(2):82-7.
17. Amaral PG, Sales GCF, Santos RL, Magalhães DBL, Gusmão ES. Influência da presença do cálcio em agentes clareadores e sua relação com a microdureza do esmalte dental humano. Rev Bras Ciência Saúde. 2010;14(2):37-44.
18. Cavalli V, Rodrigues LK, Paes-Leme AF, Brancalion ML, Arruda MA, Berger SB, et al. Effects of bleaching agents containing fluoride and calcium on human enamel. Quintessence Int. 2010;41(8):157-65.
19. Torneck, CD, Titley KC, Smith DC, Adibfar A. Effect of water leaching on the adhesion of composite resin to bleached and unbleached bovine enamel. J Endod.1991;17(4):156-60.
20. Matta ENR, Maia JAC, Chevitaresse O. Influencia do agente clareador peróxido de carbamida a 10% na resistência mecânica da colagem de braquetes ortodônticos. Rev Dental Press Ortod Ortop Facial. 2005;10(2):69-74.
21. Souza MAL. Clareamento caseiro de dentes: ação do peróxido de carbamida sobre dentes e mucosa bucal [tese]. Porto Alegre (RS): Pontifica Universidade Católica do Rio Grande do Sul; 1993.
22. Mishima FD, Valentim RG A, Araújo MTS, Ruellas ACO, Sant'Anna EF. Clareação dentária: revisão de literatura e sua interferência na colagem de braquetes ortodônticos. Rev Dental Press Estét. 2008;5(3):100-6.
23. Romano FL, Tavares SW, Nouer DF, Consani S, Magnani MBBA. Shear Bond strenght of metalic orthodontic brackets bonded to enamel prepared with Self-Etching Primer. The Angle Orthod. 2005;75(5)849-53.
24. Ajlouni R, Bishara SE, Oonsombat C, Soliman M, Laffoon J. The effect of porcelain surface conditioning on bonding orthodontic brackets. Angle Orthod. 2005;75(5):858-64.
25. Artun J, Bergland S. Clinical trials With crystal growth conditioning as an alternative to acid-etch enamel pretreatment. Am J Orthod. 1984;85(4):333-40.
26. Homewood C, Tyas M, Woods M. Bonding to previously bleached teeth. Aust Orthod J. 2001;17(1):27-34.
27. Martin JM, Almeida JB, Rosa EA, Soares P, Torno V. Rached RN, Mazur RF. Effect of fluoride therapies on the surface roughness of human enamel exposed to bleaching agents. Quintessence Int. 2010;41(1):71-8.
28. Godwin JM, Barghi N, Berry TG, Knight GT, Hummert TW. Time duration for dissipation of bleaching effects before enamel bonding. J Dent Res. 1992;71(1):179-85.
29. Van der vyver PJ, Lewis SB, Marais JT. The effect of bleaching agent on composite enamel bonding. J Dent Assoc S Afr. 1997;52(10):601-3.
30. Ruse ND, Smith DC, Torneck CD, Titley KC. Preliminary surface analysis of etched, bleached, and normal bovine enamel. J Dent Res. 1990;69(9):1610-3.
31. Miles, P. G.; Pontier JP, Bahiraei D, Close J. The effect of carbamide peroxide bleach on the tensile bond strength of ceramic brackets: an in vitro study. Am J Orthod Dentofacial Orthop. 1994;105(4):371-5.
32. Cavalli V, Reis A.F, Giannini M, Ambrosano GM. The effect of elapsed time following bleaching on enamel bond strength of resin composite. Oper Dent. 2001;26:597-602.
33. Uysal T,Basciftci A, Usumez , Sari Z, Buyukerkmen A. Can previously bleached teeth be bonded safely? Am J Orthod Dentofacial Orthop. 2003;123(6):628-32.
34. Nour El-Din AK, Miller BH, Griggs JA, Wakefied CI. Immediate bonding to bleached enamel. Oper Dent. 2006;31(1):106-14.
35. Perdigão J, Francci C, Swift EJ Jr, Ambrose WW, Lopes M. Ultra-morphological study of the interaction of dental adhesives with carbamide peroxide-bleached enamel. Am J Dent. 1998;11(6):291-301.
36. Soares FF, Sousa JAC, Maia CC, Fontes CM, Cunha LG, Freitas AP. Clareamento em dentes vitais: uma revisão literária. Rev Saúde Com. 2008;4(1):72-84.
37. Turkkahraman H, Adanir N, Gungor Y. bleaching and desensitizer application effects on shear bond strengths of orthodontic brackets. Angle Orthod. 2007;77(3):489-93.
38. Featherstone JD, Cutress TW, Rodgers BE, Dennison PJ. Remineralization of artificial caries-like lesion in vivo by a self administered mouthrinse or paste. Caries Res.1982;16(3):235-42.

6

Transversal changes in dental arches from non-extraction treatment with self ligating brackets

Liliana Avila Maltagliati[1], Yasushi Inoue Myiahira[2], Liana Fattori[3], Leopoldino Capelozza Filho[4], Mauricio Cardoso[4]

Objective: The present study aimed at analyzing, with the use of dental casts, the transverse changes of the upper and lower dental arches, after non-extraction orthodontic treatment, with self-ligating brackets. **Methods:** The sample comprised 29 patients, all presenting Class I malocclusion with upper and lower crowding of at least 4 mm and treated only with a fixed appliance, without stripping, extraction or distalization. The dental casts were obtained before and after leveling with 0.019 x 0.025-in stainless steel archwires. **Conclusion:** The results indicated that the majority of transverse changes occurred at the premolar areas, both the first and the second, as well as on the upper and lower dental arches. The intercanine distance increased 0.75 mm, on average, in the upper arch and 1.96 mm in the lower arch. The molars also demonstrated a tendency towards an increase in their transverse dimension, however, at a lower intensity comparing to premolars. All measurements presented statistically significant differences with the exception of the maxillary second molars.

Keywords: Corrective orthodontics. Dental models. Orthodontic brackets.

[1] MSc and PhD in Orthodontics, Bauru School of Dentistry, University of São Paulo (USP).
[2] MSc in Orthodontics, School of Dentistry, Methodist University of São Paulo (UMESP).
[3] Professor, Specialization Course in Orthodontics, Straight-Wire Group of Rio de Janeiro.
[4] Professor, Graduation and Post-Graduation Program and MSc in Orthodontics, Sacred Heart University.

» The authors report no commercial, proprietary or financial interest in the products or companies described in this article.

Liliana Avila Maltagliati
Rua Salete, 200 – Sala 42 – Santana – São Paulo/SP – Brazil
CEP: 02.016-001 – E-mail: lilianamaltagliati@hotmail.com

INTRODUCTION

Every orthodontic treatment has its foundation in the moment of diagnosis and planning. A correct diagnosis and a well-designed treatment plan are responsible for the success of the treatment, independent of the selected appliance to achieve the proposed objectives. There are several parameters and tests used to aid in the detection of anomalies and malocclusions affecting patients and guiding the planning, but knowledge of the effects that each appliance provides brings safety to the choice of treatment modality based on the goals set forth. Similarly, knowledge of a successful procedure and how stable it is also brings safety in using a treatment method.

Admittedly, dental malocclusion with dental crowding, can be treated by obtaining space in the arch that can occur in 5 ways: Archwire expansion, protrusion of the anterior teeth, dental extractions, stripping, or even distalization in the upper arch. In Class I malocclusion, the distal procedure presents itself as contraindicated, remaining two alternatives that reduce the arch perimeter and two others that increase the perimeter. To decide on the procedure, the orthodontist must ponder factors like facial convexity, type of mandibular growth, facial pattern, overjet and overbite, among others. Historically, it has been touted in the literature that the extraction procedures would be more stable than the expansion ones, unless through orthopedic expansion at an early age, when is possible to separate the intermaxillary suture with minimal buccal tooth movement.[1,2,3]

There are countless studies in the literature dealing with maxillary expansion caused by rapid maxillary expansion and the skeletal and dental effects resulting from this procedure.[4-9] The purely dental expansion is not accepted by orthodontists because of the alveolar limitation of this procedure, being reduced to only cases with very mild crowding or that permit a buccal tipping effect, especially on the anterior segment.

However, the literature is still not clear on this subject when it comes to stability, since the results of some studies have shown that the dimensions are more altered in the post-treatment period when extraction is performed as opposed to treating without extraction,[10-13] and still others show that post-treatment stability is compromised in both cases with and without extractions.[12,14,15,16] Walter[13] evaluated 50 cases without extractions and 50 with extractions, measuring the intercanine and intermolar widths in the pre and post-treatment periods and 1 year after removal of the retainers. A year after the removal of the retainers, there was a decrease in the intercanine and intermolar widths in cases with or without extractions, demonstrating that the canines and molars rarely remain stable after removal of the appliance, regardless of whether or not the extraction was performed. A similar outcome was found by Heiser et al.[17]

Shapiro[18] sought to identify the alterations that occur in between the intercanine, intermolar widths and the arch length in the pre- and post-treatment phases and 10 years after retention in the lower dental arch in patients orthodontically treated, with or without extractions. Lower dental casts of 80 treated subjects were evaluated, who initially presented Class I or Class II malocclusions, division 1 or 2, measuring the intercanine distance, having the cusp tips of the canines as reference, and intermolar distances, based on the cusp tips of the first molars. The results showed a strong tendency of intercanine width to return to its initial dimension and the length of the dental arch to substantially decrease in all cases during the post-retention period. The intermolar width decreased more in patients treated with extractions, in the period between the phases before treatment and after retention. Several cases where intermolar expansions were obtained during treatment were maintained in the treated group without extractions, although, they tend to return to the initial dimension.

The presence of crowding in the arch, even in mild cases, which were treated without extraction, stripping or expansion, with a fixed appliance demand flaring of the teeth that occurs with greater intensity in the anterior region of the arch, since the occlusal contact of the posterior teeth further restricts the buccal movement and the anterior teeth, besides being smaller and being just juxtaposed, are generally more crowded and therefore more likely to yield to the buccal movement to accommodate all the teeth.

Due to the incisors flaring, instead of the buccal posterior movement to accommodate the crowded teeth, the procedure for correction of crowding would only be suitable for specific cases, such as cases of incisors with lingual inclination, absence of narrow arches, or increased overjet.

When they were reintroduced in orthodontics, self-ligating brackets promised tooth movement with a significant reduction of friction. However, Damon[19] raised another possibility that would involve the passive expansion of the arches by means of tooth movement in the buccal direction, due to the freedom of the wires in the slots which would slide in the posterior direction as the crowding is being solved and thus reduce the effect of incisor flaring. In cases with completed facial growth and negative discrepancy, in which the extraction could greatly harm the patient profile, this possibility would present itself as a big advantage for orthodontic treatment. Faced with the controversy that raises this issue, we decided to evaluate in dental casts the transverse changes resulted from a non-extraction treatment with self-ligating brackets.

MATERIAL AND METHODS

Fifty-eight pairs of dental casts were used for this research, 29 pre-treatment and 29 taken at the end of leveling with 0.019 x 0.025-in stainless steel wire. The sample consisted of 29 patients, 12 to 34 years old, all presenting with Class I malocclusion, with a minimum of 4 mm crowding in both upper and lower arch. All patients used Damon 2 brackets bonded with the VA point as a reference point in the center of the clinical crown and undergone a treatment protocol with a sequence of archwires as recommended by Damon,[19] starting with the 0.014-in CuNiti archwire followed by the 0.016 x 0.025-in CuNiti archwire and finishing with the 0.019 x 0.025-in stainless steel archwire. No procedure was performed to obtain space, namely stripping, extraction, distalization or any procedure other than the sequential archwires exchange. To perform the measurements on the dental casts (Fig 1), it was used a Mitutoyo digital caliper with 150 mm capacity and a resolution of 0.01 mm, for it is a very accurate tool.

Dental measurements on cast models

The measurements were performed transversely, from the canines to the second molars in the upper and lower casts. With the caliper positioned parallel to the occlusal plane, it was measured the distance between the cusp tips of the canines, followed by the buccal cusp tips of the first and second premolars and mesiobuccal cusp tips of the first and second molars.

To compare the significance of the transversal changes, it was used the Student t test, with a significance level of 5%. Ten percent of the sample was re-measured with a mean interval of 30 days to evaluate the systematic and random errors. The systematic error was insignificant for all variables except the transverse distance of the first molars that reached a p value of 0.03 and the random error had the higher value of 0.47 mm for the width measurement of the upper first molars

RESULTS

Table 1 shows random and systematic error values of the repetitive measurements evaluated by the Student t test and the Dahlberg's formula.

The initial and final measurements obtained in the dental casts are shown in Tables 2 and 3.

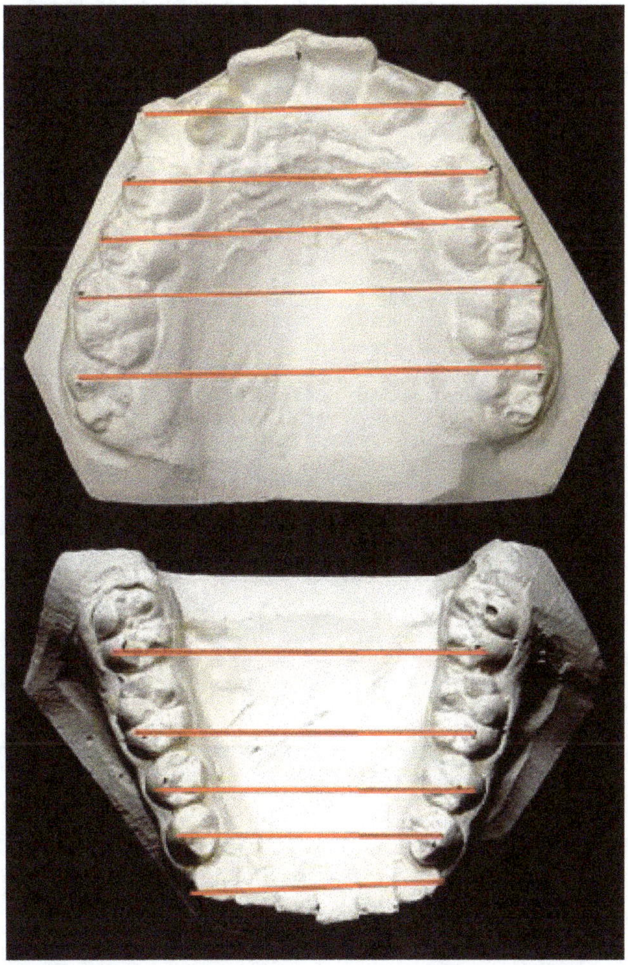

Figure 1 - Transverse measurements performed on the upper and lower casts.

DISCUSSION

By studying cases that were orthodontically treated successfully, Strang[12] noted that the initial lower intercanine and intermolar distances showed little or no variation in relation to the post-treatment values. He found that the muscle harmony should be preserved and that the forms and positions of the teeth of the upper arch are controlled by the characteristics of the lower arch, which in turn are imposed by the surrounding tissues. Thus, every effort should be made towards preservation of the muscular balance.

Grounded in such a theory as this,[12] Orthodontics understands that cases with crowding, which require space in the arch for correct alignment, should be treated by the extraction of teeth, as it is believed that, proceeding in this manner, the original arch shape is preserved, making the obtained occlusion more stable. The procedure has always been: First obtain the space and then move the displaced teeth, that is out of the arch due to the lack of space.[10,14,15]

With the introduction of nickel titanium wires in the 80s, their property of great flexibility allowed

Table 1 - Systematic and random errors tests, for the upper and lower dental arches variables.

Upper arch	Mean 1 ± SD	Mean 2 ± SD	Dahlberg	t test	p
13 x 23	36.95 ± 3.83	36.92 ± 3.79	0.27	0.23	0.82
14 x 24	42.80 ± 3.79	42.85 ± 3.78	0.32	0.33	0.74
15 x 25	50.50 ± 4.77	50.34 ± 4.74	0.23	1.67	0.12
16 x 26	55.90 ± 1.67	55.82 ± 1.88	0.47	0.24	0.82
17 x 27	52.65 ± 4.36	52.12 ± 4.42	0.35	1.11	0.28
Lower arch	**Mean 1 ± SD**	**Mean 2 ± SD**	**Dahlberg**	**t test**	**p**
33 x 43	26.66 ± 3.14	27.00 ± 3.22	0.41	1.53	0.18
34 x 44	32.70 ± 3.91	32.90 ± 3.96	0.29	1.60	0.14
35 x 45	37.00 ± 3.54	37.06 ± 3.31	0.37	0.38	0.70
36 x 46	42.31 ± 3.91	42.52 ± 3.89	0.24	2.44	0.03*
37 x 47	46.46 ± 3.94	46.44 ± 3.87	0.28	0.18	0.85

*Statistically significant at p<0.05.

Table 2 - Initial and final values, in millimeters, of the transverse measurements of the upper dental arch, standard deviations, mean difference, paired Student t test and p value.

Measurements	Initial average ± SD	Final average ± SD	Mean difference	t test	p
13 x 23	35.99 ± 2.47	36.74 ± 2.20	0.75	2.16	0.03*
14 x 24	41.59 ± 2.96	44.77 ± 2.34	3.18	7.19	0.01*
15 x 25	46.32 ± 3.31	49.66 ± 3.04	3.34	7.53	0.01*
16 x 26	52.13 ± 3.62	54.62 ± 11.24	2.49	7.08	0.01*
17 x 27	58.12 ± 4.02	58.16 ± 3.69	0.04	0.85	0.40

*Statistically significant at p<0.05.

Table 3 - Initial and final values, in millimeters, of the transverse measurements of the lower dental arch, standard deviations, mean difference, paired Student's t test and p value.

Measurements	Initial average ± SD	Final average ± SD	Mean difference	t test	p
33 x 43	26.44 ± 2.40	28.40 ± 2.37	1.96	6.08	0.01*
34 x 44	34.49 ± 2.13	37.44 ± 2.02	2.95	8.41	0.01*
35 x 45	39.43 ± 3.03	42.82 ± 2.39	3.39	11.12	0.01*
36 x 46	44.90 ± 3.73	47.13 ± 2.93	2.23	6.09	0.01*
37 x 47	50.75 ± 3.52	53.12 ± 3.15	2.37	4.09	0.01*

*Statistically significant at p<0.05.

mal-positioned teeth, even without space, to be connected to the wire. Still, this procedure continued to be contraindicated because the lack of space would require buccal movement of the teeth for aligning. It occurs because the crowding requires an increased archwire length to be ligated on the teeth, and the memory effect of these wires lead to a severe flaring. This effect, under conventional conditions, occurs mainly in the region of the incisors, because they are the teeth usually involved in crowding which have a lower resistance to movement, since there is no occlusal contact, as in the posterior teeth and are also the teeth with a smaller volume of crown and root.

Damon[19] challenged the precepts of orthodontics to indicate that this paradigm to open space before and then proceed to the leveling of mal-positioned teeth can and should be broken, assuming that self-ligating brackets provide a significant reduction in friction, and when a light archwire is used, while alignment occurs, the archwire slides posteriorly, thus avoiding excessive anterior movement of incisor teeth and obtaining spaces mainly through a lateral dentoalveolar expansion, called the "posterior transverse adaption". As the thermal active alloys release light forces, the tipping movement could also be reduced, since the moment created is reduced due to its direct relation to the force magnitude.

As stated by Bagden,[20] the tip of the system is to use light archwire in passive self-ligating brackets, giving great freedom for the wire inside the slot. With the friction and "binding" effect reduced, the teeth align more efficiently and with much less force than required for conventional brackets.

In accordance with this philosophy, the freedom of the wire causes the teeth to suffer the pressure of leveling, but without forcing the movement. Thus, the tooth tends to move towards areas of lesser resistance, i.e., where there is more space and no resistance to tooth movement. Furthermore, since there is no friction and the freedom of the wire is large, it tends to slide in the posterior direction as the teeth are leveled. This sliding allows the wire length — which is greater when inserted, since deflections must occur to fit the mal-positioned teeth — to do not cause excessive expansion of the arches, what leads the teeth to extremely buccal positions, as it easily slides through the adjacent brackets and remains on the distal of the last tooth inserted on leveling, allowing greater control in the tooth movement and less protrusive effect in cases without extractions. The purpose of this study was to evaluate, in patients treated with self-ligating brackets and thermal active nickel titanium alloy wires, if it occurs, in fact, this later expansion by offering space in the arch and therefore reducing the need for protruding incisors, and verify how this treatment interferes with the intercanine distance in the upper and lower arches that could suggest a potentially unstable treatment.

INTERCANINE DISTANCE

Recognizing the canine teeth as corresponding to a stable structure and that any significant change in its position causes post-treatment movement which result in relapse, the less changes in its position, the better is the treatment.[2] Many clinicians and researchers believe that the shape of the mandible represents a state of structural and functional balance that should not be changed with treatment, according to cited by Burke et al.[14] In this study, the upper intercanine distance presented an average expansion of 0.75 mm and the lower, 1.96 mm. This change reached a statistical significant index for both arches, although in the upper arch, on average, the change was smaller than in the lower arch. However, even if statistically significant, it is important to consider if this transverse alteration in the lower canines would be clinically important to cause, in the post-treatment period, a relapse that incurs in failure. To answer this question it is interesting to analyze the literature, and verify the expected alteration in this region with conventional orthodontic treatment. It would be interesting if it could be not modified, but the literature shows that this does not occur. Burke et al,[14] through a meta-analysis, evaluated 26 studies that investigated the longitudinal stability of the intercanine distance. The studies they evaluated had different malocclusions with respect to Angle classification, cases treated with and without extraction and different treatment modalities. This data was checked to verify the relationship in the stability in the inter-canine dimension. The results showed that the intercanine distance tends to increase in the order of 1 to 2 mm, irrespective of malocclusion, treatment modality and treatment with or without extraction, and that this alteration tends to be lost in the post-retention period. Johnson,[11] also evaluated the intercanine and intermolar distances in dental casts of cases treated with and without extractions. An average increase of 0.8 mm in the intermolar distance was found, and 0.3 mm for the intercanine distance, while the maximum increase was 1.5 mm in one case without extraction, the intercanine distance did not change. Another interesting work was published by Araújo, Leite and Brito.[10] The authors assessed the alterations in the intercanine distance in the lower arch in patients with Class I malocclusion, treated with and without extraction. The average increase in the intercanine distance observed during treatment was 1.35 mm in cases with extraction and 0.54 mm in cases without extraction. In the post-retention period, there was a reduction of this expansion in the order of 0.5 mm on average in patients treated with extraction and 0.13 mm in cases treated without extraction. In the present study, all patients were treated without extraction, with a minimum of 4 mm crowding in both arches and the changes observed during treatment, were within the parameters indicated in the literature as common in any type of treatment, making the treatment with low friction and thermal nickel titanium wires in cases of crowding, an additional option which tends to have the same degree of stability than any other protocol. Future works evaluating stability regarding the intercanine distance using this modality of treatment may bring greater clarity to the subject, as well as a correlation between the changes after retention and the degree of initial crowding or the amount of alteration observed in the active period of treatment. Once observed that the intercanine width undergoes alterations similar to other therapies, the question arises about where, indeed, there was a greater movement. For this, we also measured the transverse alterations in the premolars and molars region.

INTERPREMOLAR AND INTERMOLAR DISTANCES

In the present study, it was possible to verify that the major average transverse alterations occurred in the region of the premolars, especially in the maxillary arch. In the lower arch, there seemed to have a more uniform distribution of labial movement between the premolars and molars, but with even more intensity for the region of the premolars.

In the upper interpremolar distance, the average alterations surpassed 3 mm, reaching statistically significant values, with a value greater than three times the alteration in the intercanine distance. The molars had a smaller transverse increase, with a mean of2.49 mm for the first molars, but with a statistical significance and the second molars practically did not alter. In the lower arch, the average alteration in the region of the premolars was 2.95 mm for the first premolars and 3.39 mm for the second premolar, indicating that they were on average 1 mm and 1.43 mm, respectively, larger than the intercanine distance. The difference in expansion between the canine and premolars in the mandibular arch was not as great as in the maxillary arch, however, the lower molars also suffered expansion, far more expressive than in the maxillary arch, especially in the second molar region, where there was an expansion average of 2.37 mm. This difference found between upper and lower second molars seemed to be related to the fact that the upper second molars erupted already, typically, in a more buccal position, being, so, little influenced by the expansion treatment, once they were in a more buccal position than the other teeth of the same arch. But in the lower arch, these teeth erupt with lingual tipping, suffering the influence of the treatment with buccal tipping. All measurements in the lower arch reached a statistical significance.

This difference in expansion, between the maxilla and the mandible, was also observed by Begole, Fox and Sadowsky.[21] Evaluating 76 casts of 38 patients treated with and without extraction of the first premolars, these authors found that, in cases treated without extraction, significant differences were found between the maxillary expansion in relation to the mandible, greater for the maxilla, with the biggest increase in the region of the first and second premolars, except for the canines, which had similar expansions in both arches.

CONCLUSION

This result challenges conventional orthodontics when it proposes that the passive property of the bracket system, allowing all bonded brackets to function as tubes and applying extremely light forces due to the use of light and superelastic wires, allowing for a slow expansion of the dental arches, in many cases eliminating the need for rapid expansion, especially surgically assisted for the maxilla.

According to the results of this research, it seems clear that occurs, in fact, a lateral expansion, with buccal movement of the premolars, molars and to a lesser extent, of the canines, that provides space for leveling of initially crowded teeth, and most importantly, the alteration in the intercanine dimension was within the literature provides as normal for a conventional treatment, with or without extraction. It seems that the expansion was distributed throughout the dental arch, causing small buccal movement of all teeth, which together reached the space needed for leveling, which also justifies that the alterations are not exaggerated, although they reached statistical significance for most measurements. However, other studies evaluating the movement of the upper and lower incisors in the dental casts, as well in radiographies, can help complete the understanding of how tooth movement occurs with treatment with nickel titanium wire in a low friction system and thereby verify, in relation to the alveolar bone, which are the modifications due to movements of the posterior teeth. These topics, however, will be addressed in future publications.

REFERENCES

1. Riedel RA, Little RM, Bui TD. Mandibular incisor extraction: post retention evaluation of stability and relapse. Angle Orthod. 1992;62(2):103-16.
2. Sadowsky C, Sakols EI. Long-term assessment of orthodontic relapse. Am J Orthod. 1982;82(6):456-63.
3. Uhde MD, Sadowsky C, BeGole EA. Long-term stability of dental relationships after orthodontic treatment. Angle Orthod. 1983;53(3):240-52.
4. Sandikçioğlu M, Hazar S. Skeletal and dental changes after maxillary expansion in the mixed dentition. Am J Orthod Dentofacial Orthop. 1997;111(3):321-7.
5. Adkins MD, Nanda RS, Currier GF. Arch perimeter changes on rapid palatal expansion. Am J Orthod Dentofacial Orthop. 1990;97(3):194-9.
6. Sarver DM, Johnston MW. Skeletal changes in vertical and anterior displacement of the maxilla with bonded rapid palatal expansion appliance. Am J Orthod Dentofacial Orthop. 1989;95(6):462-6.
7. Davis WM, Kronman JH. Anatomical changes induced by splitting of the midpalatal suture. Angle Orthod. 1969;39(2):126-32.
8. Haas AJ. The treatment of maxillary deficiency by opening the midpalatal suture. Angle Orthod. 1965;35(3):200-17.
9. Haas AJ. Entrevista com Andrews Haas. Rev Dental Press Ortod Ortop Facial. 2001;6(1):1-10.
10. Araújo PRR, Leite HR, Brito HHA. Avaliação das alterações na distância intercaninos do arco inferior em pacientes com má oclusão de classe I tratados ortodonticamente Rev Dental Press Ortod Ortop. 2007;12(2):105-14.
11. Johnson KC. Cases six years postretention. Angle Orthod. 1977;47(3):210-21.
12. Strang RHW. The fallacy of denture expansion as a treatment procedure. Angle Orthod. 1949;14(1):12-22.
13. Walter DC. Comparative changes in mandibular canine and first molar widths. Angle Orthod. 1962;32(4):232-41.
14. Burke SP, Silveira AM, Goldsmith LJ, Yancey JM, Van Stewart A, Scarfe WC. A meta-analysis of mandibular intercanine width in treatment and postretention. Angle Orthod. 1998;68(1):53-60.
15. Erdinc AE, Nanda RS, Işiksal E. Relapse of anterior crowding in patients treated with extraction and nonextraction of premolars. Am J Orthod Dentofacial Orthop. 2006;129(6):775-84.
16. Rossouw PE, Preston CB, Lombard C. A longitudinal evaluation of extraction versus nonextraction treatment with special reference to the posttreatment irregularity of the lower incisors. Semin Orthod. 1999;5(3):160-70.
17. Heiser W, Richter M, Niederwanger A, Neunteufel N, Kulmer S. Association of the canine guidance angle with maxillary and mandibular intercanine widths and anterior alignment relapse: extraction vs nonextraction treatment. Am J Orthod Dentofacial Orthop. 2008;133(5):669-80.
18. Shapiro PA. Mandibular dental arch form and dimension: treatment and postretention changes. Am J Orthod. 1974;66(1):58-70.
19. Damon D. The rationale, evolution and clinical application of the self-ligating bracket. Clin Ortho Res. 1998;1(1):52-61.
20. Bagden A. The Damon system: questions and answers. Clin Impress. 2005;14(1):4-13.
21. Begole EA, Fox DL, Sadowsky C. Analysis of change in arch form with premolar expansion. Am J Orthodont Dentofaial Orthop. 1998;113(3):307-15.

7

Corrosion behavior of self-ligating and conventional metal brackets

Lúcio Henrique Esmeraldo Gurgel Maia[1], Hibernon Lopes Filho[1], Antônio Carlos de Oliveira Ruellas[2], Mônica Tirre de Souza Araújo[2], Delmo Santiago Vaitsman[3]

Objective: To test the null hypothesis that the aging process in self-ligating brackets is not higher than in conventional brackets. **Methods:** Twenty-five conventional (GN-3M/Unitek; GE-GAC; VE-Aditek) and 25 self-ligating (SCs-3M/Unitek; INs-GAC; ECs-Aditek) metal brackets from three manufacturers (n = 150) were submitted to aging process in 0.9% NaCl solution at a constant temperature of 37 ± 1°C for 21 days. The content of nickel, chromium and iron ions in the solution collected at intervals of 7, 14 and 21 days was quantified by atomic absorption spectrophotometry. After the aging process, the brackets were analyzed by scanning electron microscopy (SEM) under 22X and 1,000X magnifications. **Results:** Comparison of metal release in self-ligating and conventional brackets from the same manufacturer proved that the SCs group released more nickel ($p < 0.05$) than the GN group after 7 and 14 days, but less chromium ($p < 0.05$) after 14 days and less iron ($p < 0.05$) at the three experimental time intervals. The INs group released less iron ($p < 0.05$) than the GE group after 7 days and less nickel, chromium and iron ($p < 0.05$) after 14 and 21 days. The ECs group released more nickel, chromium and iron ($p < 0.05$) than the VE group after 14 days, but released less nickel and chromium ($p < 0.05$) after 7 days and less chromium and iron ($p < 0.05$) after 21 days. The SEM analysis revealed alterations on surface topography of conventional and self-ligating brackets. **Conclusions:** The aging process in self-ligating brackets was not greater than in conventional brackets from the same manufacturer. The null hypothesis was accepted.

Keywords: Corrosion. Orthodontic brackets. Metal.

[1] PhD resident of Orthodontics, Federal University of Rio de Janeiro (UFRJ).
[2] Associate professor, Department of Pediatric Dentistry and Orthodontics, UFRJ.
[3] Adjunct professor, Department of Analytical Chemistry, LaDA - IQ/UFRJ.

» The authors report no commercial, proprietary or financial interest in the products or companies described in this article.

Mônica Tirre de Souza Araújo
Avenida Professor Rodolpho Paulo Rocco, 325 – Ilha do Fundão – Departamento de Ortodontia / UFRJ. CEP: 21941-590 – Rio de Janeiro/RJ – Brazil
E-mail: monicatirre@uol.com.br

INTRODUCTION

Metal alloys are frequently used in Orthodontics to fabricate brackets, bands, wires and tubes. These alloys are made of austenitic stainless steel,[1,2] such as AISI 303, 304 and 316L,[3] and have nickel, chromium and iron in their composition.

When exposed to the oral environment, metal orthodontic accessories are subjected to degradation, such as corrosion by pits, fracture due to fatigue, increase in the coefficient of friction or microbiological degradation.[4,5] When the corrosive process occurs, metal ions are released into the oral medium or transformed into oxides.[2]

Self-ligating brackets have been widely used during the last decade by supposing that they have advantages[6] such as reduced treatment time as a result of reduced friction, and a more irregular morphology due to the connection system and larger volume in comparison with conventional brackets. For this reason, it is possible that they are more susceptible to corrosion.

Orthodontic appliance biodegradation is undesirable, and can hinder sliding mechanics,[7] cause reactions of hypersensitivity due to the release of nickel and chromium,[8,9] stain the enamel as a result of incorporating metal ions,[10] or even damage the appliance.[2] In self-ligating brackets, corrosion is also capable of altering the connection system and reducing its effectiveness.[11] In the active ligation system, it may hinder the capacity of pressing the wire into the slot.[11] Conversely, in the passive one, it may hamper opening or closing of the connection system.[12]

The aim of this study was to assess the aging process in conventional and self-ligating metal brackets. To this end, the null hypothesis assumed that the aging process in self-ligating brackets is not greater than in conventional brackets.

MATERIAL AND METHODS

Table 1 shows the distribution of the analyzed samples. The sample consisted of 150 metal brackets, 75 self-ligating and 75 conventional for maxillary right central incisors, from three different manufacturers (3M Unitek, Aditek and GAC) (25 brackets each). The conventional brackets were Gemini (3M/Unitek, Monrovia, CA, USA), Generus (GAC, Islandia, NY, USA) and Vector (Aditek, Cravinhos, SP, Brazil); whereas the self-ligating brackets were Smart Clip (3M/Unitek), In Ovation R (GAC) and Easy Clip (Aditek).

The 25 brackets of each group were divided into five subgroups, with an equal number of samples each, numbered from one to five.

The brackets of each subgroup were stored in previously sterilized Petri dishes, without coming into contact with one another. They were subjected to corrosion in 20 ml of sterile 0.9% NaCl solution[13,14] for a period of 21 days. The Petri dishes were kept in an incubator (Quimis - Quimis Aparelhos Científicos LTDA., Diadema-SP, Brazil) at an unchanged temperature of 37 ± 1°C.[15] Every 7 days ± 1 hour, the brackets were removed and transferred to another container filled with a new solution.[1,13]

At the end of each experimental time interval (7 days, 14 days and 21 days), the solution remaining in each container was analyzed by atomic absorption spectrophotometry in a Varian spectrophotometer, Model AA-1475 (Varian Indústria e Comércio Ltda., São Paulo/SP, Brazil) with a view to determining their nickel, chromium and iron contents.

At the end of the experiment, five brackets from each group (one from each subgroup) were randomly selected and their surface topography was analyzed by scanning electron microscopy – SEM (Jeol JSM 6460 LV, Japan) and compared with the surface of new brackets.

Table 1 - Distribution of samples.

Bracket	n	Group	Ligation system	Manufacturer	Reference	Lot
Gemini	25	GN	Conventional	3M / Unitek	119-713	019329500
Generus	25	GE		GAC	31-212-32	B479
Vector	25	VE		Aditek	12.32.411	100329
Smart clip	25	SCs	Self ligating	3M / Unitek	004-302	016560600B
In Ovation R	25	INs		GAC	89-112-00	B3Y7
Easy clip	25	ECs		Aditek	13.32.011	090303

SEM was operated at 20 kV, and readouts were taken under 22X and 1,000X magnification. The 22X magnification allowed a complete view of the bracket. The 1,000X magnification was performed at the slot of each bracket with the connection system opened so as to analyze the area for wire insertion. No treatment was performed on the brackets at the end of the experiment in order to prevent any possible oxides, deposited on the bracket surface as a result of the corrosion process, from being removed. Energy-dispersive X-ray spectroscopy (EDS) was used to identify atypical depositions on bracket surface.

In each group and at each time interval, nickel, chromium and iron concentrations as well as the total amount released during the experiment were statistically assessed. The Kolmogorov-Smirnov test was used to verify the

Table 2 - Nickel content (PPM) after the different experimental time intervals.

Nickel release (PPM)											
	7 days			14 days			21 days			Total	
Group	**Mean ± SD**	**Intra. Sig.**	**Inter. Sig.**	**Mean ± SD**	**Intra. Sig.**	**Inter. Sig.**	**Mean ± SD**	**Intra. Sig.**	**Inter. Sig.**	**Mean ± SD**	**Inter. Sig.**
GN	0.00	a	A	0.00	a	A	0.00	a	A	0.0 (0.0)	A
GE	0.14 ± 0.28	a	ABC	0.92 ± 0.03	b	B	0.68 ± 0.02	b	B	1.74 ± 0.27	B
VE	0.53 ± 0.03	a	B	0.00 ± 0.01	b	A	0.00 ± 0.01	b	A	0.54 ± 0.03	C
SCs	0.11 ± 0.03	a	C	0.07 ± 0.01	b	C	0.00	c	A	0.18 ± 0.01	D
INs	0.14 ± 0.01	a	C	0.39 ± 0.02	b	D	0.00 ± 0.01	c	A	0.54 ± 0.03	C
ECs	2.79 ± 0.03	a	D	1.24 ± 0.03	b	E	0.00 ± 0.01	c	A	4.03 ± 0.03	E

Identical letters reveal no statistical difference ($p > 0.05$). Intragroup significance - Comparison of the different time intervals in each group with ANOVA test and Tukey post hoc-test. Intergroup Significance - Comparison among the groups in each time interval with Kruskal-Wallis test and Wilcoxon post hoc-test.

Table 3 - Chromium content (PPM) after the different experimental time intervals.

Chromium release(PPM)											
	7 days			14 days			21 days			Total	
Group	**Mean ± SD**	**Intra. Sig.**	**Inter. Sig.**	**Mean ± SD**	**Intra. Sig.**	**Inter. Sig.**	**Mean ± SD**	**Intra. Sig.**	**Inter. Sig.**	**Mean ± SD**	**Inter. Sig.**
GN	0.50 ± 0.11	a	AB	1.03 ± 0.01	b	A	1.68 ± 0.03	c	A	3.21 ± 0.12	AB
GE	0.89 ± 0.10	a	C	1.29 ± 0.02	b	B	1.95 ± 0.03	c	B	4.13 ± 0.10	C
VE	1.15 ± 0.02	a	D	1.03 ± 0.05	b	A	1.95 ± 0.06	c	B	4.13 ± 0.11	C
SCs	0.45 ± 0.01	a	A	0.30 ± 0.03	a	C	2.05 ± 0.35	b	AB	2.81 ± 0.33	D
INs	0.76 ± 0.02	a	C	1.03 ± 0.08	b	A	1.42 ± 0.02	c	C	3.21 ± 0.09	A
ECs	0.63 ± 0.02	a	B	1.55 ± 0.03	b	D	1.16 ± 0.03	c	D	3.34 ± 0.05	B

Identical letters indicate no statistical difference ($p > 0.05$). Intragroup significance - Comparison of the different time intervals in each group with ANOVA test and Tukey post hoc-test. Intergroup Significance - Comparison among the groups in each time interval with Kruskal-Wallis test and Wilcoxon post hoc-test.

Table 4 - Iron content (PPM) after the different experimental time intervals.

Iron release (PPM)											
	7 days			14 days			21 days			Total	
Group	**Mean ± SD**	**Intra. Sig.**	**Inter. Sig.**	**Mean ± SD**	**Intra. Sig.**	**Inter. Sig.**	**Mean ± SD**	**Intra. Sig.**	**Inter. Sig.**	**Mean ± SD**	**Inter. Sig.**
GN	0.35 ± 0.03	a	A	0.44 ± 0.03	b	A	1.02 ± 0.02	c	A	1.81 ± 0.04	A
GE	0.93 ± 0.05	a	B	1.02 ± 0.02	b	B	1.28 ± 0.02	c	B	3.23 ± 0.08	B
VE	1.01± 0.05	a	B	0.77 ± 0.04	b	C	1.02 ± 0.02	a	A	2.80 ± 0.09	CD
SCs	0.00 ± 0.01	a	C	0.01 ± 0.02	a	D	0.94 ± 0.02	b	C	0.96 ± 0.04	E
INs	0.77 ± 0.02	a	D	0.94 ± 0.02	b	E	1.01 ± 0.03	c	A	2.72 ± 0.02	C
ECs	1.02 ± 0.03	a	B	0.94 ± 0.02	b	E	0.94 ± 0.04	b	D	2.90 ± 0.08	D

Identical letters indicate no statistical difference ($p > 0.05$). Intragroup significance - Comparison of the different time intervals in each group with ANOVA test and Tukey post hoc-test. Intergroup Significance - Comparison among the groups in each time interval with Kruskal-Wallis test and Wilcoxon post hoc-test.

sample normality of distribution. As normal distribution was not found, the non-parametric ANOVA test with Tukey post-test were applied for intragroup assessment, whereas the Kruskal-Wallis test with Wilcoxon post-test were applied for intergroup assessment. The data were statistically analyzed using SPSS 17.0 software (Statistical Package for Social Sciences, SPSS Inc., Chicago, IL, USA). The significance level was set at 5%.

RESULTS

During the experimental period, the release of nickel, chromium and iron metal ions was observed in all groups, except for nickel ion in the GN group, which was not detected at any of the time intervals (Tables 2, 3 and 4).

There was greater release of nickel in the initial period of the experiment, both for conventional and self-ligating brackets, with a trend towards no release of this ion at the end of the experiment ($p < 0.05$). Only group GN and group GE behaved differently with greater release of nickel on the 14th and 21st days. The experimental groups revealed a trend towards increasing release of ions, such as chromium and iron, from the first to the third week of the experiment ($p < 0.05$). The only exception was group VE, in which a great amount of iron release was found in the first week. Metal release was similar in self-ligating and conventional brackets from the same manufacturer. Group SCs released more nickel ($p < 0.05$) than group GN after 7 and 14 days, but group GN released more chromium ($p < 0.05$) after 14 days and more iron ($p < 0.05$) at the three experimental time intervals. Group INs released less iron ($p < 0.05$) than group GE after 7 days; and less nickel, chromium and iron ($p < 0.05$) after 14 and 21 days. Group ECs released more nickel, chromium and iron ($p < 0.05$) than group VE after 14 days, but released less nickel and chromium ($p < 0.05$) after 7 days and less chromium and iron ($p < 0.05$) after 21 days.

At the end of the experiment, the SEM analysis revealed that the surface topography of all brackets changed, with signs of aging when compared with the surface of new brackets (Figs 1 to 4).

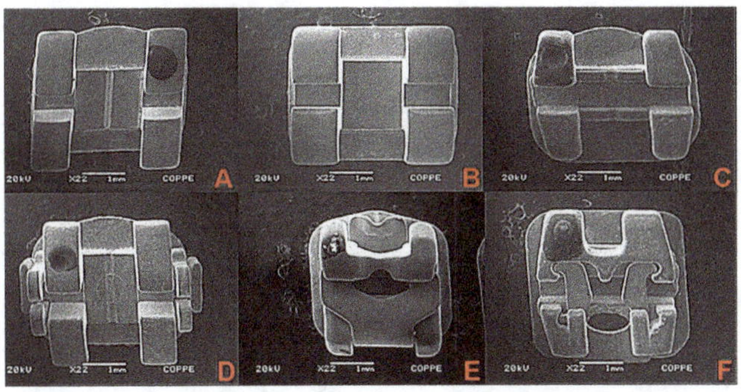

Figure 1 - Surface topography of new brackets visualized by SEM under 22X magnification. **A)** GN; **B)** GE; **C)** VE; **D)** SCs; **E)** INs; **F)** ECs.

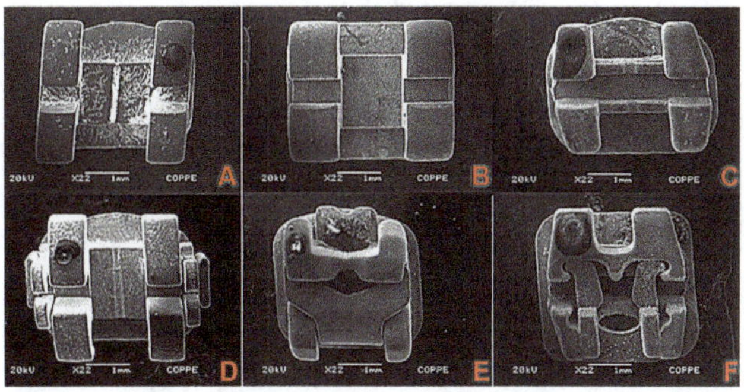

Figure 2 - Surface topography of brackets visualized by SEM under 22X magnification after 21 days. **A)** GN; **B)** GE; **C)** VE; **D)** SCs; **E)** INs; **F)** ECs.

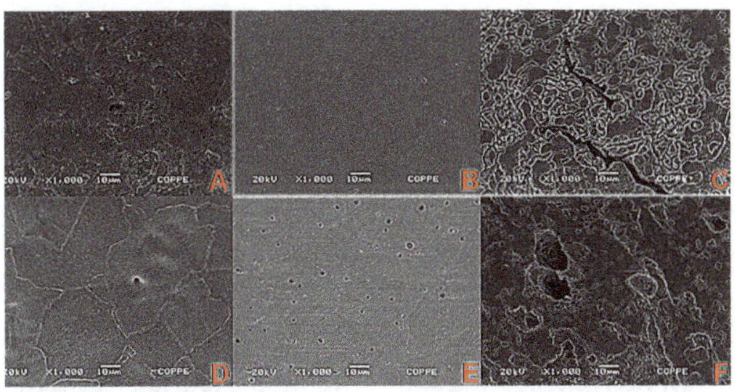

Figure 3 - Surface topography of new brackets visualized by SEM under 1000X magnification. **A)** GN; **B)** GE; **C)** VE; **D)** SCs; **E)** INs; **F)** ECs.

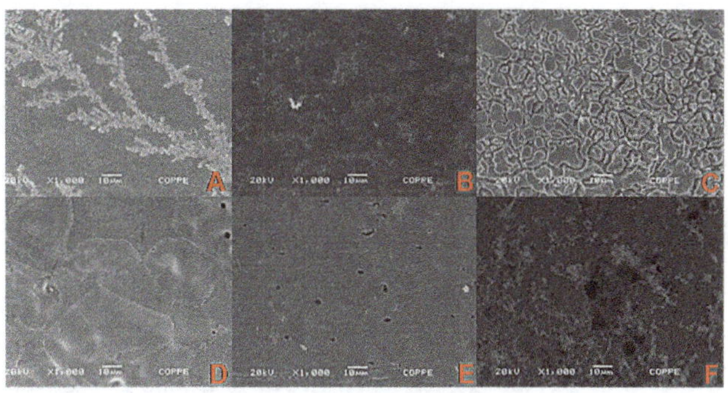

Figure 4 - Surface topography of brackets visualized by SEM under 1000X magnification after 21 days. **A)** GN; **B)** GE; **C)** VE; **D)** SCs; **E)** INs; **F)** ECs.

DISCUSSION

Bracket corrosion with consequent release of metal ions during orthodontic treatment may hinder orthodontic mechanics,[2] trigger hypersensitivity reactions with hyperplasia and gingival tissue inflammation,[4,8,9] and contribute to iatrogenic staining of the enamel with the incorporation of metals.[10,16]

A corroded bracket often presents a more irregular surface and can accumulate products resulting from corrosion (Fig 4). Thus, friction between the bracket and wire during sliding mechanics increases, making it necessary to apply force of greater magnitude to overcome the friction and produce physiologic tooth movement.[7,17,18] When excessive force is applied to the bracket, there is loss of mechanical control and increased probability of root resorption.[5,9,19,21]

One of the advantages attributed to self-ligating brackets is the lower degree of friction that the ligation system imposes on the orthodontic wire when compared with conventional tying.[6,22,24] However, if the bracket has an increased corrosion potential, friction also increases,[25] affecting this advantage.

In the present study, SEM analysis under 22X magnification (Fig 2) revealed that, in general, self-ligating brackets showed more areas with altered surface topography due to corrosion, when compared with conventional brackets from the same manufacturer, possibly due to their geometry with larger retentive areas. Thus, brackets in the INs group had a more irregular surface than the brackets in the GE group, while the brackets in the ECs group presented greater alterations in comparison to those in the VE group. The self-ligating brackets of the SCs group and the conventional brackets in group GN did not present significant alterations in their surface topography. Energy-dispersive X-ray spectroscopy (EDS) revealed NaCl deposition on the surfaces of the brackets in group GN.

Analysis of the images obtained by SEM under 1000X magnification (Figs 3 and 4) suggests that new brackets with more irregular surfaces were more susceptible to corrosion. Thus, the brackets in group ECs, which presented a surface topography with deficient smoothness and porosity at the beginning of the experiment, presented a considerably more irregular surface at the end of it. The brackets in group VE also presented considerably altered surfaces at the end of the experiment, due to the formation of oxides. Moreover, the brackets in group INs, which presented irregularities at the beginning of the experiment, were significantly subjected to pitting corrosion. Quantification of the metal ions released during the experiment corroborates these data. These groups had great release of nickel, chromium and iron ions.

The release of metal ions into the oral environment may trigger hypersensitivity reactions.[4,5,8,9,26] Nickel and chromium are present in the composition of brackets with the goal of increasing resistance to corrosion.[2,4,16,27] These elements are largely responsible for the aforementioned adverse reactions. Nickel is strongly responsible for triggering more allergic reactions than any other metal.[8,26]

Under the conditions of this experiment, the release of nickel was considerably lower than the daily ingestion of this metal through food (300 to 600 μg/day).[13] However, it is worth noting that susceptible patients in contact with small concentrations of this metal are more likely to suffer hypersensitivity reactions.[29]

The oral reaction of allergy to nickel is difficult to diagnose, since its clinical signs and symptoms are similar to those of gingivitis caused by poor oral hygiene. The low number of reports of hypersensitivity to nickel is possibly due to this difficulty in diagnosis. Epidemiological data point towards an incidence of sensitivity to this metal of approximately 20% in the general population.[28,30]

Similarly to other *in vitro* studies,[1,15,31] the release of nickel in this experiment was higher in the first two weeks, with a trend towards no further release during the third week. The exception was group GE which continued to release nickel ions during the last week (Table 2).

Similarly to previous studies,[1,13] chromium and iron ions had a trend towards increasing release throughout the experiment in all groups, except for group ECs (Tables 3 and 4). In this group, there was a greater release of chromium in the second week, and greater release of iron in the first week, although the concentration of these ions remained high at the end of the third week.

Within the limitations and conditions of this experiment, it is reasonable to conclude that metal release was similar in self-ligating and conventional brackets from the same manufacturer.

When self-ligating and conventional brackets from the same manufacturer were compared, group SCs proved to release more nickel ($p < 0.05$) than group GN after

7 and 14 days, whereas group GN released more chromium ($p < 0.05$) after 14 days and more iron ($p < 0.05$) at the three experimental time intervals. Group INs released less iron ($p < 0.05$) than group GE after 7 days and less nickel, chromium and iron ($p < 0.05$) after 14 and 21 days. Group ECs released more nickel, chromium and iron ($p < 0.05$) than group VE after 14 days, but released less nickel and chromium ($p < 0.05$) after 7 days and less chromium and iron ($p < 0.05$) after 21 days.

Metal ions released by metal brackets and bands during orthodontic treatment may be incorporated into tooth enamel, causing iatrogenic color alteration and stains.[10,16] In cases of severe pigmentation, restorative treatment of the vestibular surface of the stained tooth proves necessary.[32,33] Special care must be given to patients with poor oral hygiene, since altered oral environment, with reduced pH and presence of acidogenic microorganisms potentiates the corrosion of metal accessories. Additionally, enamel demineralization and remineralization processes may influence the incorporation of metals.[4,10]

CONCLUSIONS

» The null hypothesis was accepted.

» The SEM analysis revealed that self-ligating and conventional brackets presented signs of aging.

» Metal ions release in self-ligating brackets was similar to conventional brackets from the same manufacturer.

Acknowledgements

We deeply thank Dr. Cláudia Trindade Mattos for helping us with statistical analysis of data.

REFERENCES

1. Barrett RD, Bishara SE, Quinn JK. Biodegradation of orthodontic appliances. Part I. Biodegradation of nickel and chromium in vitro. Am J Orthod Dentofacial Orthop. 1993;103(1):8-14.
2. Toms AP. The corrosion of orthodontic wire. Eur J Orthod. 1988;10:87-97.
3. Zinelis S, Annousaki O, Eliades T, Makou M. Elemental composition of brazing alloys in metallic orthodontic brackets. Angle Orthod. 2004;74(3):394-9.
4. Eliades T, Athanasiou AE. In vivo aging of orthodontic alloys: implications for corrosion potential, nickel release, and biocompatibility. Angle Orthod. 2002;72(3):222-37.
5. House K, Sernetz F, Dymock D, Sandy JR, Ireland AJ. Corrosion of orthodontic appliances--should we care? Am J Orthod Dentofacial Orthop. 2008;133(4):584-92.
6. Pizzoni L, Ravnholt G, Melsen B. Frictional forces related to self-ligating brackets. Eur J Orthod. 1998;20(3):283-91.
7. Andreasen GF, Quevedo FR. Evaluation of friction forces in the 0.022 x 0.028 edgewise bracket in vitro. J Biomech. 1970;3(2):151-60.
8. Menezes LM, Campos LC, Quintão CC, Bolognese AM. Hypersensitivity to metals in orthodontics. Am J Orthod Dentofacial Orthop. 2004;126(1):58-64.
9. Hwang CJ, Shin JS, Cha JY. Metal release from simulated fixed orthodontic appliances. Am J Orthod Dentofacial Orthop. 2001;120(4):383-91.
10. Maia LHEG, Lima Filho HL, Araujo MVA, Ruellas ACO, Araujo MTS. Incorporation of metal and color alteration of enamel in the presence of orthodontic appliances. Angle Orthod. 2012;82(5):889-93.
11. Pandis N, Bourauel C, Eliades T. Changes in the stiffness of the ligating mechanism in retrieved active self-ligating brackets. Am J Orthod Dentofacial Orthop. 2007;132(6):834-7.
12. Eliades T. Self-ligating brackets malfunction: is it due to corrosion? Orthod Mat Insider. 2009;21:4-7.
13. Grimsdottir MR, Gjerdet NR, Hensten-Pettersen A. Composition and in vitro corrosion of orthodontic appliances. Am J Orthod Dentofacial Orthop. 1992;101(6):525-32.
14. Kerosuo H, Moe G, Kleven E. In vitro release of nickel and chromium from different types of simulated orthodontic appliances. Angle Orthod. 1995;65(2):111-6.
15. Park HY, Shearer TR. In vitro release of nickel and chromium from simulated orthodontic appliances. Am J Orthod. 1983;84(2):156-9.
16. Maijer R, Smith DC. Corrosion of orthodontic bracket bases. Am J Orthod. 1982;81(1):43-8.
17. Angolkar PV, Kapila S, Duncanson MG Jr, Nanda RS. Evaluation of friction between ceramic brackets and orthodontic wires of four alloys. Am J Orthod Dentofacial Orthop. 1990;98(6):499-506.
18. Kapila S, Angolkar PV, Duncanson MG Jr, Nanda RS. Evaluation of friction between edgewise stainless steel brackets and orthodontic wires of four alloys. Am J Orthod Dentofacial Orthop. 1990;98(2):117-26.
19. Drescher D, Bourauel C, Schumacher HA. Frictional forces between bracket and arch wire. Am J Orthod Dentofacial Orthop. 1989;96(5):397-404.
20. Lin MC, Lin SC, Lee TH, Huang HH. Surface analysis and corrosion resistance of different stainless steel orthodontic brackets in artificial saliva. Angle Orthod. 2006;76(2):322-9.
21. Reitan K. Initial tissue behavior during apical root resorption. Angle Orthod. 1974;44(1):68-82.
22. Berger JL. The influence of the SPEED bracket's self-ligating design on force levels in tooth movement: a comparative in vitro study. Am J Orthod Dentofacial Orthop. 1990;97(3):219-28.
23. Thorstenson GA, Kusy RP. Resistance to sliding of self-ligating brackets versus conventional stainless steel twin brackets with second-order angulation in the dry and wet (saliva) states. Am J Orthod Dentofacial Orthop. 2001;120(4):361-70.
24. Thomas S, Sherriff M, Birnie D. A comparative in vitro study of the frictional characteristics of two types of self-ligating brackets and two types of pre-adjusted edgewise brackets tied with elastomeric ligatures. Eur J Orthod. 1998;20(5):589-96.
25. Marques IS, Araujo AM, Gurgel JA, Normando D. Debris, roughness and friction of stainless steel archwires following clinical use. Angle Orthod. 2010;80(3):521-7.
26. Bishara SE, Barrett RD, Selim MI. Biodegradation of orthodontic appliances. Part II. Changes in the blood level of nickel. Am J Orthod Dentofacial Orthop. 1993;103(2):115-9.
27. Maijer R, Smith DC. Biodegradation of the orthodontic bracket system. Am J Orthod Dentofacial Orthop. 1986;90(3):195-8.
28. Bass JK, Fine H, Cisneros GJ. Nickel hypersensitivity in the orthodontic patient. Am J Orthod Dentofacial Orthop. 1993;103(3):280-5.
29. Prystowsky SD, Allen AM, Smith RW, Nonomura JH, Odom RB, Akers WA. Allergic contact hypersensitivity to nickel, neomycin, ethylenediamine, and benzocaine. Relationships between age, sex, history of exposure,

and reactivity to standard patch tests and use tests in a general population. Arch Dermatol. 1979;115(8):959-62.

30. Kerosuo H, Kullaa A, Kerosuo E, Kanerva L, Hensten-Pettersen A. Nickel allergy in adolescents in relation to orthodontic treatment and piercing of ears. Am J Orthod Dentofacial Orthop. 1996;109(2):148-54.
31. Menne T, Brandup F, Thestrup-Pedersen K, Veien NK, Andersen JR, Yding F, et al. Patch test reactivity to nickel alloys. Contact Dermatitis. 1987;16(5):255-9.
32. Romano FS, Correr Sobrinho L, Consani S, Araújo MBB, Nouer DF. Oxidação de bráquetes metálicos. Rev Dental Press Ortod Ortop Facial. 2005;10(6):24-5.
33. Hodges SJ, Spencer RJ, Watkins SJ. Unusual indelible enamel staining following fixed appliance treatment. J Orthod. 2000;27(4):303-6.

8

Color stability of ceramic brackets immersed in potentially staining solutions

Bruna Coser Guignone[1], Ludimila Karsbergen Silva[1], Rodrigo Villamarim Soares[2], Emilio Akaki[2], Marcelo Coelho Goiato[3], Matheus Melo Pithon[4], Dauro Douglas Oliveira[5]

Objective: To assess the color stability of five types of ceramic brackets after immersion in potentially staining solutions. **Methods:** Ninety brackets were divided into 5 groups (n = 18) according to brackets commercial brands and the solutions in which they were immersed (coffee, red wine, coke and artificial saliva). The brackets assessed were Transcend (3M/Unitek, Monrovia, CA, USA), Radiance (American Orthodontics, Sheboygan, WI, USA), Mystique (GAC International Inc., Bohemia, NY, USA) and Luxi II (Rocky Mountain Orthodontics, Denver, CO, USA). Chromatic changes were analyzed with the aid of a reflectance spectrophotometer and by visual inspection at five specific time intervals. Assessment periods were as received from the manufacturer (T_0), 24 hours (T_1), 72 hours (T_2), as well as 7 days (T_3) and 14 days (T_4) of immersion in the aforementioned solutions. Results were submitted to statistical analysis with ANOVA and Bonferroni correction, as well as to a multivariate profile analysis for independent and paired samples with significance level set at 5%. **Results:** The duration of the immersion period influenced color alteration of all tested brackets, even though these changes could not always be visually observed. Different behaviors were observed for each immersion solution; however, brackets immersed in one solution progressed similarly despite minor variations. **Conclusions:** Staining became more intense over time and all brackets underwent color alterations when immersed in the aforementioned solutions.

Keywords: Orthodontic brackets. Optical properties. Color instability.

[1] MSc in Orthodontics, Pontifícia Universidade Católica de Minas Gerais (PUC Minas), Belo Horizonte, Minas Gerais, Brazil.
[2] Associate professor, Pontifícia Universidade Católica de Minas Gerais (PUC Minas), Belo Horizonte, Minas Gerais, Brazil.
[3] Full professor, Universidade Estadual Paulista Júlio de Mesquita Filho (UNESP), Araçatuba, São Paulo, Brazil.
[4] Adjunct professor of Orthodontics, Universidade Estadual do Sudoeste da Bahia (UESB), Jequié, Bahia, Brazil.
[5] Director of Orthodontics Program, Pontifícia Universidade Católica de Minas Gerais (PUC Minas), Belo Horizonte, Minas Gerais, Brazil.

Dauro Douglas Oliveira
Av. Dom José Gaspar, 500 – Prédio 46, Sala 106
Belo Horizonte, MG, Brazil, CEP: 30535-610 - E-mail: dauro.bhe@gmail.com

INTRODUCTION

The increasing number of adult patients seeking orthodontic treatment has reinforced the need for esthetic orthodontic appliances.[1] The orthodontic industry, aiming to profit from this demand, has invested in the development of different types of esthetic material, striving to meet the expectations of patients and clinicians.[1,2] Ceramic brackets are a result os this process.[3,4]

Ceramic brackets may be manufactured with polycrystalline ceramic or monocrystalline sapphire.[3,4,5] These brackets are inert to the oral environment[1] and have become the most commonly used esthetic fixed orthodontic appliances worldwide due to superior esthetics and mechanical resistance when compared to plastic brackets.[1,3-6]

Despite remarkable quality improvement since the introduction of the first ceramic brackets in the 80's, ceramic brackets currently available on the market still present significant limitations, such as high friability; increased friction with orthodontic wires, when compared to metallic brackets; the possibility of causing wear on antagonist teeth; and the risk of damaging the enamel structure during debonding.[7,8,9] Although their color features are their major advantage over metallic brackets, there is a limited number of reports analyzing their optical properties over time.[10] Lack of such studies may be related to technical difficulties in measuring brackets color, given that their geometry may hinder accurate color measurement with a spectrophotometer or colorimeter.[12]

Therefore, the objective of this study was to assess the color stability of different ceramic brackets exposed to potentially staining solutions during a period of time.

MATERIAL AND METHODS

Ninety maxillary central incisor ceramic brackets of five different types and commercial brands (Table 1) were assessed (n = 18). Prior to immersion in potentially staining solutions, all brackets had their bases leveled by 180-grain water sandpapers (Doble A®, Argentine Abrasives S.A.I.C, Argentina) in a polishing machine (Knuth-Rotor®, Struers, Denmark) under constant irrigation. Subsequently, all brackets were cleaned with acetone to remove any speck adhered to their surface.

Staining analysis

Brackets were immersed in four potentially staining solutions: red wine (Miolo Terranova 2006, Bento Gonçalves, Brazil), coffee (Café Três Corações, Três Corações, Brazil), coke (Coca-Cola, Belo Horizonte, Brazil) and artificial saliva (control group). Each solution was distributed into five small black plastic containers, so as to eliminate light interference. Each container had six brackets of the same brand and was stored at room temperature. Solutions were changed every 24 hours. All brackets were divided into four groups, according to the solution in which they were immersed (n = 6).

Before immersion (T_0), all brackets had color measured (baseline – T_0). Subsequently, color was analyzed after a period of 24 (T_1), and 72 hours (T_2), as well as after 7 (T_3) and 14 days (T_4) of immersion.

Color readings were assessed with the aid of a reflectance spectrophotometer (UV-visible spectrophotometer UV-2450, Shimadzu, Kyoto, Japan), according to the Commission Internationale de l´Eclairage (CIE) L★, a★, b★ (LAB) color scale.[15] The CIELAB system of color assessment quantitatively assess the color features of an object, based on three parameters (L★, a★ e b★): L★ is the measurement of brightness quantified on a scale in which black has an L★ value equal to zero, whereas a totally reflected light has an L★ value equal to 100; a★ measures the amount of red (+a★) and green (-a★); and b★ measures the amount of yellow (+b★) and blue (-b★). Total color

Table 1 - Ceramic brackets evaluated.

Commercial brand	Composition	Manufacturer
Clarity	Polycrystalline alumina, stainless steel slot	3M/Unitek, Monrovia, CA, USA
Transcend	Polycrystalline alumina	3M/Unitek, Monrovia, CA, USA
Radiance	Monocrystalline alumina	American Orthodontics, Sheboygan, WI, USA
Mystique	Polycrystalline alumina	GAC International Inc., Bohemia, NY, USA
Luxi II	Polycrystalline alumina, gold slot	Rocky Mountain Orthodontics, Denver, CO, USA

changes (Δ E★ab) were calculated by the following equation:[16] $\Delta E^\star ab = [(\Delta L^\star)^2 + (\Delta a^\star)^2 + (\Delta b^\star)^2]^{1/2}$.

Changes in color parameters (Δ L★, Δ a★ and Δ b★) were calculated by subtraction (i.e. $T_1 - T_0$). Prior to each measurement carried out with the reflectance spectrophotometer, all brackets were washed with distilled water, so as to remove any staining solution residue from their surface.

Visual assessment

Visual analysis of brackets was performed at the same time intervals previously described and by two different operators. One bracket from each group was washed with distilled water, air-dried and placed on a white surface beside a similar bracket, which had not been immersed in any staining solution, for comparison.

This analysis aimed to visually detect potential bracket staining and relate it to the time of immersion in different solutions. Whenever any visible color change was detected, it was recorded as described by Mancuso et al.[11]

Statistical analysis

Data were analyzed by means of SPSS 15.0, Microsoft Excel and Gpower 3.0. Multivariate profile analysis, analysis of variance (ANOVA) and t test for independent paired samples, with significance level set at 5%, were used to compare intra and intergroup mean values obtained in the reflectance spectrophotometer after immersion of brackets in different solutions during specific time intervals.

ANOVA was used to investigate differences between groups and when significant differences were found, Bonferroni correction was used to verify in which group such differences had occurred (Table 2). Multivariate profile analysis (Table 3) was used to analyze time effect not considering brackets brand. It was also used to test whether the staining pattern and the tested brackets brands were similar or different over time.

RESULTS

After being immersed in artificial saliva for 24 hours, Radiance brackets presented statistically significant color alteration when compared to Transcend brackets which were the most stable group (Table 2).

ANOVA results (Table 2) revealed that, when immersed in coke, Radiance brackets presented statistically significant ($p < 0.05$) color alterations in comparison to other bracket brands after 24 and 72 hours, as well as after 7 days of immersion. However, there were no statistically significant differences ($p > 0.05$) regarding color changes between brackets brands in this solution after 14 days (Table 2). Immersion in coffee only caused statistically significant color alterations in Transcend brackets compared to Mystique brackets after 14 days of immersion (Table 2). When immersed in red wine for 24 hours, Radiance brackets presented statistically higher ($p < 0.05$) color alterations in comparison to Luxi II. The same interval of red wine immersion promoted statistically higher ($p < 0.05$) color alterations in Radiance brackets in comparison to Clarity, Luxi II and Transcend brackets. However, after 72 hours, the color alterations observed in Radiance brackets were only higher than Luxi II brackets (Table 2), and differences between bracket brands after this period of immersion were not found.

Multivariate analysis results (Table 3) revealed that, during a specific time period (from 7 to 14 days),there were significant color changes ($p = 0.000$) in all brackets immersed in coke. Immersion in the same solution led to similar staining patterns after 24 to 72 hours ($p = 0.486$), and from 72 hours to 7 days ($p = 0.525$), although a different staining pattern occurred from 7 to 14 days ($p = 0.002$). A time effect ($p = 0.004$) was also observed on brackets exposed to coffee solution, since there were significant color alterations for specific time periods (24 to 72 hours – $p = 0.007$; 72 hours to 7 days – $p = 0.002$). Immersion in the same solution led to a similar staining pattern on bracket brands only from 24 to 72 hours ($p = 0.478$). Finally, immersion in red wine also revealed a time effect ($p = 0.000$), since significant color alterations at all time intervals (24 to 72 hours – $p = 0.000$; 72 hours to 7 days – $p = 0.002$; 7 to 14 days – $p = 0.000$) were observed in the brackets tested. Exposure to this solution also led to different ($p = 0.004$) staining patterns on bracket brands at all time intervals (24 to 72 hours, $p = 0.018$; 72 hours to 7 days, $p = 0.012$; 7 to 14 days, $p = 0.005$).

Visual inspection

After seven days of immersion in staining solutions, chromatic changes were found in all types of brackets analyzed. Thereafter, there was progressive staining of brackets until 14 days of immersion. Brackets immersed

Table 2 - Mean values of color alteration of brackets immersed in different solutions and over different periods of time.

		ΔE_1 (24h)	ΔE_2 (72h)	ΔE_3 (7d)	ΔE_4 (14d)
Clarity	Saliva	126.93	126.93	126.93	126.93
	Coke	117.53	104.93	98.06	46.38
	Coffee	109.86	90.31	54.93	42.24
	Red wine	40.5	50.84	72.94	135.31
Luxi II	Saliva	142.3	142.3	142.3	142.3
	Coke	88.41	108.6	98.19	29.68
	Coffee	78.16	48.88	74.13	58.15
	Red wine	26.84	43.42	65.63	140.72
Mystique	Saliva	116.47	116.47	116.47	116.47
	Coke	120.81	135.18	129.67	36.67
	Coffee	78.19	67.65	59.67	37.43
	Red wine	58.61[b]	65.71	73.39	112.14
Radiance	Saliva	155.07[e]	155.07[e]	155.07[e]	155.07[e]
	Coke	173.45[be]	166.85[abe]	175.58[abce]	55.92
	Coffee	96.95	74.78	40.79	85.03
	Red wine	80.52[abe]	75.39[b]	65.96	97.34
Transcend	Saliva	111.65	111.65	111.65	111.65
	Coke	75.57	93.5	96.78	50.92
	Coffee	44.74	45.6	44.12	94.18[c]
	Red wine	40.56	67.13	61.98	126.09

ANOVA and Bonferroni correction. Statistically significant differences ($p < 0.05$) between bracket brands are represented by letters.

Table 3 - Multivariate analysis of brackets exposed to different staining solutions: time and brand factors.

	Significance		
	Coke	Coffee	Wine
Time (initial)	0.000	0.004	0.000
24 hours - 72 hours	0.363	0.007	0.000
72 hours - 7 days	0.801	0.002	0.002
7 days - 14 days	0.000	0.650	0.000
Time by brand (parallelism)	0.020	0.002	0.004
24 hours - 72 hours	0.486	0.478	0.018
72 hours - 7 days	0.525	0.009	0.012
7 days - 14 days	0.002	0.014	0.005
Brands	0.000	0.424	0.354

Coke: 1) Mauchly's sphericity test ($p = 0.152$); 2) non-significant Levene's test [ΔE_1 (24 h) ($p = 0.03$); ΔE_2 (72 h) ($p = 0.08$); ΔE_3 (7 d) ($p = 0.22$); ΔE_4 (14 d) ($p = 0.79$)].
Coffee: 1) Mauchly's sphericity test ($p = 0.001$); 2) non-significant Levene's test [ΔE_1 (24 h) ($p = 0.58$); ΔE_2 (72 h) ($p = 0.37$); ΔE_3 (7 d) ($p = 0.32$);ΔE_4 (14 d) ($p = 0.98$)].
Wine: 1) Mauchly's sphericity test ($p < 0.001$); 2) non-significant Levene's test [ΔE_1 (24 h) ($p = 0.02$); ΔE_2 (72 h) ($p = 0.82$); ΔE_3 (7 d) ($p = 0.97$); ΔE_4 (14 d) ($p = 0.18$)].

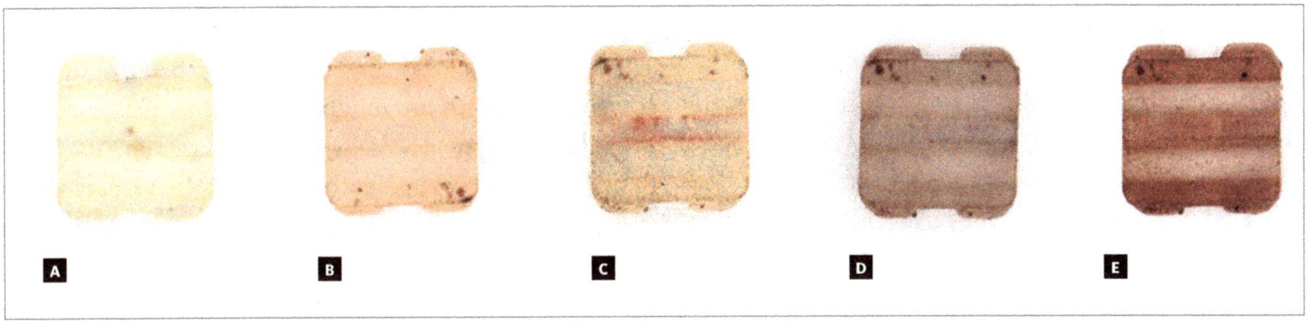

Figure 1 - Brackets after immersion in red wine: **A)** baseline, **B)** after 24 hours, **C)** after 72 hours, **D)** after 7 days, and **E)** after 14 days of immersion.

in artificial saliva revealed no visible color changes after 24 hours of immersion (Fig 1).

DISCUSSION

Ceramic brackets are used in Orthodontics when patients require an esthetic alternative to metallic brackets. Although color stability throughout orthodontic treatment is a very important characteristic of this type of material,[12] very little is found in the literature about this property. Therefore, the aim of the present study was to assess color stability of different ceramic brackets immersed in potentially staining solutions.

Assessment of orthodontic material color stability may be performed with equipment especially designed to analyze the reflective characteristics of an object or by means of comparative visual assessment.[12] Reflectance spectrophotometer and colorimeter are usually used for color analysis because these instruments provide consistent numerical evaluation of color characteristics.[13,14]

Previous studies have tried to correlate numeric color alteration readings ($\Delta E^\star$) provided by a spectrophotometer to the visual perception of staining of composite resin or prosthetic restorations.[15-19] In visual perception, a threshold of color alteration reflected in esthetic restorations with a mean $\Delta E^\star$ value greater than 2.0 is noticed by all observers, while $\Delta E^\star$ values ranging between 1.0 and 2.0 are not often perceived.[18] Nevertheless, other authors have proposed $\Delta E^\star$ values as from 3.3[20] and 3.7[21] for clinical perception of color changes involving composite resin restorations. Thus, research in the orthodontic field can use these references to assess color stability of esthetic brackets and elastics.

Faltermeier et al[22] investigated color stability of esthetic brackets after ultraviolet light irradiation and exposure to staining solutions.[13] The authors considered $\Delta E^\star$ mean alues ≥ 3.3 as clinically unacceptable. However, Lee[23] assessed color changes in reflected and transmitted color, in addition to color parameters of esthetic brackets after thermocycling, and suggested $\Delta E^\star$ equal to 3.7 was the threshold for clinical perception of color alteration.

Importantly, the $\Delta E^\star$ values used as reference in previous studies may not be compared to those used in the present study, since in addition to using different types of brackets, our spectrophotometric assessment was performed on bracket worn bases, while the others measured it on bracket buccal surfaces. Assessment on bracket buccal surface may be influenced by the shadows of the bracket slot and wings. These areas also present greater potential for accumulation of staining pigments, which may camouflage the actual staining of the ceramic brackets structure. We decided to level the bracket bases to increase the precision of spectrophotometer assessment, since this equipment was developed to analyze the characteristics of light reflected on flat surfaces.

In addition to assessment carried out with the aid of a spectrophotometer, two calibrated operators also performed a visual analysis. Staining of all ceramic brackets was observed in all three staining solutions after the seventh day of immersion. Thereafter, a progressive staining of these brackets was visually observed by the end of the 14-day period. Red wine was the solution that caused the most intense staining of all brackets tested, followed by coffee and coke, respectively. Despite presenting the lowest pH levels among the three staining solutions tested and potentially affecting a given material surface, coke did not cause as much color alteration as coffee and red wine, probably due to lack of yellow pigment in its composition.[22,25]

As previously mentioned, the literature on color stability of orthodontic material is limited.[22,25] However, several techniques have been described to study the staining of dental material. Methods of aging acceleration, such as thermocycling, immersion in artificial saliva, coffee, tea, grape juice and chlorhexidine, have been used in *in vitro* simulations.[14] It has been demonstrated that the type of solution as well as total exposure time influenced the degree of color alteration of these types of material.[26] These results are in accordance with our findings.

Ertas et al[15] assessed color stability of five types of composite resins immersed in tea, coke, coffee, red wine and water. Similarly to the present study, these solutions were used because they are the potentially staining solutions frequently consumed by adults. The authors also established 14 days as the total immersion time due to believing it would initially resemble the environmental color stability challenge that composite resins must face in the oral cavity.

Although Radiance brackets showed greater ΔE★ mean values of color alteration when compared to the other brackets after 24 and 72 hours and 7 days of immersion in coke, this difference was not statistically significant after 14 days. Bracket brand staining in coffee solution was similar, since only one single statistically significant difference was detected (14 days, Transcend *versus* Mystique, $p = 0.9418$). After 24 hours of immersion in red wine, Mystique brackets presented with significant color alteration in comparison to Luxi II. After the same period of time, as well as after 72 hours and 7 days of immersion in this solution, Radiance brackets stood out statistically with a higher color alteration in comparison to other bracket brands (Table 2). It was also possible to observe that, in general, time significantly affected color alteration of these brackets, and the pattern of color change in specific solutions and time periods was similar or different (Table 3).

Regarding the staining potential of each solution, an interesting fact was observed. Coke, which was the solution that caused the least color alteration during visual inspection, yielded the highest ΔE★ values in the spectrophotometric analysis. A possible explanation for this ob servation is that, due to its acidic properties, this solution has the ability of altering the material surface, leading to greater absorption of coloring pigments from the solution by the porcelain, which can be detected accurately by the spectrophotometer while not detected by the human eye. In agreement with previous studies, it was visually observed in the present study that red wine caused more color alterations than coffee, which was also confirmed by the spectrophotometric analysis.

It is important to point out that these results should not be extrapolated to clinical reality, given that methodological limitations are inevitable when assessing color alterations of brackets *in vitro*. Reproducibility of the conditions present in the oral cavity is quite complex due to several factors, including the intricate flora and its by-products, in addition to biofilm deposition in the tested material. Therefore, further clinical studies investigating orthodontic material color stability should be conducted in order to keep up with orthodontic patients' demand.

CONCLUSION

Ceramic brackets displayed color changes after immersion in staining solutions, and the period of exposure to red wine influenced the amount of staining registered in the ceramic brackets assessed. When immersed in coke and red wine for specific periods of time, Radiance brackets generally presented statistically higher color alterations in comparison to other bracket brands.

Author contributions

Conceived and designed the study: BCG. Acquisition, analysis or interpretation: BCG. Data collection: MCG. Wrote the article: BCG, LKS, RVS, MCG. Critical revision of the article: MMP, DDO. Final approval of the article: EA, DDO.

REFERENCES

1. Gkantidis N, Zinelis S, Karamolegkou M, Eliades T, Topouzelis N. Comparative assessment of clinical performance of esthetic bracket materials. Angle Orthod. 2012;82(4):691-7.
2. Faltermeier A, Burgers R, Rosentritt M. Bacterial adhesion of Streptococcus mutans to esthetic bracket materials. Am J Orthod Dentofacial Orthop. 2008;133(4 Suppl):S99-103.

3. Dostalova T, Jelinkova H, Sulc J, Nemec M, Jelinek M, Fibrich M, et al. Ceramic bracket debonding by TM: YAP laser irradiation. Photomed Laser Surg. 2011;29(7):477-84.
4. Sarp AS, Gulsoy M. Ceramic bracket debonding with ytterbium fiber laser. Lasers Med Sci. 2011;26(5):577-84.
5. Falkensammer F, Freudenthaler J, Pseiner B, Bantleon HP. Influence of surface conditioning on ceramic microstructure and bracket adhesion. Eur J Orthod. 2012;34(4):498-504.
6. Pithon MM, Oliveira MV, Ruellas AC, Bolognese AM, Romano FL. Shear bond strength of orthodontic brackets to enamel under different surface treatment conditions. J Appl Oral Sci. 2007;15(2):127-30.
7. Pereira BR, Tanaka OM, Lima AA, Guariza-Filho O, Maruo H, Camargo ES. Metal and ceramic bracket effects on human buccal mucosa epithelial cells. Angle Orthod. 2009;79(2):373-9.
8. Bishara SE, Ostby AW, Laffoon J, Warren JJ. Enamel cracks and ceramic bracket failure during debonding in vitro. Angle Orthod. 2008;78(6):1078-83.
9. Lindauer SJ, Macon CR, Browning H, Rubenstein LK, Isaacson RJ. Ceramic bracket fracture resistance to second order arch wire activations. Am J Orthod Dentofacial Orthop. 1994;106(5):481-6.
10. Ozcan M, Finnema K, Ybema A. Evaluation of failure characteristics and bond strength after ceramic and polycarbonate bracket debonding: effect of bracket base silanization. Eur J Orthod. 2008;30(2):176-82.
11. Mancuso DN, Goiato MC, Dekon SF, Gennari-Filho H. Visual evaluation of color stability after accelerated aging of pigmented and nonpigmented silicones to be used in facial prostheses. Indian J Dent Res. 2009;20(1):77-80.
12. Lopes Filho H, Maia LE, Araujo MV, Ruellas AC. Influence of optical properties of esthetic brackets (color, translucence, and fluorescence) on visual perception. Am J Orthod Dentofacial Orthop. 2012;141(4):460-7.
13. Faltermeier A, Behr M, Mussig D. Esthetic brackets: the influence of filler level on color stability. Am J Orthod Dentofacial Orthop. 2007;132(1):5.e13-6.
14. Haselton DR, Diaz-Arnold AM, Dawson DV. Color stability of provisional crown and fixed partial denture resins. J Prosthet Dent. 2005;93(1):70-5.
15. Ertas E, Guler AU, Yucel AC, Koprulu H, Guler E. Color stability of resin composites after immersion in different drinks. Dent Mater J. 2006;25(2):371-6.
16. Drubi-Filho B, Garcia Lda F, Cruvinel DR, Sousa AB, Pires-de-Souza FC. Color stability of modern composites subjected to different periods of accelerated artificial aging. Braz Dent J. 2012;23(5):575-80.
17. Bayindir F, Kurklu D, Yanikoglu ND. The effect of staining solutions on the color stability of provisional prosthodontic materials. J Dent. 2012;40 Suppl 2:e41-46.
18. Gonulol N, Yilmaz F. The effects of finishing and polishing techniques on surface roughness and color stability of nanocomposites. J Dent. 2012;40 Suppl 2:e64-70.
19. Erdemir U, Yildiz E, Eren MM. Effects of sports drinks on color stability of nanofilled and microhybrid composites after long-term immersion. J Dent. 2012;40 Suppl 2:e55-63.
20. Ruyter IE, Nilner K, Moller B. Color stability of dental composite resin materials for crown and bridge veneers. Dent Mater. 1987;3(5):246-51.
21. Johnston WM, Kao EC. Assessment of appearance match by visual observation and clinical colorimetry. J Dent Res. 1989;68(5):819-22.
22. Faltermeier A, Behr M, Mussig D. In vitro colour stability of aesthetic brackets. Eur J Orthod. 2007;29:354-358.
23. Lee YK. Changes in the reflected and transmitted color of esthetic brackets after thermal cycling. Am J Orthod Dentofacial Orthop. 2008;133(5):641.e1-6.
24. Um CM, Ruyter IE. Staining of resin-based veneering materials with coffee and tea. Quintessence Int. 1991;22(5):377-86.
25. Eliades T, Kakaboura A, Eliades G, Bradley TG. Comparison of enamel colour changes associated with orthodontic bonding using two different adhesives. Eur J Orthod. 2001;23(1):85-90.
26. Yannikakis SA, Zissis AJ, Polyzois GL, Caroni C. Color stability of provisional resin restorative materials. J Prosthet Dent. 1998;80(5):533-9.
27. Stober T, Gilde H, Lenz P. Color stability of highly filled composite resin materials for facings. Dent Mater. 2001;17(1):87-94.
28. Khokhar ZA, Razzoog ME, Yaman P. Color stability of restorative resins. Quintessence Int. 1991;22(9):733-7.

Mechanical properties of NiTi and CuNiTi shape-memory wires used in orthodontic treatment - Part 1: Stress-strain tests

Marco Abdo Gravina[1], Ione Helena Vieira Portella Brunharo[2], Cristiane Canavarro[3], Carlos Nelson Elias[4], Cátia Cardoso Abdo Quintão[5]

Objective: This research aimed to compare, through traction tests, eight types of superelastic and heat-activated NiTi archwires, by six trade companies (GAC, TP, Ormco, Masel, Morelli and Unitek) to those with addition of copper (CuNiTi 27°C and 35°C, Ormco). **Methods:** The tests were performed in an EMIC mechanical testing machine, model DL10000, capacity of 10 tons, at the Military Institute of Engineering (IME). **Results:** The results showed that, generally, heat-activated NiTi archwires presented slighter deactivation loadings in relation to superelastic. Among the archwires that presented deactivation loadings biologically more adequate are the heat-activated by GAC and by Unitek. Among the superelastic NiTi, the CuNiTi 27°C by Ormco were the ones that presented slighter deactivation loadings, being statistically (ANOVA) similar, to the ones presented by the heat-activated NiTi archwires by Unitek. When compared the CuNiTi 27°C and 35°C archwires, it was observed that the 27°C presented deactivation forces of, nearly, ⅓ of the presented by the 35°C. **Conclusion:** It was concluded that the CuNiTi 35°C archwires presented deactivation loadings biologically less favorable in relation to the other heat-activated NiTi archwires, associated to lower percentage of deformation, on the constant baselines of deactivation, showing less adequate mechanical behavior, under traction, in relation to the other archwires.

Keywords: Orthodontic archwires. Dental movement. Copper. Nickel. Titanium. Physical properties.

[1] Assistant Professor of Orthodontics, UFJF.
[2] Visiting Professor of Orthodontics, FOUERJ.
[3] Substitute Professor of Orthodontics, FOUERJ.
[4] Assistant Professor of the Military Institute of Engineering (IME).
[5] Assistant Professor of Orthodontics, FOUERJ.

» The authors report no commercial, proprietary or financial interest in the products or companies described in this article.

Marco Abdo Gravina
Av. Barão do Rio Branco, 2595 – Sala 1204 – Juiz de Fora/MG – Brazil
CEP: 36010-011 – E-mail: marcoabdogravina@yahoo.com.br

INTRODUCTION

The tooth alignment and leveling constitute the preliminary clinical phase of any orthodontic procedure with fixed appliances.[8] It has been accepted in orthodontics the principle that slight and continuous forces would be desirable for obtainment of physiologic and controlled tooth movement. For this purpose, it has been suggested the superelastic and heat-activated nickel-titanium (NiTi) archwires, which offer a force-bending curve with a defined baseline and a larger activation range.[5,6,11]

Despite the small number of available alloys for manufacture of orthodontic archwires, there is a large number of trade brands of available archwires. The manufacturing companies invest in advertising calling the archwires superior (superelastic and heat-activated NiTi) and emphasize that they provide better performance due to the appropriate mechanical properties. However, these properties not always are described on the product package. Thus, the variety of brands, the large number of manufacturing companies and the lack of information about the material properties make it difficult for the professional to choose the most adequate material and with better cost-benefit for use.[11,22]

Some mechanical properties of orthodontic archwires, such as high resilience, low elasticity module, high flexibility, high elastic recovery, low coefficient of attrition and biocompatibility, are necessary in order to stimulate the adequate tissue response[1,4,15,17,19] and promote slight and continuous forces during the tooth leveling and alignment.[9,30] However, to quantify the ideal force becomes difficult due to individual variations on the tissue response, to root morphology and to type of induced movement.[9] Rock and Wilson[23] asserted that there is a consensus that the ideal orthodontic forces should vary between 15 and 500 gf.

The superelastic NiTi archwires were commercially launched in 1986 (Japanese NiTi and Chinese NiTi). *In vitro* studies showed that such alloys had excellent elastic properties and generated constant forces, when subjected to loadings, even before the increase on deformation. This made the archwires extremely popular for the use in tooth leveling and alignment.[8] The heat-activated NiTi alloys emerged commercially in the 90's. Besides the properties of maintenance of constant loadings during loading and unloading, the heat dynamic NiTi archwires showed shape memory thermally induced, presenting ductility and malleability in lower temperatures returning to the initial configuration, when heated to higher temperatures than their transition temperature.[16,20]

According to Sachdeva,[25] NiTi archwires with addition of copper (CuNiTi) appeared in the 90's and are composed, basically, of nickel, titanium, copper and chromium. For presenting addition of copper (efficient heat conductor) to nickel and titanium, they would present better defined transition temperatures, which would ensure the generation of more homogeneous loadings from arch to arch and from end to end, increasing the effectiveness on tooth movement. They were introduced in the market by Ormco Corporation with three transition temperatures: 27°C, 35°C and 40°C, enabling to clinicians the quantification and application of levels of adequate loadings to the initial purposes of the orthodontic treatment. When compared to the conventional heat-activated and superelastic NiTi archwires, the CuNiTi archwires would present, still, lower elasticity module, i.e., they would experience similar deformations, before lower activation loadings, presenting a high capacity to fit to brackets of misplaced teeth, with less discomfort to the patient and lower potential to generate tooth resorption. Besides, they would present reduced hysteresis, which would ensure the production of more constant forces and for longer periods of time during deactivation, factors biologically favorable to tooth movement.[25]

Because of existing gaps in publications related to comparison of mechanical behavior of NiTi and CuNiTi archwires, it is the objective of the present work to determine and compare some of the mechanical properties, in tests of resistance to traction, presented by the conventional superelastic and heat-activated orthodontic archwires, by different trade brands, to the presented by the NiTi archwires with addition of copper (CuNiTi 27°C and 35°C).

MATERIAL AND METHODS

Sixty orthodontic archwires were used, 0.018-in, precontoured and with the same arch shape. According to the mechanical properties provided by the manufacturers, the archwires were divided into two groups (Table 1).

The mechanical properties of the archwires were determined from the tests of resistance to traction, performed in EMIC mechanical testing machine, model DL10000, capacity of 10 tons (EMIC International Corp., Garland, USA) (Fig 1A), at the Military Institute of Engineering (IME), Rio de Janeiro. It was used a 500 N cell (50 kgf) and testing speed of 1 mm of deformation per minute.

The archwires were positioned in the testing machine, as obtained at the store. Initially, it was applied a slight force so the portion of wire positioned between the machine's nails became straight (Fig 1B).

First, three specimens from each subgroup of archwires were stretched until break to determine their yield stress and constant baselines of activation. The obtained results enabled that the following tests, of loading and unloading (three specimens from each subgroups of archwires) were performed with maximum activation loadings immediately inferior to the respective yield stress (Fig 3). With this methodology the mechanical properties of clinical interest from the several subgroups of archwires could be calculated, without permanent deformations, which could invalidate the tests. On the testing, it were obtained the curves that allowed to determine the stress applied on the wire (MPa) versus the deformation (mm).

All tests of resistance to traction were performed at 37 ± 1°C (average oral temperature) to point the possible shape memory effect (SME), according to methodology of Gravina et al.[12] The temperature was controlled with a precision digital heat meter, calibrated by INMETRO (Fig 1C). The testing environment in which the archwires were attached to the machine was isolated with styrofoam plates and the temperature was kept constant (≅ 37°C) using three lamps of 60 watts. The lamps were used to simulate a greenhouse, so the temperature could be controlled through a thermostat (Fig 1C).

Every force-bending curve is constituted of a large number of points, and each one of them is numerically

Table 1 - Orthodontic archwires used in this work.

I – SUPERELASTIC GROUP (36 archwires)		II – HEAT-ACTIVATED GROUP (24 archwires)	
GAC	6 NiTi (REF. 03-018-53T)	GAC Sentalloy	6 NiTi (REF. 02-511-132)
TP Reflex	6 NiTi (REF.381-264)	TP Reflex	6 NiTi (REF. 381-825)
Ormco NiTi	6 NiTi (REF. 219-3204)	Ormco 35OC	6 CuNiTi (REF. 219-4204)
Ormco 27°C	6 CuNiTi (REF. 205-0048)	Unitek Nitinol	6 NiTi (REF. 4286-981)
Masel Elastinol	6 NiTi (REF. 4828-018)		
Morelli	6 NiTi (REF. 50.70.014)		

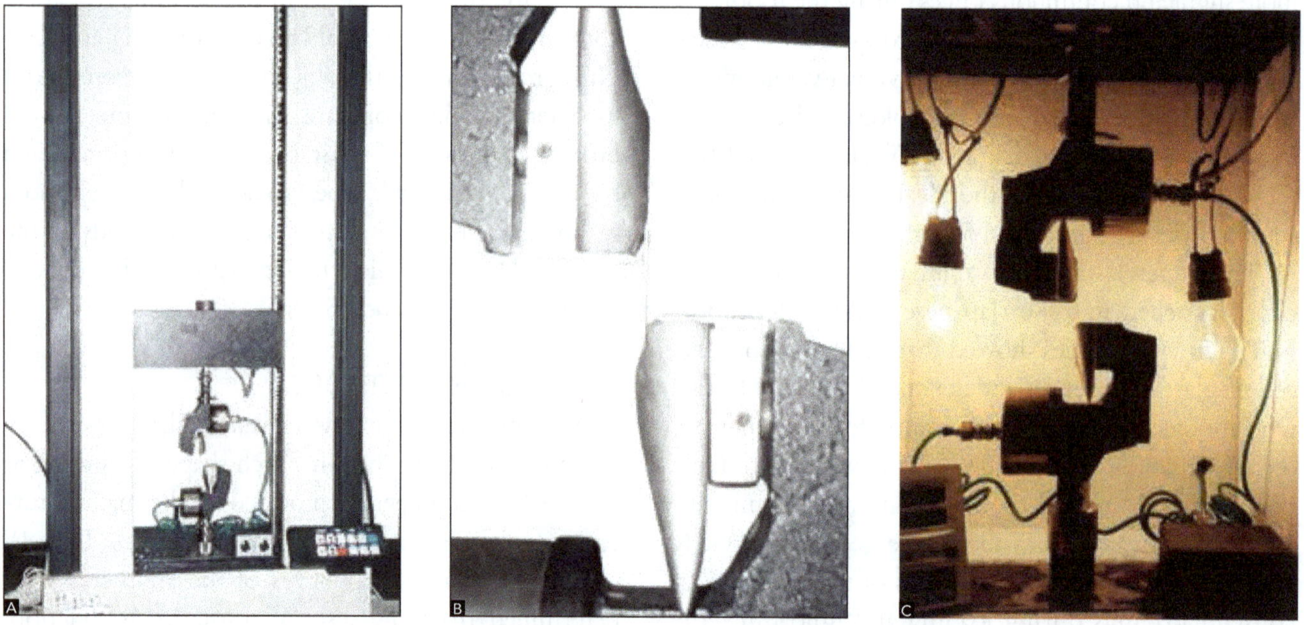

Figure 1 - **A)** Machine used on the performance of traction resistance tests, **B)** Detail of the wire tied by its ends to the machine's nails, **C)** Device used on the performance of tests at oral temperature (37°C).

represented by a value where the ordinate (y axis) express the applied force (MPa) and the abscissa (x axis) express the deformation occurred (mm). To calculate the mechanical properties of the several subgroups of archwires, all points component of the curve, obtained during performance of the tests, by the program Tesc 3.04 (São José dos Pinhais, PR, Brasil), were exported to Microsoft Excel (Microsoft Corporation®, Redmond, WA, USA). From this on, the curves were obtained on Excel (Fig 2A) and the mechanical properties were calculated (Fig 2B) and, statistically analyzed to verify the inter-groups differences (significance) as for the maximum break stress, yield stress, percentage of deformation on constant baselines of deactivation, loadings released during deactivations, permanent deformations and resilience. For so, it were used the analysis of variance (ANOVA) and the Tukey test, both parametric tests, through OriginPro 7.0 and Tesc 3.04 (São José dos Pinhais, PR, Brasil), developed for Windows.

RESULTS

Results are shown in Table 1.

DISCUSSION

Several types of laboratorial tests were suggested on the attempt to obtain the mechanical properties of orthodontic archwires, from the test of resistance to traction[27,28,29] to the flexion and bending tests.[3,28] In 1977, the American Dental Association (ADA) released a specification[18] to standardize the laboratorial tests for classification of orthodontic archwires, being chosen the flexion and bending tests. However, the obtained results were controversial in relation to the test of resistance to traction, especially, as for the

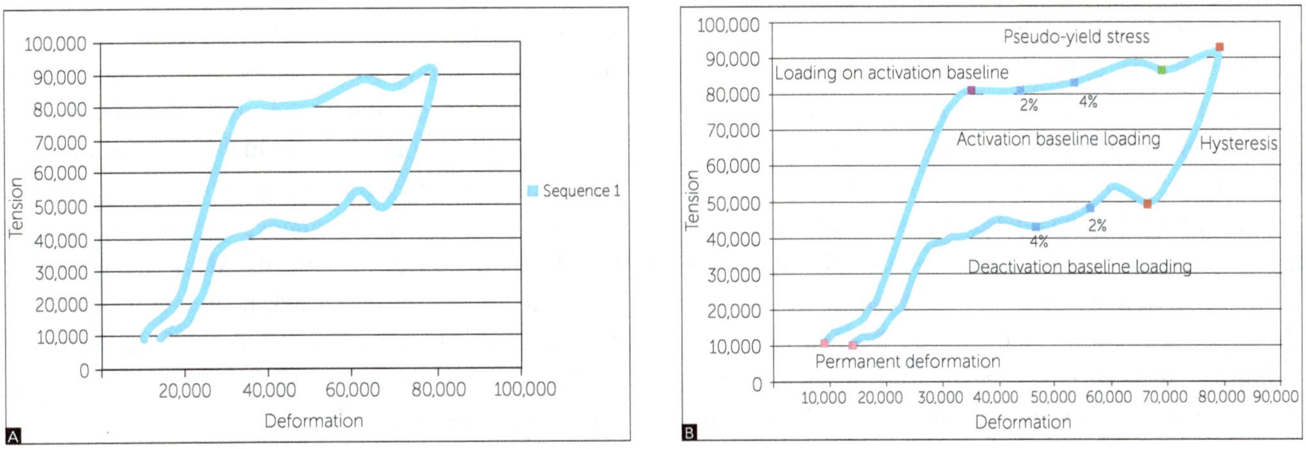

Figure 2 - **A)** Curve initially obtained on Microsoft Excel. **B)** Mechanical properties obtained from the curves.

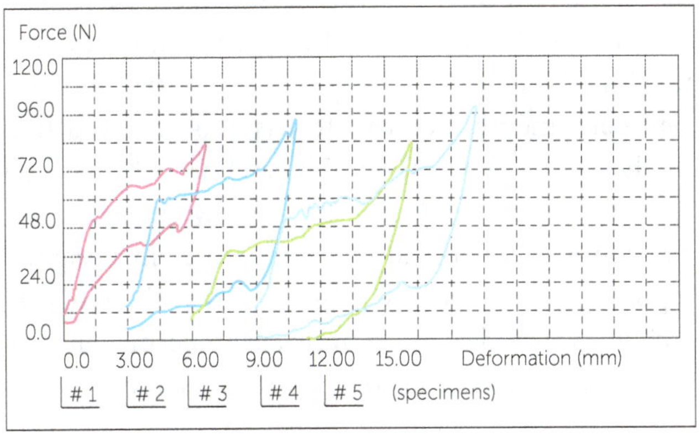

Figure 3 - Stress-strain curve obtained on the tests of heat-activated NiTi and CuNiTi archwires during their loading until their respective limits of flow followed by unloading.

Table 1 - Values obtained for mechanical properties of the subgroups of tested archwires, where similar symbols indicate similar statistics.

	Mean									
Mechanical properties	**GAC NiTi Super**	**TP NiTi Super**	**Ormco CuNiTi 27°C**	**Ormco NiTi Super**	**Masel NiTi Super**	**Morelli NiTi Super**	**GAC NiTi Heat**	**TP NiTi Heat**	**Ormco CuNiTi 35°C**	**Unitek NiTi Heat**
Maximum break stress (MPa)	1447.67 ■	1432.49 ■	1458.68 ■	1286.31 +	1267.45 +	1523.25 #	1415.13 ■	1171.78 •	1444.03 ■	1011.44 °
Yield stress (MPa)	604.44 ■#	546.66 ■	450.00 °	555.00 ■	455.60 °	653.55 #	530.00 ■	454.44 °	438.88 °	448.36 °
Deformation deact. bas. (%)	8.23 °	7.64 °	8.84 °	8.64 °	12.83 #	12.32 #+	9.56 +°	7.61 °	8.88 °	12.84 #
Force (N) deactivation baseline	27.62 ■	27.81 ■	11.53 °	35.56 #	16.91 +	41.70 #	3.71 °	0.95 •	29.82 ■	7.59 °
% perm. deformation	6.64 °	4.65 °	10.22 °	12.41 °	4.34 °	6.29 °	17.40 °+	72.67 #	8.80 °	28.52 +

Similar symbols indicate statistical similarities. Heat = heat-activated. Super = superelastic.

values found for the elasticity module. Rantley et al[3] and Asgharnia and Brantley,[2] criticized the precision of the tests suggested by ADA, especially for archwires of gauge lower than 0.020-in, choosing the tests of resistance to traction as the most reliable to obtain the materials mechanical properties, which explains the choice in this present work.

Analyzing the data on Table 2, representative of the mean values for maximum break stress (N) of the subgroups of tested archwires, it was possible to find that the superelastic NiTi archwires by Morelli presented maximum resistance to fracture, for resistance to traction, statistically superior to all others. Among the archwires that presented the lowest resistance to traction are the heat-activated NiTi archwires by Unitek, followed by the heat-activated NiTi archwires by TP. It is also noticed that even for archwires that presented lower fracture loadings, they were extremely high when compared to the clinically used.[4,16] This way, it could be presumed that none of the tested archwires would be clinically used with risk of fracture.

In relation to the yield stress of the NiTi and CuNiTi archwires, it was observed that, initially, the stress and deformation were proportional and abided Hooke's law ($\sigma = E \times \varepsilon$). From this on, the deformation did not increase proportionally to the stress increase. On the contrary, the stress was kept constant while the deformation increased (constant baseline of activation, Fig 2B). Such baseline represents the pseudoplastic deformation behavior, since, when the loading was removed, the metal did not present expressive permanent or residual deformation, being capable to return to its initial configuration. This behavior is clinically favorable, for constant forces would be supposedly accumulated as the wire was activated. In the present work it was considered the loadings corresponding to the end of the constant baselines of activation as equivalent to the yield stress of the tested archwires (Fig 2B).

It was observed that, generally, the superelastic NiTi archwires presented superior yield stress than the heat-activated (Table 2). Among the archwires that presented the highest yield stress, are the superelastic NiTi by Morelli and by GAC, and they suffered the highest stress, for resistance to traction, before permanently deform. It was also observed that the heat activate CuNiTi 35°C archwires by Ormco were the ones that presented the lowest yield stress and consequently the lowest work limits, meeting the report by Sachdeva,[25] who asserted that the CuNiTi archwires would be more resistant to permanent deformation and would show better elastic recovery.

Regarding the percentage of deformation on constant baselines of deactivation (in relation to original length of 50 mm archwires) it was observed that the superelastic NiTi archwires by Masel and heat-activated archwires by Unitek were the ones that presented, statistically, the highest values (Table 2). Regarding the NiTi archwires with addition of copper (CuNiTi 27°C and 35°C), it was observed percentage of deformation statistically inferior on baselines of deactivation in relation to heat-activated NiTi archwires by Unitek and superelastic archwires by Masel and by Morelli (Table 2). Such results do not confirm the findings by Sachdeva,[25] who asserted that CuNiTi archwires, for presenting reduced hysteresis, would present their plateaus constant of loadings superior in extension, during the unloading, favorable factors to tooth movement. On the other hand, the percentage of deformation found for CuNiTi archwires, on constant baselines of deactivation, were statistically similar to the presented by the superelastic NiTi archwires by GAC, TP and Ormco, which presented the lowest percentage of deformation among all tested archwires (Table 2).

Among all mechanical properties of orthodontic archwires, the strength released during deactivation is the one that expresses the most and it relates to the archwires clinical behavior. It was observed that, generally, the heat-activated NiTi archwires presented slighter loadings of deactivation in relation to superelastic. Among superelastic NiTi archwires, the CuNiTi 27°C by Ormco were the ones that presented the slightest deactivation loadings. Among the heat-activated NiTi archwires, the CuNiTi 35°C were the ones that presented the highest deactivation loadings, being statistically similar to the ones presented by the superelastic NiTi archwires by GAC and by TP (Table 2). Such results meet the report by Sachdeva[25] who asserted that the CuNiTi archwires, for having lower elasticity module, would suffer deformations similar to the conventional superelastic and heat-activated NiTi archwires, before lower activation loadings. Among the archwires that presented the highest deactivation loadings are the superelastic by Morelli and by Ormco, being statistically superior to the presented by the other tested NiTi and CuNiTi archwires. Among the archwires that presented the lowest deactivation loadings are the heat-activated by GAC and by Unitek and the superelastic CuNiTi 27°C by Ormco, with statistically similar deactivation loadings. Although the heat-activated NiTi archwires by TP presented slight deactivation loadings, they presented significant percentage of permanent deformation on most unloading tests at 37°C, which would disable its mechanical properties and explain the obtainment of such loadings.

When compared the CuNiTi 27°C and 35°C archwires, it was observed that the first presented deactivation forces of about ⅓ of the presented by the last ones. This data meets the recommendations from the manufacturer (Ormco Corp.), which supported by the works of Sachdeva,[25] stated that the CuNiTi 27°C archwires should be used in cases where high and biologically acceptable loadings were required and the CuNiTi 35°C archwires should be used to obtain mild loadings. The result of the present work are in agreement to the findings by Dalstra and Melsen,[6] which asserted that some patients reported greater discomfort when using the CuNiTi 40°C archwires, when ingesting warm mouth rinses, in relation to the CuNiTi 27°C archwires, since the loading generated by those, during unloading, would be superior to the produced by these.

In the present work, it was demonstrated that the loading released on constant baselines of deactivation were extremely high when compared to the ones used intraorally, which should vary between 15 and 500 gf.[21,23] From this principle, in the present work, only the heat-activated NiTi archwires by GAC could be clinically used since they released loading corresponding to 3.71 N (371 gf), being the other loadings released by the tested NiTi and CuNiTi archwires, above this baseline (Table 2). Gurgel et al[13] asserted, however, that although the tests of resistance to traction, bending, torsion and deflection do not completely reproduce the clinical situation, they establish adequate values for comparison between archwires of similar or different metallic alloys. Ibe and Segner,[14] however, emphasized that the comparison or extrapolation of values obtained in laboratorial tests, to the clinically obtained, should be done very carefully.[14]

The results of the present work were different from the ones found by Fisher-Brandies et al,[10] which through the deflection test in 3 points, reported that the CuNiTi 35°C archwires (Ormco) and the Neo Sentalloy F80 (GAC), both heat-activated, presented plateaus of unloading under lower loadings related to the Rematitan Lite (Dentaurum) and Titanol SE S (Forestadent) archwires, both superelastic. In the present work, the CuNiTi 35°C archwires presented deactivation loadings statistically superior to the other heat-activated NiTi archwires and similar to the superelastic NiTi archwires by GAC and TP (Table 2).

Still contrary to the results obtained in the present work, Gurgel et al,[13] through artificial models of dental arches, showed that the CuNiTi 35°C (Ormco) and Neo Sentalloy F200 (GAC) archwires, presented intermediate deactivation loadings, without statistical difference between them, while the Elastinol 35°C (Masel), heat-activated NiTi (Morelli) and Nitinol heat-activated (3M Unitek) archwires presented the slightest deactivation loadings. It is worth emphasizing however that Gurgel et al[13] used the Neo Sentalloy F200, while the authors of this present work used the Neo Sentalloy F80, both by GAC. In relation to the CuNiTi 27°C archwires (Ormco), Gurgel et al[13] asserted that they presented deactivation loadings statistically higher to the presented by heat-activated archwires by Unitek and CuNiTi 35°C by Ormco,[13] not confirming the results of the present work (Table 2).

On the other hand, the results of the present work were consistent with the found by Sakima et al,[26] which through Force System Identification (FSI), showed that the CuNiTi 40°C (Ormco) and Neo Sentalloy F200 (GAC) archwires were the ones that presented the unloading plateaus under the lowest loadings, followed by CuNiTi 35°C archwires (Ormco); while the superelastic NiTi by Ormco, presented plateaus of unloading under the highest loadings, becoming the most inflexible archwires in this work. Also in the present work the heat-activated NiTi archwires by GAC presented the slightest deactivation loadings among the tested archwires and the CuNiTi 35°C archwires presented deactivation loadings statistically lower to the presented by superelastic NiTi archwires by Ormco, which presented the second highest deactivation loadings among the tested archwires.

Table 2 shows that, generally, the superelastic NiTi archwires presented lower percentage of permanent deformations in relation to the heat activate NiTi archwires. Among the tested superelastic NiTi and CuNiTi archwires it were not observed statistically significant differences between the percentage of permanent deformation. Among the heat-activated NiTi archwires, it was observed that the ones by TP presented the highest percentage of permanent deformation in the work, statistically superior to the ones presented by all other tested NiTi and CuNiTi archwires. However, it was observed, in a pilot trial, that the mean percentage of permanent deformation was reduced from 72.67 to 28.50%, with the increase of testing temperature from 37 to 40°C. As these archwires were not subjected to activation loadings higher than their respective pseudo-yield stress, which could have invalidated the tests and generated permanent deformations, it was concluded that the transition temperature of the heat-activated NiTi archwires by TP was superior to 37°C. For this reason, such archwires presented deactivation loadings extremely reduced.

Confirming the results of the present work, Parvizi and Rock[20] asserted that the complete recovery of the initial configuration after unloading is not always obtained for superelastic and heat-activated NiTi archwires, being kept between baselines of 89 and 94%.[20] The present work showed that, at 37°C, all tested NiTi and CuNiTi archwires presented some degree of permanent deformation, being significantly expressive only for heat-activated NiTi archwires by TP (Table 2). Among the tested superelastic NiTi and CuNiTi archwires, the complete recovery of the initial configuration was kept between 88 and 96%, while for heat activated NiTi archwires, it was kept between 71 and 82% (Table 2).

The results of the present work were against the findings by Damon,[7] who proved the efficiency of the application of slight loadings during the phase of tooth alignment with insertion of the CuNiTi 35°C wire (Ormco). According to the same author, the word "system" (Damon system) would be used to define the combination of self-ligating brackets and high technology orthodontic archwires, carefully selected so the applied loading is kept within the great levels of force or biozone. He recommended for such purpose, the sequential use of CuNiTi 35°C orthodontic arches of diameter 0.014-in, 0.014 x 0.025-in and 0.018 x 0.025-in, being the reduction of the generated attrition the key to a more efficient and fast orthodontic treatment, with reduction of up to 70% on the number of necessary visits to orthodontists.[7] In the present work, the CuNiTi 35°C archwires were the less recommended for clinical use, among the heat activated, because of the loadings released during deactivation and of the percentage of deformation of the unloading baselines. It is recommended, however, a new work that evaluates the attrition of such archwires in relation to the other superelastic and heat activated NiTi and CuNiTi archwires.

CONCLUSION

1) Among the tested superelastic NiTi and CuNiTi archwires, the CuNiTi 27°C presented mechanical properties superior to the others, releasing lower deactivation loadings. The superelastic NiTi archwires by Morelli were the less recommended for use, for presenting deactivation loadings statistically superior to the presented by the other tested archwires.

2) Among the tested heat activated NiTi and CuNiTi archwires, the ones by GAC and Unitek presented mechanical properties superior to the others, releasing lower deactivation loadings and presenting superior percentage of deformation on the deactivation baselines. In relation to the CuNiTi 35°C archwires, they did not present mechanical properties, under traction resistance, that justified its clinical choice.

REFERENCES

1. Andreasen GF, Morrow RE. Laboratory and clinical analysis of Nitinol wire. Am J Orthod. 1978;73 (2) :142-51.
2. Asgharnia MK, Brantley WA. Comparison of bending and tension tests for orthodontic wires. Am J Orthod. 1986;89 (3) :228-36.
3. Brantley WA, Augat WS, Myers CL, Winders RV. Bending deformation studies of orthodontic wires. J Dent Res. 1978;57 (4) :609-15.
4. Burstone CJ, Goldberg AJ. Beta titanium: a new orthodontic alloy. Am J Orthod. 1980;77 (2) :121-32.
5. Cobb NW 3rd, Kula KS, Phillips C, Proffit WR. Efficiency of multi-strand steel, superelastic Ni-Ti and ion-implanted Ni-Ti archwires for initial alignment. Clin Orthod Res. 1998;1 (1) :12-9.
6. Dalstra M, Melsen B. Does the transition temperature of Cu-NiTi archwires affect the amount of tooth movement during alignment? Orthod Craniofac Res. 2004;7 (1) :21-5.
7. Damon DH. The Damon low-friction bracket: a biologically compatible straight-wire system. J Clin Orthod. 1998;32 (11) :670-80.
8. Evans TJW, Durning P. Orthodontic products update. Aligning archwires. The shape of things to come? A forth and fifth phase of force delivery. Br J Orthod. 1996;23 (3) :269-75.
9. Evans TJ, Jones ML, Newcombe RG. Clinical comparison and performance perspective of three aligning arch wires. Am J Orthod Dentofacial Orthop. 1998;114 (1) :32-9.
10. Fischer-Brandies H, Es-Souni M, Kock N, Raetzke K, Bock O. Transformation behavior, chemical composition, surface topography and bending properties of five selected 0.016" X 0.022" NiTi archwires. J Orofac Orthop. 2003;64 (2) :88-99.
11. Gravina MA, Motta TS, Almeida AAO, Quintão CCA. Fios ortodônticos: propriedades mecânicas relevantes e aplicação clínica. Rev Dental Press Ortod Ortop Facial. 2004;9 (1) :113-28.
12. Gravina MA, Quintão CA, Koo D, Elias CN. Mechanical properties of nickel titanium and steel alloys under stress-strain test. Korean J Orthod. 2003;33 (6) :465-74.
13. Gurgel JA, Kerr S, Powers JM, LeCrone V. Force-deflection properties of superelastic nickel-titanium archwires. Am J Orthod Dentofacial Orthop. 2001;120 (4) :378-82.
14. Ibe DM, Segner D. Superelastic materials displaying different force levels within one archwire. J Orofac Orthop. 1998;59 (1) :29-38.
15. Kapila S, Sachdeva R. Mechanical properties and clinical applications of orthodontic wires. Am J Orthod Dentofacial Orthop. 1989;96 (2) :100-9.
16. Miura F, Mogi M, Ohura Y, Hamanaka H. The super-elastic property of the Japanese NiTi alloy wire for use in orthodontics. Am J Orthod Dentofacial Orthop. 1986;90 (1) :1-10.
17. Mohlin B, Müller H, Odman J, Thilander B. Examination of Chinese Ni-Ti wire by a combined clinical and laboratory approach. Eur J Orthod. 1991;13 (5) :386-91.
18. Council on Dental Materials and Devices. New American Dental Association specification no. 32 for orthodontic wires not containing precious metals. J Am Dent Assoc. 1977;95:1169-71.
19. O'Brien WJ, Ryge G. An outline of dental materials and their selection. Philadelphia: W.B. Saunders; 1973.
20. Parvizi F, Rock WP. The load/deflection characteristics of thermally activated orthodontic archwires. Eur J Orthod. 2003;25 (4) :417-21.
21. Proffit W. Contemporary orthodontics. St. Louis: Mosby; 1986.
22. Quintão CCA, Elias CN. Fios utilizados em fase inicial de tratamento ortodôntico: propriedades mecânicas e desempenho clínico [tese]. Rio de Janeiro (RJ) : Universidade Federal do Rio de Janeiro; 2000.
23. Rock WP, Wilson HJ. Forces exerted by orthodontic aligning archwires. Br J Orthod. 1988;15 (4) :255-9.
24. Rygh P. Orthodontic forces and tissue reaction. In: Thilander B, Rönning O. Introduction to orthodontics. Stockholm: Tandläkarförlaget; 1985. p. 205-24.
25. Sachdeva R. Sure-Smile: Technology-driven solution for orthodontics. Tex Dent J. 2002;119 (7) :608-15.
26. Sakima MT, Dalstra M, Melsen B. How does temperature influence the properties of rectangular nickel-titanium wires? Eur J Orthod. 2006;28 (3) :282-91.
27. Souza SA. Ensaios mecânicos de materiais metálicos. 3ª ed. São Paulo: Edgard Blücher; 1974.
28. Thurow RC. Edgewise orthodontics. 3rd ed. Saint Louis: Mosby; 1979.
29. Twelftree CC, Cocks GJ, Sims MR. Tensile properties of orthodontic wires. Am J Orthod. 1977;72 (6) :683-7.
30. West AE. A clinical comparison of two initial aligning archwires [thesis]. Cardiff: University of Wales; 1992.

10

Mechanical properties of NiTi and CuNiTi wires used in orthodontic treatment - Part 2: Microscopic surface appraisal and metallurgical characteristics

Marco Abdo Gravina[1], Cristiane Canavarro[2], Carlos Nelson Elias[3], Maria das Graças Afonso Miranda Chaves[4], Ione Helena Vieira Portella Brunharo[5], Cátia Cardoso Abdo Quintão[6]

Objective: This research aimed at comparing the qualitative chemical compositions and the surface morphology of fracture regions of eight types of Nickel (Ni) Titanium (Ti) conventional wires, superelastic and heat-activated (GAC, TP, Ormco, Masel, Morelli and Unitek), to the wires with addition of copper (CuNiTi 27°C and 35°C, Ormco) after traction test. **Methods:** The analyses were performed in a scanning electronic microscope (JEOL, model JSM-5800 LV) with EDS system of microanalysis (energy dispersive spectroscopy). **Results**: The results showed that NiTi wires presented Ni and Ti as the main elements of the alloy with minimum differences in their composition. The CuNiTi wires, however, presented Ni and Ti with a significant percentage of copper (Cu). As for surface morphology, the wires that presented the lowest wire-surface roughness were the superelastic ones by Masel and Morelli, while those that presented the greatest wire-surface roughness were the CuNiTi 27°C and 35°C ones by Ormco, due to presence of microcavity formed as a result of pulling out some particles, possibly of NiTi.[4] The fracture surfaces presented characteristics of ductile fracture, with presence of microcavities. The superelastic wires by GAC and the CuNiTi 27°C and the heat-activated ones by Unitek presented the smallest microcavities and the lowest wire-surface roughness with regard to fracture, while the CuNiTi 35°C wires presented inadequate wire-surface roughness in the fracture region. **Conclusion:** CuNiTi 35°C wires did not present better morphologic characteristics in comparison to the other wires with regard to surfaces and fracture region.

Keywords: Physical properties. Orthodontic wires. Scanning electron microscopy. Nickel. Titanium. Copper.

[1] Adjunct professor, Department of Orthodontics, UFJF.
[2] Assistant professor, Department of Orthodontics, FOUERJ.
[3] Assistant professor, Military Institute of Engineering (IME).
[4] Adjunct professor, Department of Pathology, UFJF.
[5] Assistant professor, Department of Orthodontics, FOUERJ.
[6] Adjunct professor, Department of Orthodontics, FOUERJ.

» The authors report no commercial, proprietary or financial interest in the products or companies described in this article.

Marco Abdo Gravina
Av. Barão do Rio Branco, 2595 – Sl. 1204 – Juiz de Fora/MG – Brazil
CEP: 36.010-011
E-mail: marcoabdogravina@yahoo.com.br

INTRODUCTION

Since NiTi wires were first supplied in the orthodontic market, over thirty years ago, improvements have been obtained in order to enhance its performance in dental leveling and alignment. In 1963, the NiTi alloys were developed at the Naval Ordinance Laboratory of Silver Springs, Maryland, USA. In orthodontic practice, Andreasen et al[1,2] were attracted by the unique properties inherent to these alloys, such as high elastic limit, high resilience and low module of elasticity and rigidity. For this reason, they developed the first commercial NiTi alloys aimed at orthodontic purposes.[1] Subsequently, Unitek Corporation produced the stabilized NiTi alloy for clinical use under the trade name Nitinol (Nickel Titanium Naval Ordinance Laboratory). It was developed on the weight percentage of 55% of nickel and 45% of titanium, and clinically used for the first time in 1972. Despite its excellent property of elastic recovery, Nitinol did not have, by that time, shape memory or superelasticity.

Superelastic NiTi alloys (SE NiTi) were initially produced in 1978 by Furukawa Eletric Co. (Japan). Thereafter, several studies were carried out in the attempt to produce wires with similar properties for orthodontic purposes, which was achieved in 1986, with the development of the Japanese NiTi wire. Concomitantly to this discovery, another NiTi alloy with similar characteristics was developed specially for orthodontic purposes by Tien Hua Cheng at the General Research Institute for Non-Ferrous Metals (Beijing, China).[6] These alloys, named Chinese NiTi, had unique characteristics of constant maintenance of forces during activation and deactivation.[6,12] The austenitic crystal structure obtained during the manufacturing process significantly differs them from stabilized NiTi wires.[6]

Heat-activated NiTi alloys emerged, for commercial purposes, in the 90's. In addition to the property of maintaining the constant load of superelastic wires, thermodynamic NiTi wires had the additional characteristic of being thermally activatable, a property that is responsible for shape memory.[12] Since 1963, Buehler[4] has observed the shape memory effect[15], asserting that, in low temperatures, the NiTi alloys were easily deformed and, when heating them above their transition temperatures, their original configurations were re-established. However, the complexity of the thermic treatment of NiTi alloys made it impossible, at that time, to manufacture heat-activated wires.[8,17] NiTi wires with copper (CuNiTi) emerged, commercially, in the mid 90's and were manufactured in three transition temperatures, one of which was superelastic (CuNiTi 27°C) and two heat-activated (CuNiTi 35°C and CuNiTi 40°C). Due to having copper (efficient heat conductor) added to nickel and titanium, these wires present better defined transition temperatures, which not only ensures the generation of more homogeneous loadings from arch to arch and from end to end, but also increases the effectiveness of tooth movement.[16]

Fischer-Brandies et al[10] compared the chemical composition and the superficial topography of five trade brands of rectangular superelastic NiTi wires (Dentaurum, Forestadent and Lancer) and heat-activated wires (GAC and CuNiTi 35°C). The results showed that all tested wires presented minimum differences in their chemical composition, with nearly 58% of nickel and 42% of titanium, except for the CuNiTi wire which, besides nickel (50.7%) and titanium (42.4%), presented 6.9% of copper in its composition. With regard to superficial topography, all wires presented inclusion and manufacturing residue (particles of Si and Al), chemical immunogeneicities and superficial slots. Superelastic wires presented smoother surfaces in comparison to the heat-activated ones. Such characteristics are important because they are associated with the intensity of bracket-wire attrition, biocompatibility and resistance to corrosion, given that the release of ions and the fractures caused by fatigue start on the spot of inclusion and corrosion.[10]

Damon[7] stated that the specific use of CuNiTi 35°C orthodontic wires associated with self-bonding brackets (Damon system) would significantly reduce the coefficient of attrition generated in conventional mechanics, which is the key to an efficient treatment. As a result, there would be significant reduction in the mean period of chair time, the number of visits paid to the orthodontist and in patient's degree of discomfort.

In this context, the present study aimed at: (1) carrying out and comparing qualitative analyses of the chemical composition of superelastic and heat-activated NiTi and CuNiTi wires of different trade brands, through scanning electron microscopy (SEM) with EDS system of microanalysis (energy dispersive spectroscopy);

and (2) analyzing and comparing by means of SEM and the technique of secondary electrons analysis, the surface finishing as well as the fracture region of these wires, given that such characteristics could affect the clinical performance of these alloys and, more specifically, the coefficient of attrition, the biocompatibility and the adequate resistance to corrosion and to fracture under orthodontic forces.[3,5,11,13]

MATERIAL AND METHODS

Twenty orthodontic 0.018" gauge precontoured wires were used, all of which had the same arch shape and were commercialized by six different companies. The wires were divided into two groups (superelastic and heat-activated) according to their mechanical properties which were informed by the manufacturers. Groups and subgroups of the analyzed samples are shown in Table 1. The wires were subjected to traction tests of which results are presented in part 1 of this work.[18]

The semiquantitative chemical composition was determined by the same methodology used by Fischer-Brandies et al.[10] Surface morphology and fracture regions of the wires were analyzed by scanning electron

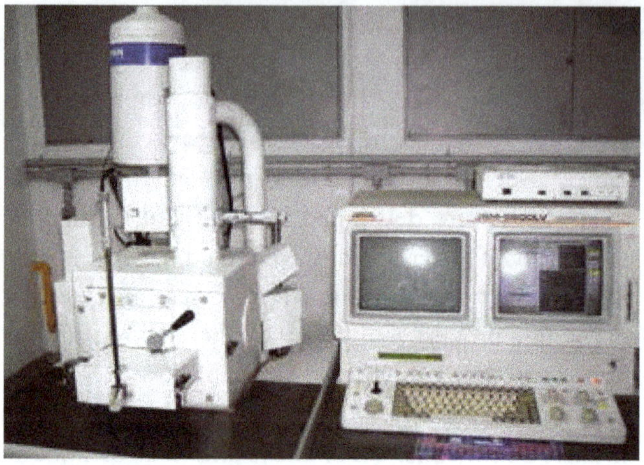

Figure 1 - Scanning electronic microscope used with EDS system of microanalysis.

microscopy (JEOL, model JSM-5800 LV with EDS system of microanalysis) (Fig 1). To analyze the surface morphology of the fracture region and wire-surface roughness of the wires, the technique of secondary electrons analysis was used, by means of which the images of inclusions, manufacturing residue and superficial heterogeneity were obtained. To carry out these tests, two samples of each wire subgroup were used.

Table 1 - Orthodontic wires used in this study: GAC (GAC Int. Inc. New York, USA); TP (TP Orthodontics, La Porte, USA); Ormco (Ormco Corp. Glendora, USA); 3M Unitek (Unitek Corporation, Monrovia, USA); Masel (Masel, Bristol, USA); Morelli (Dental Morelli, São Paulo, Brazil).

SUPERELASTIC GROUP (12 archwires)		HEAT-ACTIVATED GROUP (08 archwires)	
GAC	2 NiTi SE (REF. 03-018-53T)	GAC Sentalloy	2 NiTi Heat (REF. 02-511-132)
TP Reflex	2 NiTi SE (REF. 381-264)	TP HA	2 NiTi Heat (REF. 381-825)
Ormco Ni-Ti	2 NiTi SE (REF. 219-3204)	Ormco 35°C	2 CuNiTi Heat (REF. 219-4204)
Ormco 27°C	2 CuNiTi SE (REF. 205-0048)	Unitek Nitinol HA	2 NiTi Heat (REF. 4286-981)
Masel Elastinol	2 NiTi SE (REF. 4828-018)	-	-
Morelli	2 NiTi SE (REF. 50.70.014)	-	-

Table 2 - Chemical composition of tested NiTi and CuNiTi wires (EDS).

Chemical composition %	Nickel (Ni) NiO	Titanium (Ti) TiO_2	Copper (Cu) CuO	Aluminium (Al) Al_2O_3	Calcium (Ca) CaO	Bromine (Br) Br	Silicon (Si) SiO_2
NiTi SUPER GAC	53.33%	43.52%	-	0.19%	-	-	-
NiTi SUPER TP	52.50%	45.44%	-	1.61%	0.16%	-	0.20%
CuNiTi 27°C Ormco	46.87%	43.70%	6.72%	2.31%	-	-	-
NiTi SUPER Ormco	50.99%	42.27%	-	-	3.50%	0.54%	1.98%
NiTi SUPER Masel	49.22%	39.40%	-	5.08%	0.27%	4.26%	1.42%
NiTi SUPER Morelli	53.84%	42.96%	-	2.11%	-	-	0.58%
NiTi Heat GAC	52.84%	41.61%	-	1.13%	0.27%	-	1.59%
NiTi Heat TP	53.48%	43.26%	-	0.86%	-	-	-
CuNiTi 35°C Ormco	43.82%	45.79%	5.09%	2.40%	0.99%	-	0.69%
NiTi Heat Unitek	54.08%	45.14%	-	0.32%	-	-	0.23%

RESULTS

Semiquantitative chemical composition

Chemical analyses revealed that all samples basically have Ni and Ti with minor differences in percentage. CuNiTi wires presented significant percentage of copper in addition to Ni and Ti in their composition. Microanalyses results shown in Table 2 indicate the oxides present on the surface of the analyzed wires.

Wire-surface roughness

Figures 2 and 3 show, respectively, the surface morphology of superelastic and heat-activated wires before traction tests. It can be observed that superelastic NiTi wires presented lower wire-surface roughness than the heat-activated ones.

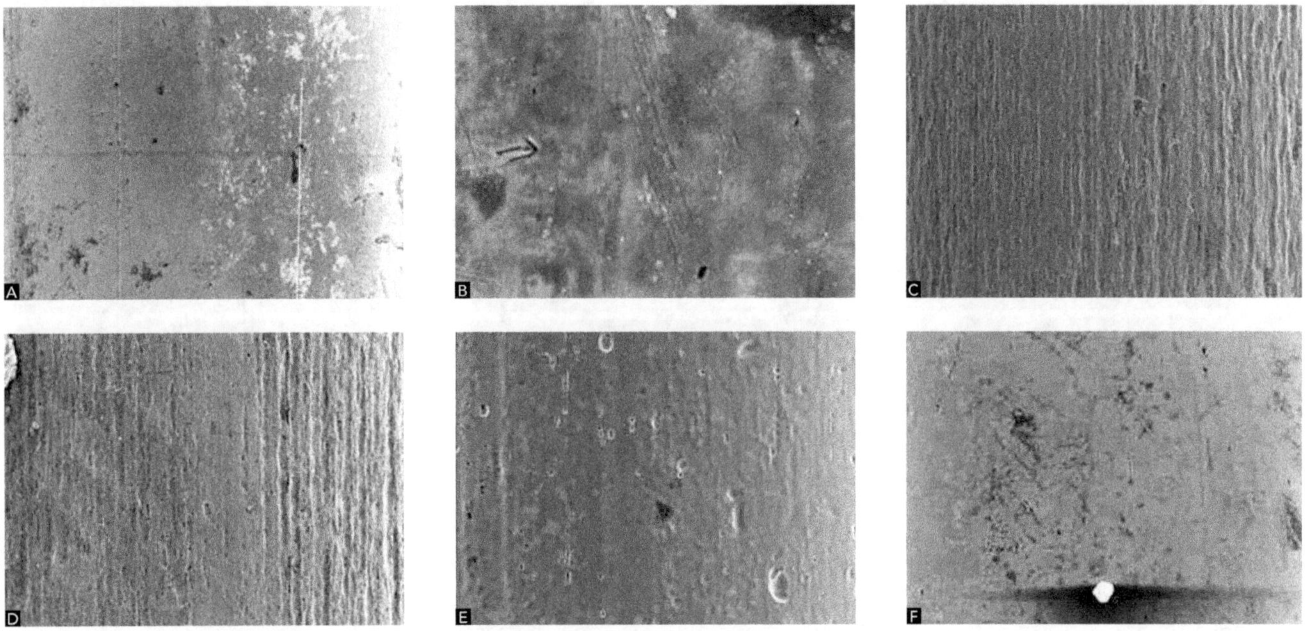

Figure 2 - Surface morphologies of superelastic NiTi and CuNiTi wires: **A)** superelastic NiTi by GAC; **B)** superelastic NiTi by TP; **C)** superelastic NiTi by Ormco; **D)** CuNiTi 27°C by Ormco; **E)** superelastic NiTi by Masel; **F)** superelastic NiTi by Morelli (X 500).

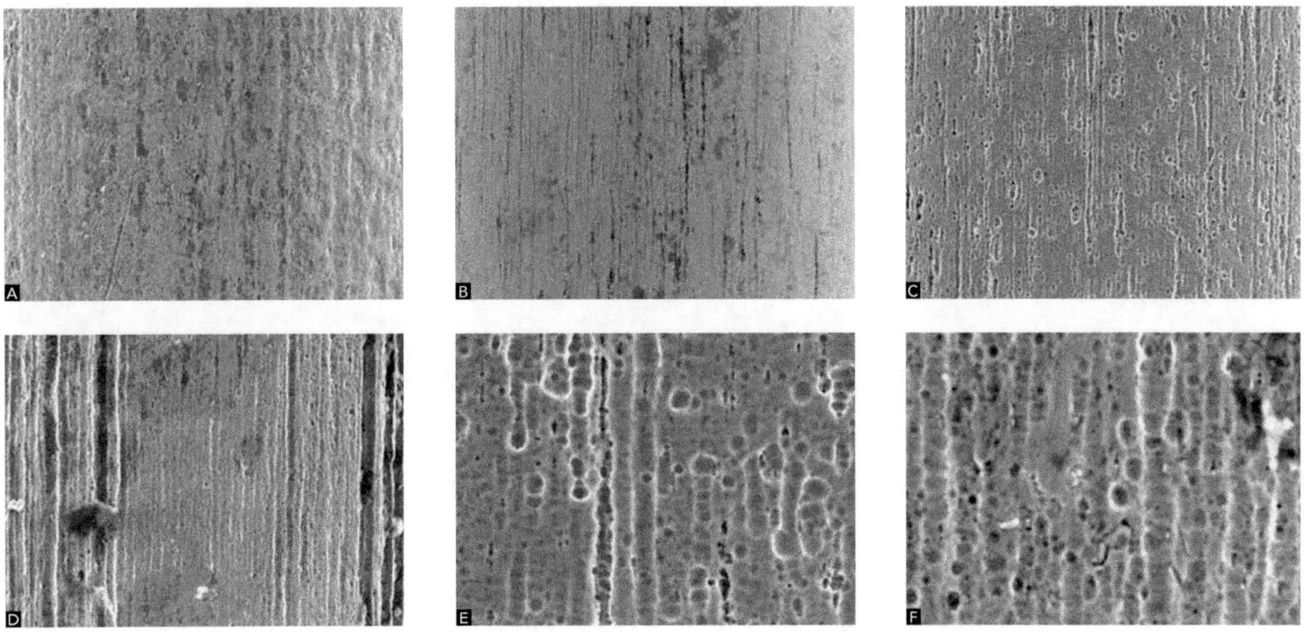

Figure 3 - Surface morphologies of heat-activated NiTi and CuNiTi wires: **A)** heat-activated NiTi by GAC; **B)** heat-activated NiTi by TP; **C)** CuNiTi 35°C by Ormco; **D)** heat-activated NiTi by Unitek (X500); **E)** CuNiTi 35°C by Ormco; **F)** heat-activated NiTi by Unitek (X 2000).

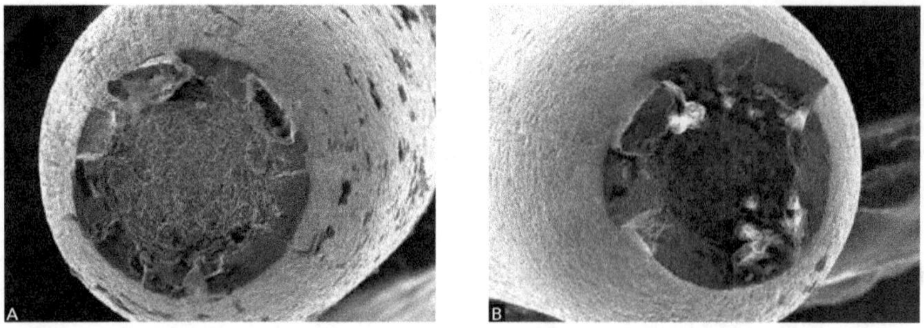

Figure 4 - Scanning electron microscopy of the fracture region on **A**) CuNiTi 27°C by Ormco and **B**) heat-activated NiTi by GAC (X 250).

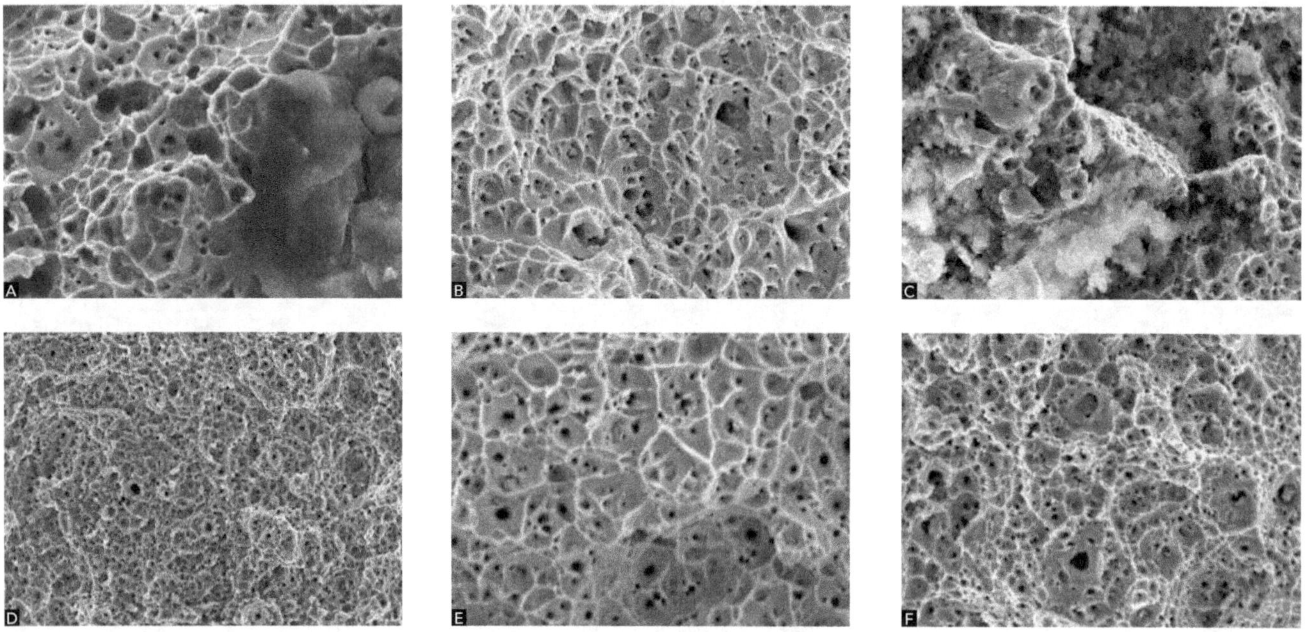

Figure 5 - Surface morphology of fracture of superelastic NiTi and CuNiTi wires: **A**) NiTi superelastic by GAC; **B**) NiTi superelastic by TP; **C**) NiTi superelastic by Ormco; **D**) CuNiTi 27°C by Ormco; **E**) NiTi superelastic by Masel; **F**) NiTi superelastic by Morelli (X 2000).

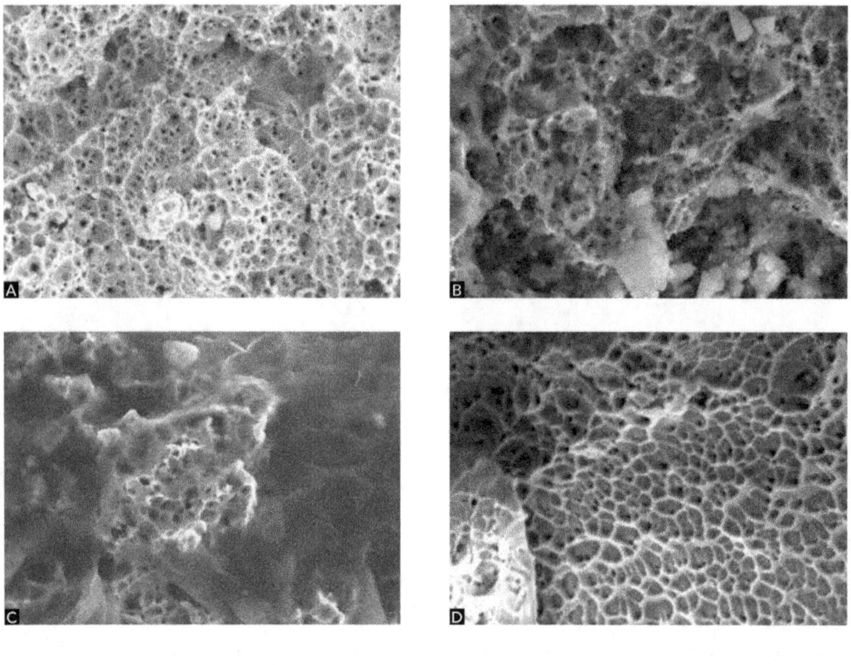

Figure 6 - Surface morphology of fracture of heat-activated NiTi and CuNiTi wires: **A**) heat-activated NiTi by GAC; **B**) heat-activated NiTi by TP; **C**) CuNiTi 35°C by Ormco; **D**) heat-activated NiTi by Unitek (X 2000).

Surface morphology of wire fracture

Figures 4 to 6 show the surface morphology of fractured NiTi and CuNiTi wires subjected to traction tests. The wires presented macroscopic plastic deformation with significant reduction in diameter. The fracture was cup-cone type, which is typical of high-ductility materials. This occurred to all subgroups of wires, implying that they underwent permanent deformations before fracturing, since they were subjected to tension and traction that were greater than their respective yield value. The analyses of fractured surfaces with greater increase (Figs 5 and 6)demonstrate the presence of microcavities, proving that the fracture is of ductile type.

DISCUSSION

With regard to the chemical composition of the tested wires, we observed that, generally, the tested NiTi wires presented Ni and Ti as the main elements of the alloy with minor differences in their composition. We also observed the presence of other chemical elements, especially Al, Si and Ca. Superelastic wires (Masel) presented a slightly lower percentage of Ni and Ti associated with a significative percentage of aluminum oxide. Superelastic wires (Ormco) presented a slightly lower percentage of Ni with higher percentage of calcium. Fischer-Brandies et al[10] suggested that all wires present inclusions, chemical immunogenicity and manufacturing residue, such as silicon oxide (SiO_2) and aluminum oxide (Al_2O_3), which was also observed in the present work.

The present work demonstrated that CuNiTi wires have a significant percentage of copper (Cu) in addition to Ni and Ti in their composition, as reported by Fischer-Brandies et al.[10] According to Parvizi and Rock,[14] adding between 5 and 6% of copper in the composition of superelastic NiTi wires would increase mechanical resistance and reduce the percentage of permanent deformation after deactivation, all of which are considered favorable characteristics. However, such benefits would be associated with an increase in the transition temperature of these wires for values greater than the ones found intraorally. An addition of 0.5% of chromium would be made with the purpose of avoiding such an increase and, thus, maintain the temperature at around 27°C. But, in the present work, no percentage of chromium was found in the composition of CuNiTi wires.

As for the surface morphology of wires, the manufacturing process is carried out by drawing. Drawing is the process in which wires with larger cross-sections (wire rod) pass through tools (spinnerets) to have their dimensions reduced, thus, being transformed into another wire with adequate diameter and which can be used for several purposes, for instance, as round, square and rectangle orthodontic wires. The presence and intensity of drawing marks on the surface of the wires depend on the period of use and on the spinneret finishing, on the alloy composition and on the thermodynamic state of the wire rod. Thus, the longer the period of use of the spinneret, the greater the chance of it making slots and imperfections on the surface of the wires during the process. The following is among the consequences of drawing marks: greater concentration of tension on the wires, reduction in the material capacity of being longitudinally deformed, reduction in the limit of traction resistance, increase in the coefficient of attrition and increase in biofilm adhesion.[8]

In the present work, superelastic wires presented smoother surfaces in relation to the heat-activated ones, as reported by Fischer-Brandies et al.[10] Among the superelastic wires, those by Masel and Morelli (Figs 2E and 2F) presented the lowest wire-surface roughness, with evidence of polishment after the drawing process. TP and GAC wires (Figs 2A and 2B) presented intermediate wire-surface roughness. Superelastic NiTi and CuNiTi 27°C wires by Ormco (Figs 2C and 2D) presented the greatest wire-surface roughness, with deep spinneret marks, which led us to believe that they had not been subjected to any chemical or mechanical treatment after drawing.

Among the heat-activated wires (Fig 3), those by GAC, TP and Unitek as well as the CuNiTi 35°C by Ormco presented inadequate characteristics regarding wire-surface roughness, with very visible drawing marks and slots seen at any degree of magnification. Such marks were more evident and deeper in wires by Unitek and in the CuNiTi 35°C by Ormco (Figs 3C and 3D). When those wires were evaluated under magnification of 2000x (Figs 3E and 3F), they presented, in addition to drawing marks and slots, microcavities formed due to pullout of particles, possibly of NiTi,[4] which was also observed in superelastic NiTi and CuNiTi 27°C wires by Ormco. NiTi[4] precipitation depends on the amount of Ni in solid solution, since it could have been altered by the presence of copper in the composition of CuNiTi wires. Variations in 0.1% of Ni would already be significant to induce the formation and precipitation of NiTi4. As for the superelastic NiTi wires by Ormco, they presented a slightly lower percentage of Ni in comparison to the other tested NiTi wires (Table 2), which could have induced the formation of a higher percentage of precipitation and pullout of particles of NiTi4.

With regard to the morphology of the fracture region of superelastic and heat-activated wires seen under magnification of 2000x (Figs 5 and 6), we observed the presence of microcavities which are a characteristic of ductile fractures, with the largest microcavities being formed by pullout of particles, possibly of NiTi4. Additionally, we observed that, in general, the size of the microcavities found for superelastic NiTi wires was larger than that found for heat-activated NiTi wires. Among the superelastic NiTi wires, those that presented the smallest microcavities were the CuNiTi 27°C ones (Fig 5D). Wires by GAC, TP, Masel and Morelli (Figs 5A, 5B, 5E and 5F) presented microcavities of similar sizes. Among the heat-activated wires, those by GAC and Unitek (Figs 6E and 6H) presented smaller microcavities in comparison to wires of other samples.

The results of the present work showed that CuNiTi 35°C wires presented inadequate characteristics regarding superficial topography, which could predispose a higher coefficient of attrition during tooth movement. Damon,[7] however, asserted that the sequential use of orthodontic wires of CuNiTi 35°C 0.014", 0.014" X 0.025" and 0.018" X 0.025" in self-bonding brackets would significantly reduce the coefficient of attrition generated in conventional mechanics, which would be the key to a more efficient treatment, with significant reduction in the mean period of chair time, in the number of visits paid to the orthodontist and in patient's degree of discomfort.

Nevertheless, a new research should be carried out in order to evaluate the attrition of such wires in relation to other superelastic and heat-activated NiTi and CuNiTi wires, given that through scanning electron microscopy, the present work, in agreement to results obtained by Fischer-Brandies et al,[10] proved that CuNiTi 35°C wires by Ormco presented not only very visible drawing marks and slots seen under any degree of magnification, but also microcavities formed due to pullout of particles of NiTi4, which could generate a higher coefficient of attrition.

CONCLUSION

1. With regard to chemical composition, the tested NiTi wires presented predominance of Ni and Ti with a small percentage of Al, Ca, and Si. CuNiTi wires presented a significant percentage of copper in addition to Ni and Ti in their compositions.
2. With regard to surface morphology, the superelastic NiTi wires by Masel and Morelli presented the lowest wire-surface roughness, while the superelastic and heat-activated NiTi and CuNiTi wires by Ormco presented the greatest wire-surface roughness.
3. With regard to the morphology of fracture regions, CuNiTi 27°C wires by Ormco and the heat-activated wires by GAC and Unitek presented the smallest microcavities, while CuNiTi 35°C by Ormco presented the largest.
4. All wires presented fractured surfaces under ductile traction.
5. CuNiTi 35°C wires did not present better morphologic characteristics on surfaces and fracture regions in comparison to the other wires.

REFERENCES

1. Andreasen GF, Hilleman TB. An evaluation of 55 cobalt substituted nitinol wire for use in orthodontics. J Am Dent Assoc. 1971;82(6):1373-5.
2. Andreasen GF, Hilleman TB. An evaluation of 55 cobalt substituted Nitinol wire for use in orthodontics. J Am Dent Assoc. 1971;82(6):1373-5. Igual a referencia acima
3. Andreasen GF, Morrow RE. Laboratory and clinical analysis of Nitinol wire. Am J Orthod. 1978;73(2):142-51.
4. Buehler WJ. Proceedings of the 7th Navy Symposium ONR-16 Office of Technical Services. 1963. Washington, DC; 1963. v. 1, p. 1-30.
5. Burstone CJ, Goldberg AJ. Beta Titanium: a new orthodontic alloy. Am J Orthod. 1980;77(2):121-32.
6. Burstone CJ, Qin B, Morton JY. Chinese NiTi wire: a new orthodontic alloy. Am J Orthod. 1985;87(6):445-52.
7. Damon DH. The Damon low-friction bracket: a biologically compatible straight-wire system. J Clin Orthod. 1998;32(11):670-80.
8. Elias CN, Lopes HP. Materiais dentários: ensaios mecânicos. São Paulo: Ed. Santos; 2007.
9. Evans TJW, Durning P. Orthodontic products update. Aligning archwires, the shape of things to come? A forth and fifth phase of force delivery. Brit J Orthod. 1996;23(3):269-75.

10. Fischer-Brandies H, Es-Souni M, Kock N, Raetzke K, Bock O. Transformation behavior, chemical composition, surface topography and bending properties of five selected 0.016" X 0.022" NiTi archwires. J Orofac Orthop. 2003;64(2):88-99.
11. Kapila S, Sachdeva R. Mechanical properties and clinical applications of orthodontic wires. Am J Orthod Dentofacial Orthop. 1989;96(2):100-9.
12. Miura F, Mogi M, Ohura Y, Hamanaka H. The super-elastic property of the Japanese NiTi alloy wire for use in orthodontics. Am J Orthod Dentofacial Orthop. 1986;90(1):1-10.
13. Mohlin B, Müller H, Odman J, Thilander B. Examination of chinese Ni-Ti wire by a combined clinical and laboratory approach. Eur J Orthod. 1991;13(5):386-91.
14. Parvizi F, Rock WP. The load/deflection characteristics of thermally activated orthodontic archwires. Eur J Orthod. 2003;25(4):417-21.
15. Perkins J, Hodgson D. The two-way shape memory effect. London: Jeff Perkings Plenum Press; 1975.
16. Sachdeva RC. Sure-Smile: technology: driven solution for orthodontics. Texas Dent J. 2002;119(7):608-15.
17. West AE. A clinical comparison of two initial aligning archwires [thesis]. Cardiff (UK): University of Wales; 1992.
18. Gravina MA, Brunharo IHVP, Canavarro C, Elias CN, Quintão CCA. Mechanical properties of NiTi and CuNiTi wires used in orthodontic treatment. Part 1: Stress-strain tests. Dental Press J Orthod. 2013;18(4):35-42.

11

Photoelastic analysis of stress generated by wires when conventional and self-ligating brackets are used

Guilherme Caiado Sobral[1], Mário Vedovello Filho[2], Viviane Veroni Degan[2], Milton Santamaria Jr[3]

Objective: By means of a photoelastic model, this study analyzed the stress caused on conventional and self-ligating brackets with expanded arch wires. **Method:** Standard brackets were adhered to artificial teeth and a photoelastic model was prepared using the Interlandi 19/12 diagram as base. Successive activations were made with 0.014-in and 0.018-in rounded cross section Nickel-Titanium wires (NiTi) and 0.019 x 0.025-in rectangular stainless steel wires all of which made on 22/14 Interlandi diagram. The model was observed on a plane polariscope — in a dark field microscope configuration — and photographed at each exchange of wire. Then, they were replaced by self-ligating brackets and the process was repeated. Analysis was qualitative and observed stress location and pattern on both models analyzed. **Conclusions:** Results identified greater stress on the region of the apex of premolars in both analyzed models. Upon comparing the stress between models, a greater amount of stress was found in the model with conventional brackets in all of its wires. Therefore, the present pilot study revealed that alignment of wires in self-ligating brackets produced lower stress in periodontal tissues in expansive mechanics.

Keywords: Orthodontic brackets. Dental arch. Corrective orthodontics.

[1] MSc in Orthodontics, School of Dentistry — University of Araras (UNIARARAS).
[2] Professor, Department of Orthodontics, UNIARARAS.
[3] Professor, Postgraduate program in Orthodontics, UNIARARAS.

» The authors report no commercial, proprietary or financial interest in the products or companies described in this article.

Milton Santamaria Jr
Av. Maximiliano Baruto, 500 – Jd. Universitário Araras – São Paulo/SP — Brazil.
CEP: 13607-339 – E-mail: santamariajr@ig.com.br

INTRODUCTION

Nowadays, orthodontists have many techniques and methods available for treatment planning. There is a great variety of brackets, with different prescriptions and forms that allow the orthodontist to individualize each case according to patient's needs.[1]

These needs make the scientific community endeavor to innovate in orthodontic appliances. Innovation, in turn, leads to better control of dental movement, given that one of the greatest challenges faced by the orthodontist is to come up with mechanical solutions to stimulate biological reactions of the periodontium without compromising treatment outcomes.[2]

Correct management of orthodontic forces depends on a series of factors, including friction generated between wires and brackets. In orthodontic sliding mechanics, friction poses clinical difficulties to the orthodontist. High levels of friction could decrease bracket efficiency, thereby reducing the speed of dental movement and hindering anchorage control.[3]

The concern of producing less friction, i.e., lower attrition between wires and brackets, contributed to the development of self-ligating brackets in which the tooth moves with the wires serving as a guide, since it does not involve the use of elastic ligatures which significantly increase friction between wires and the slot.[4]

The difference between conventional and self-ligating brackets system is the absence of elastic or metallic ligatures in the latter. In other words, brackets have a closing system that leaves the wire free inside the slot.[5]

One of the purposes of orthodontic mechanics is gaining space in the arch before alignment of crowded teeth. Including badly-positioned teeth in the wire without previous space gain leads to unwanted displacements of adjacent teeth.[6] On the other hand, according to Damon,[5] lower friction treatment provides transversal adaptation that prevents potential side-effects of alignment, thereby providing treatment of crowded teeth without previous mechanic space gain.

In addition to treating crowding cases, this transversal adaptation might be used in favor of the orthodontist. For instance, in cases aiming at transversal expansion of one or both arches, Maltagliati[6] showed that treatment with self-ligating brackets significantly increased the transversal dimensions. This unique behavior of the self-ligating system in comparison to the conventional one seems to derive from lower friction associated with heat activated nickel-titanium wires of small diameter acting as adjuvant in treatment results.[6]

One of the methods used to study the way forces manifest on bodies is by means of photoelasticity. The principle of photoelasticity is based on the fact that most materials turn birefringent (separation of light into two rays with different velocity and refraction indexes) when subjected to mechanical stress.[7,8]

Birefringence is manifested by colored fringes in areas of induced stress. Orthodontic material reproduces resilience of the periodontium.[9] Monochromatic tones are used for analysis of force quantity, while colored fringes provide more information on stress direction and distribution.[10]

By means of photoelasticity, the present study analyzed the stress caused on conventional and self-ligating brackets when combined with nickel-titanium wires.

MATERIAL AND METHODS

Photoelastic model

Only one photoelastic model was made. Initially, with conventional brackets (Kirium, Abzil Indústria e Comércio Ltda, São José do Rio Preto, Brazil) which were afterwards replaced by self-ligating brackets (Portia, Abzil Indústria e Comércio Ltda, São José do Rio Preto, Brazil) bonded with cyanoacrylate (Superbonder glue Loctite, Barueri, SP) to lower artificial teeth (B2-306, Kilgore-Nissin, Kilgore International, USA).

The photoelastic model of the lower arch was manufactured on a wax roller based on Interlandi 19/12 diagram.[11] The wax was cut so as to have a constant thickness throughout the model. A mold was made with the wax pressed on a muffle furnace.

The wax was thus removed with hot water, detergent and Remox (Vipi, Pirassununga, Brazil). The epoxy flexible photoelastic resin (Polipox, Ind. e Com. Ltda, São Paulo, Brazil) was handled in accordance with the manufacturer's specifications and placed on the space created by the wax until teeth roots were completely submerged. After 72 hours, the model was removed from the mold.

Plane polariscope characteristics

The polariscope was assembled with the following components: a light source, a polarizer, the Photoelastic model and the analyzer (Keyko). The camera (SX120 IS, Canon Inc., Tokyo, Japan) was mounted on a tripod and positioned in front of the analyzer. The photoelastic model was placed on a rotating platform with measurement markings to ensure consistency in placing the model.

Prior to applying stress, the model was observed and photographed in frontal view, profile view (both left and right) and occlusal view. The objective was to assess absence of residual stress on the material and the initial conditions of the photoelastic resin (Fig 1).

Mechanical trial

In conventional brackets with elastic ligatures, 0.014-in and 0.018-in rounded cross section Nickel-Titanium (NiTi) wires and 0.019 x 0.025-in rectangular stainless steel wires were successively placed in the 22/14 Interlandi diagram. The photoelastic model was made on the bases of dimensions corresponding to 19/12 Interlandi diagram. Thus, it aimed at exerting expansive forces during wire changes.

After each exchange of wire, the photoelastic model was photographed and analyzed for fringe standards. Self-ligating brackets were analyzed by the same means.

Photographs were taken based on the same criteria for both groups so as to avoid potential interference from other variables. All polariscope components remained within the same distance. Angling with the camera lenses and the photoelastic model also remained the same throughout the experiment.

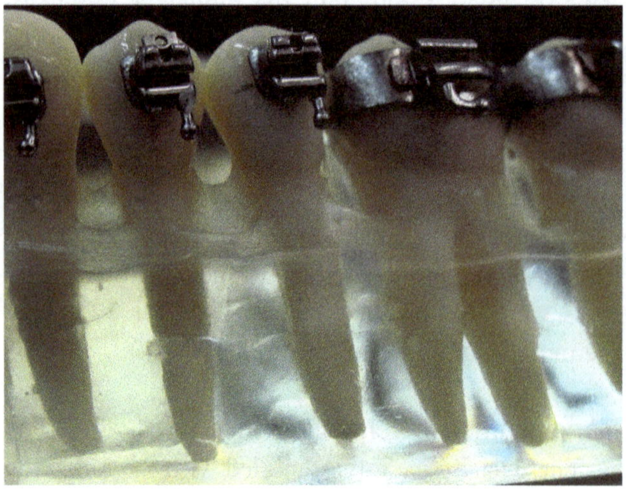

Figure 1 - Photoelastic model without residual tension.

In order to ensure that the model would be positioned in the exact same place after archwire placement, markings from the rotating platform were used. Photographs were taken at the same location under the same lighting conditions in the room.

Qualitative assessment of photoelastic model

In photograph analysis, the value of fringes depends on the type of material used, its width, length of light wave impacting and temperature of the model.[10] Therefore, this study assessed — by qualitative means — stress distribution on photoelastic models.[12]

Qualitative assessment was carried out by assessing stress pattern on the model, expressed by different fringe colors on the root surface of premolars and marked in scores, as follows:

Results evolve from lack of stress (-) to a small whitish halo (+), a bigger white halo (++), followed by a yellow (+++), violet or magenta halo (++++) and a cyan or light blue halo(+++++). Assessment was conducted in the apical region and middle third of lower premolar roots.

Results are presented in tables according to groups, either with conventional or passive self-ligating brackets. Moreover, results were determined via descriptive statistics by categorizing the scores according to the colors of fringes.

RESULTS

Figure 2 illustrates photographs of premolars and molars under activation with conventional and self-ligating brackets. Figures A, B and C show the photoelastic model with conventional brackets associated to 0.014-in and 0.018-in NiTi wires as well as 0.019 x 0.025-in stainless steel wires respectively. Figures D, E and F show the photoelastic model with self-ligating brackets activated with 0.014-in and 0.018-in NiTi wires and 0.019 x 0.025-in stainless steel wires, respectively.

Results revealed that activations with either conventional or self-ligating brackets show the presence of stress in the apex of the premolars (Fig 2). However, conventional brackets produced higher stress due to greater concentration of blue and violet colored fringes, especially in activations with 0.018-in NiTi wires and 0.019 x 0.025-in stainless

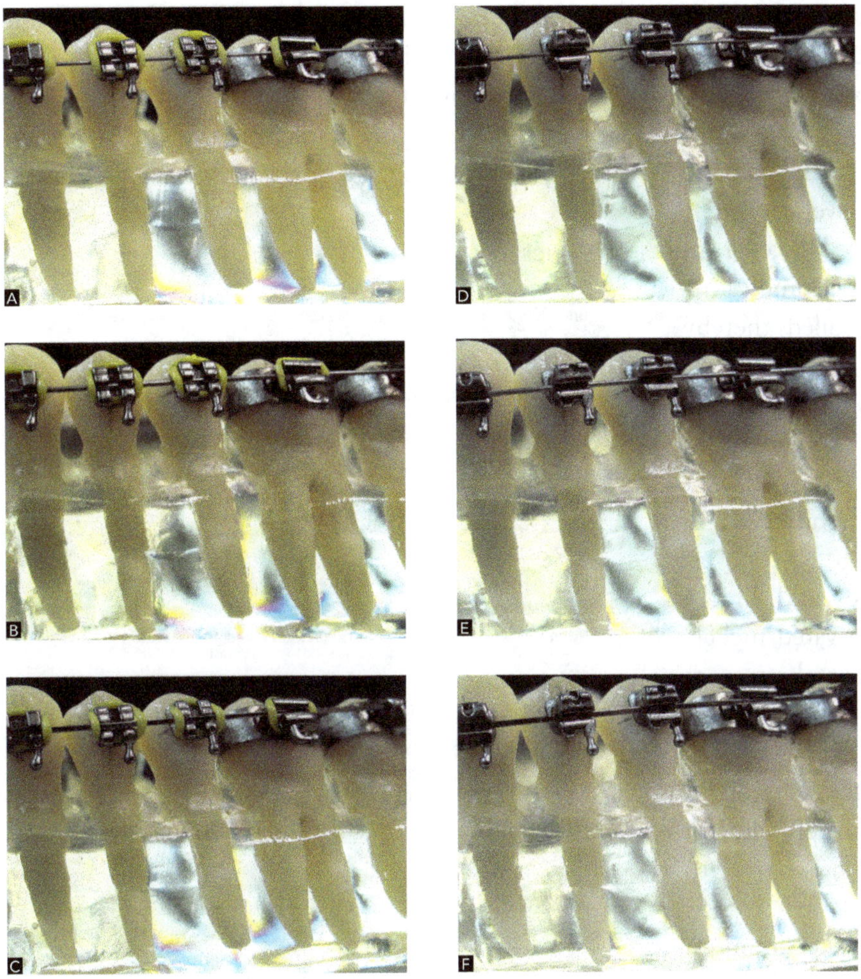

Figure 2 - A, B, C) Conventional brackets; D, E, F) Self-ligating brackets.

Table 1 - Qualitative analysis of the apical region of premolar roots expressed in scores according to the colors of the fringes on the photoelastic model.

WIRE	SELF-LIGATING BRACKETS	CONVENTIONAL BRACKETS
0.014-in NiTi	++++	+++
0.018-in NiTi	+++++	+++
0.019 x 0.021-in Stainless steel	+++++	+++

Table 2 - Qualitative analysis of the middle third of premolar roots expressed in scores according to the colors of the fringes on the photoelastic model.

WIRE	SELF-LIGATING BRACKETS	CONVENTIONAL BRACKETS
0.014-in NiTi	+++	-
0.018-in NiTi	+++	-
0.019 x 0.021-in Stainless steel	+++	-

steel wires (Figs 2A, B and C; Table 1). In the middle third, stress was only found in activations with conventional brackets, as yellow fringes were found in the three activations (Figs 2A, B and C; Table 2). The same was not found in self-ligating brackets (Figs 2D, E and F; Table 2).

DISCUSSION

This study reveals that both self-ligating and conventional brackets produce photoelastic stress under conditions of alignment with expansive forces, since diagramming of wires was larger than the size of the photoelastic model dental arch. It also found that stress concentrated in the apical region of premolars in both models, but with greater stress concentration in conventional brackets models.

Furthermore, lower periodontal forces, seen in the photoelastic model, allow more physiological expansive treatment. Pandis[13] conducted a study comparing the intercanine and intermolar distance after treatment with conventional and passive self-ligating brackets. In the self-ligating group, intermolar distance was greater. However, buccal tipping of lower incisors was the same in both groups.

The system of self-ligating brackets can increase buccal tipping of incisors and the transverse dimension of the maxilla and the mandible.[14] However, in patients with muscular balance, buccal tipping of incisors might be desired and better controlled, thereby not changing patient's facial profile.

Table 1 compares the stress observed in the apical region of premolar roots subjected to conventional and self-ligating systems. Greater concentration of photoelastic stress is observed in conventional brackets.

Lower friction between the wires and brackets,[4,6] associated with resilient heat-activated nickel-titanium wires[5] produce lower periodontal stress, as seen in the photoelastic study mode, thereby favoring expansive mechanics in crowding resolution. This treatment modality is indicated, for example, to patients with mainly horizontal growth, presence of muscular balance and some freedom for incisors to tip forward.

In this study, no heat-activated nickel-titanium wires were used. Additionally, all study models tested were free of crowding. Moreover, the self-ligating brackets used herein were passive. In active self-ligating brackets, the more the diameter of wires increase, the greater the friction which can be higher than conventional brackets.[15]

Therefore, according to the present results and the growing development of self-ligating brackets systems, it is reasonable to assert that much has to evaluate with regards to stress produced by the use of self-ligating brackets compared to conventional brackets in expansive mechanics.

CONCLUSION

Based on the results of the current study, it is suggested that both bracket systems produced stress when activated. However, conventional brackets produced greater stress in comparison to passive self-ligating brackets. Therefore, the present pilot study reveals that self-ligating brackets produce softer forces in periodontal tissues in alignment expansive mechanics.

ACKNOWLEDGMENTS

Special thanks is dedicated to the Department of Dental Material at the School of Orthodontics – State University of Campinas/Piracicaba (UNICAMP), especially to Professor Dr. Américo Bortolazzo Correr.

REFERENCES

1. Brito Júnior VS, Ursi WJS. O aparelho pré-ajustado: sua evolução e suas prescrições. Rev Dental Press Ortod Ortop Facial. 2006;11(3):104-56.
2. Picchioni MS. Análise comparativa dos níveis de atrito em braquetes e autoligados [dissertação]. São Bernardo do Campo (SP): Universidade Metodista de São Paulo; 2007.
3. Frank C. A comparative study of frictional resistances between orthodontic bracket and arch wire. Am J Orthod. 1980;78(6):593-609.
4. Voudouris JC. Interactive edgewise mechanisms: form and function comparison with conventional edgewise brackets. Am J Orthod Dentofacial Orthop. 1997;111(2):119-40.
5. Damon DH. The Damon low-friction bracket: a biologically compatible straight-wire system. J Clin Orthod. 1998;32(11):670-80.
6. Maltagliati L. Sistema autoligado: quebrando paradigmas. Ortodontia SPO. 2009;42(5):360-1.
7. Rocha JET, Fuziy A, Tukasan PC, Oliveira RCG. Fotoelasticidade: aplicabilidade na mecânica ortodôntica. Braz Oral Res. 2006;20(Spec issue1):81.
8. Vuolo JH. Polarização da luz e displays TN. São Paulo: IFUSP; 1998. p. 1-16.
9. Rossato C. Estudo fotoelástico das áreas de pressão, produzidas no periodonto, por forças ortodônticas, na distalização do canino pelos métodos convencionais e com "Power arm". [dissertação]. Bauru (SP): Unicersidade de São Paulo; 1982.
10. Glickman I, Roeber FW, Brion M, Pameijer JH. Photoelastic analysis of internal stresses in the periodontium created by occlusal forces. J Periodontol. 1970;41(1):30-5.
11. Interlandi S. Diagrama de contorneamento ortodôntico para a técnica do arco contínuo (Straight Wire). Ortodontia. 2002;35(4):91-105.
12. Dobranszki A. Estudo fotoelástico do controle vertical com arco de dupla chave na técnica Straight wire. Rev Dental Press Ortod Ortop Facial. 2009;14(4):123-8.
13. Pandis N. Self ligating vs conventional brackets in the treatment of mandibular crowding: a prospective clinical trial of treatment duration and dental effects. Am J Orthod Dentofacial Orthop. 2007;132(2):208-15.
14. Kochenborger R. Avaliação das alterações dentárias e do perfil facial obtidas no tratamento ortodôntico com braquetes autoligáveis [dissertação]. São Bernardo do Campo (SP): Universidade Metodista de São Paulo; 2009.
15. Lorenz M. Active and passive self-ligation: a myth? Angle Orthod. 2011;81(2):312-8.

12

Are self-ligating brackets related to less formation of *Streptococcus mutans* colonies?

Leonard Euler Andrade Gomes do Nascimento[1], Margareth Maria Gomes de Souza[2], Angela Rita Pontes Azevedo[3], Lucianne Cople Maia[4]

Objective: To verify, by means of a systematic review, whether the design of brackets (conventional or self-ligating) influences adhesion and formation of *Streptococcus mutans* colonies. **Methods:** Search strategy: four databases (Cochrane Central Register of Controlled Trials, Ovid ALL EMB Reviews, PubMed and BIREME) were selected to search relevant articles covering the period from January 1965 to December 2012. Selection Criteria: in first consensus by reading the title and abstract. The full text was obtained from publications that met the inclusion criteria. Data collection and analysis: Two reviewers independently extracted data using the keywords: conventional, self-ligating, biofilm, *Streptococcus mutans*, and systematic review; and independently evaluated the quality of the studies. In case of divergence, the technique of consensus was adopted. **Results:** The search strategy resulted in 1,401 articles. The classification of scientific relevance revealed the high quality of the 6 eligible articles of which outcomes were not unanimous in reporting not only the influence of the design of the brackets (conventional or self-ligating) over adhesion and formation of colonies of *Streptococcus mutans*, but also that other factors such as the quality of the bracket type, the level of individual oral hygiene, bonding and age may have greater influence. Statistical analysis was not feasible because of the heterogeneous methodological design. **Conclusions:** Within the limitations of this study, it was concluded that there is no evidence for a possible influence of the design of the brackets (conventional or self-ligating) over colony formation and adhesion of *Streptococcus mutans*.

Keywords: Biofilms. Orthodontic brackets. *Streptococcus mutans*. Review.

[1] Visiting professor, Federal University of Piauí (UFPI).
[2] Full professor, Department of Pediatric Dentistry and Orthodontics, Federal University of Rio de Janeiro (UFRJ).
[3] Doctorate student in Orthodontics, UFRJ.
[4] Full Professor, Department of Pediatric Dentistry and Orthodontics, UFRJ.

» The authors report no commercial, proprietary or financial interest in the products or companies described in this article.

Lucianne Cople Maia
Disciplina de Odontopediatria da Faculdade de Odontologia da Universidade Federal do Rio de Janeiro – Caixa Postal 68066 – Universitária – CCS
CEP: 21.941-971 – Rio de Janeiro/RJ – Brazil – E-mail: leonardeuler@hotmail.com

INTRODUCTION

Increased oral microbiota of *Streptococcus mutans* and *Lactobacillus* is associated with the onset of tooth demineralization and periodontal disease, especially in orthodontic patients who present greater risk of colonization by these microrganisms.[1-4] It seems that the main factor behind the increase in the accumulation of dental plaque and inflammatory response is the appearance of new locations of retention around the components of fixed orthodontic appliance.[5] The devices used in orthodontic appliances (bands, wires, ligatures or brackets) can promote changes in the oral environment, such as pH, amount of *Streptococcus mutans*, biofilm[6-9] and enamel decalcification.[10-16] The clinical characteristics and the physical properties of the bracket types are very different,[17] and, thus, can directly influence the amount of biofilm adhesion and, consequently, gingivitis.[5,18-22] The characteristics of both the surface of the teeth and the gingiva influence the spontaneous formation of plaque, not only in quantity, but also in quality.[18,23-30] Saliva composition and secretion rate also influence plaque formation.[27]

Conventional brackets (C) are associated with the use of either elastomeric or stainless steel ligature to keep the orthodontic wire inside the slot.[8] In Orthodontics, the term self-ligating (SL) refers to orthodontic brackets that have their own mechanism for opening and closing the slot, and do not require any metal or elastomeric ligature as a method for wire ligation.[31,32] All these methods have advantages and disadvantages, but in relation to biofilm retention, the literature[8,33] suggests that it is greater with elastomeric ligatures. Orthodontic treatment with C brackets usually presents some periodontal changes as side effects caused by difficulty in periodontal hygiene and also by greater accumulation and qualitative alteration of plaque.[3,5,6,8,19,20] Thus, in order to improve the deficiency of conventional brackets systems, SL were developed so as to, according to the manufacturers and some studies,[8,34-38] allow better hygiene. They claim that SL brackets are less susceptible to bacterial colonization due to their shape and absence of elastomeric and metal ligatures.[33] It is questionable, however, if the adhesion of microorganisms and the development of biofilm is reduced by the removal of ligatures of conventional brackets and with the use of the opening and closing mechanism of SL systems. Even with the changes in modern bracket types, the problem of plaque accumulation around the brackets is still persistent in daily orthodontic practice.[37,39]

Over the years, many publications[6-11,33,34,38-41] have reported different results concerning microorganism adhesion and biofilm development for C and SL brackets. Biofilm adhesion on brackets is measured by different systems, which hinders the evaluation of scientific quality. Therefore, it was proposed to verify, through a systematic review, whether bracket design (conventional or self-ligating) influences adhesion and formation of *Streptococcus mutans* colonies. Additionally, the methodological soundness of the studies included in the review was assessed in terms of quality.

MATERIAL AND METHODS

Search strategy

The strategy of this review was based on the National Health Service Center for Reviews and Dissemination.[42] Four databases (Cochrane Central Register of Controlled Trials; Ovid ALL EMB Reviews, PubMed and Bireme) were selected to find relevant articles published between January 1965 and December 2012. The search used the keywords "conventional" and/or "self-ligating" crossed with combinations of the terms biofilm and / or *Streptococcus mutans* and / or systematic review. Two reviewers separately sought additional relevant publications, which may not have been in the searched databases, by manually searching for papers in libraries and contacting authors. There were no language restrictions. As a first step, the reviewers selected the articles by reading titles and abstracts. Full texts were obtained from publications that met the inclusion criteria. After the articles were selected, their scientific relevance was independently assessed by the reviewers, and in case of divergence, the technique of consensus was adopted. This review used the PICO (Population Intervention Comparator Outcomes) strategy[43] to develop both the research and the bibliography (Table 1).

Inclusion and exclusion criteria

The inclusion criteria for the selected studies initially aimed at human beings, only: those who were periodontally healthy before the study began and who were at 11 years of age or older. The randomized and controlled clinical trials had to involve conventional edgewise and/or self-ligating brackets prescriptions. Case reports, review articles, abstracts and letters to the Editor were also included. The exclusion criteria comprised studies carried out with animals, *in vitro*

Table 1 - Description of the PICO (Population Intervention Comparator Outcomes) strategy used to develop the research and the bibliography.

Acronym	Description
Population	Patients with fixed orthodontic appliance with conventional or self-ligating edgewise brackets.
Intervention	Assessment of the amount of biofilm and microbiota attached to conventional or self-ligating brackets.
Comparison	Through the levels of biofilm accumulation on conventional or self-ligating brackets.
Outcomes	Measurement of colonies of *Streptococcus mutans* and/or their effects on periodontal tissues.

studies, treatment plans that included extractions of premolars as well as studies that included patients younger than 11 years of age, with periodontal problems, who were users of antibiotics and oral antiseptic solutions, alcoholics and smokers. Articles mentioning patients who used mechanical and anchoring devices, as well as Hyrax, were also excluded.

Assessment of the scientific relevance of the eligible studies

The following data were collected from each one of the papers selected: author/year of publication, journal, study design, age, teeth involved, bracket type and brand, ligature type, objective and method of analysis, follow-up, statistical analysis and outcome. A quality assessment[44] was performed on each article, according to the following ten criteria:

1) Study design (randomized clinical trials [RCT], prospective [P] or controlled clinical trials [CCT]) = 2 points.
2) Adequate study description = 1 point.
3) Adequate sample size = 1 point.
4) Adequate sample selection description = 1 point.
5) Drop outs description = 1 point.
6) Adequate description of biofilm measurement method = 0.5 point.
7) Blind study = 0.5 point.
8) Adequate statistics = 1 point.
9) Confounding factors considered = 1 point; and
10) Clinical significance = 1 point.

The ten criteria specified above were used to identify the scientific relevance of the methodological quality of the reviewed papers. The rating was "low" when the points given were less than or equal to 4, "medium" from 5 to 8 points and "high" for 9 or 10 points.

RESULTS

Search strategy outcomes

The search strategy resulted in 1,401 articles, out of which 195 were repeated references. The exclusion criteria used by both independent reviewers excluded 1,194 articles, which were not considered as relevant to the review, thus, totalizing twelve potentially relevant articles.[33,45-55] They were chosen for retrieval and evaluation of the full text, for which a summarized data extraction sheet was used (Table 2). Out of the twelve full-text articles that were retrieved, 6 were excluded because: one article[45] presented premolar extractions in its sample, three[47,49,51] were *in vitro* studies, and two[50,53] did not provide a direct comparison between C and SL brackets systems. This resulted in six articles[33,46,48,52,54,55] that were suitable for the final analysis as they evaluated periodontal and clinical variables originating from bacterial adhesion in patients with C and SL brackets (Fig 1).

Assessment of the scientific relevance of the eligible studies

The six articles[33,46,48,52,54,55] included in this review (Table 3) met the inclusion criteria, although with differences among their methods of study, sampling, analysis and follow-up. All the eligible studies[33,46,48,52,54,55] compared both systems: conventional and self-ligating edgewise brackets. Pandis[46] also made reference to gingival plaque and calculus index, whereas the article by van Gastel[48] examined the amount of gingival fluid and anaerobic and aerobic colonies. Another study carried out by Pandis[54] collected saliva 2-3 months after orthodontic appliances had been bonded. *Mitis salivarius* culture medium (MS), specific for *Streptococcus mutans*, was used to count the colony forming units (CFU). Pithon[52] collected the plaque samples directly from SL and C brackets of different brands, and 3

Table 2 - Search data, search strategies and number of results for each database.

Database	Search strategies	Results	Selected papers
Cochrane C.R.C. Trials	conventional OR self-ligating	160	2
Ovid ALL EMB Reviews	exp Orthodontic Appliances / OR edgewise.mp. AND exp Orthodontic Appliance Design/ OR exp Orthodontic Brackets/ OR self-ligating.mp. OR exp Orthodontic Appliances/ AND biofilm.mp. OR exp Dental Biofilm Index/ AND streptococcus mutans.mp. OR exp Streptococcus mutans/	53	4
PubMed (NLM)	conventional AND self-ligating, OR biofilm OR Streptococcus mutans	788	5
Bireme	conventional OR self-ligating	400	1
TOTAL		1,401	12

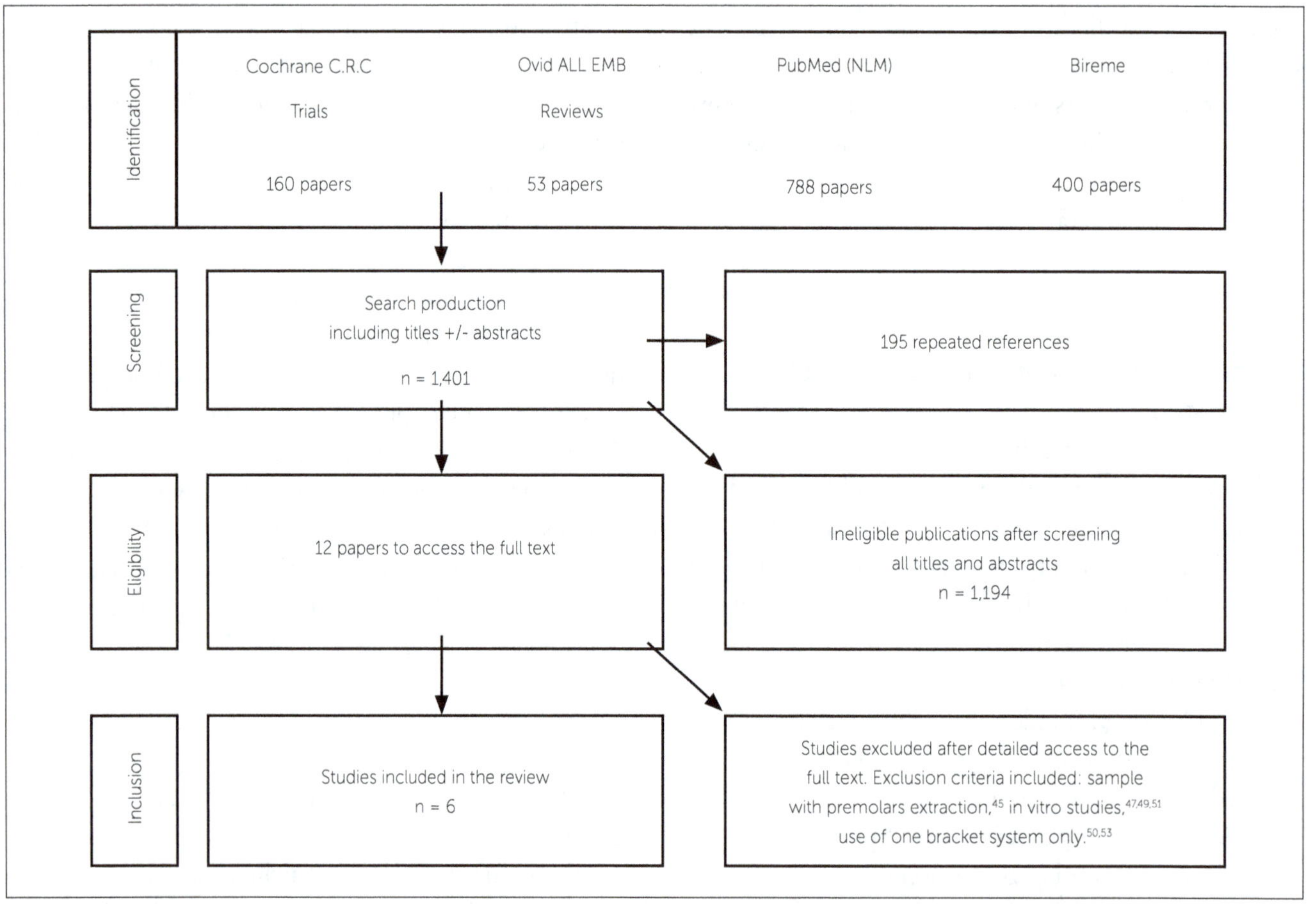

Figure 1 - Review flowchart.

weeks after bonding, the CFU was carried out in the following culture medium: MS, specific for *S. mutans,* and BHI (Brain Heart Infusion), not specific for bacteria and fungi. In this study,[52] CFU was visually performed after 24, 48 and 72 hours of incubation. Pejda et al[54] collected the plaque samples of subgingival sulcus after 18 weeks of treatment, counting 5 periodontal pathogens by PCR, while Pellegrini et al[33] collected the samples from tooth surfaces surrounding the brackets after 5 weeks of bonding, and the CFU was analyzed by MS and bioluminescence of ATP (adenosine triphosphate).

When evaluating the scientific relevance of the six eligible articles,[33,46,48,52,54,55] we found that the description of the sample selection was appropriate, however, the number of drop outs was declared in studies by Pellegrini,[33] Pandis,[46] van Gastel[48] and Pejda[54]. All studies[33,48,52,54] provided the approval of the Institutional Review Board, except for the articles by Pandis,[46,55] who asked for the consent of patients / parents before starting the study, only. Considering the confounding factors, similar oral routine and hygiene instructions were given to the subjects taking part in these six studies.[33,46,48,52,54,55]

Table 3 - Summarized data of the six studies included in the review.

Author Year Journal	Pellegrini et al[33] 2009 AJODO	Pandis et al[46] 2008 Orthod Craniofac Res	van Gastel et al[48] 2007 Journal of Clinical Periodontology	Pithon et al[52] 2011 Braz J Oral Sci.	Pejda et al[54] 2012 Angle Orthod	Pandis et al[55] 2010 Eur J Orthod
Type of study	Randomized controlled trial	Prospective cohort	Randomized controlled trial	Randomized controlled trial	Randomized controlled trial	Randomized controlled trial
Number of patients	18	100	16	5	38	32
Age	11-17 y	12-17 y	17-27 y	20-30 y	11-18 y	11-17 y
Teeth involved	Lateral incisors	Maxilla and mandible	1st and 2nd premolars	Canines; 1st and 2nd premolars and molars (lower)	Maxilla and mandible	Maxilla and mandible
Bracket type/brand	14 p: C – Mini Ovation 14 p: SL – Innovation – R GAC	50 p: C – GAC 50 p: SL – In-Ovation – R – GAC	16 C – GAC 16 SL – Speed	10 C – Morelli 40 SL: GAC; Aditek; Ormco; 3M Unitek	19 p: C – Sprint Forestadent 19 p: SL – Damon 3MX, Ormco	16 p: C – GAC 16 p: SL – In-Ovation R – GAC
Ligature type	Elastomeric ligatures for the C brackets	Elastomeric ligatures for the C brackets	Elastomeric ligatures for the C brackets	Elastomeric ligatures for the C brackets	Metal ligatures for the C brackets	Elastomeric ligatures for the C brackets
Objective of analysis	Accumulation of bacterial plaque around the brackets. To determine if ATP by bioluminescence may be useful in assessing the plaque index	Index of gingival plaque and calculus of the pocket depth	Crevicular fluid and pocket depth. Aerobic (An) colonies	*S. mutans* and other microorganisms attachment to C and SL.	Accumulation of different microorganisms on C and SL.	Effect of the type of bracket (C or SL) on the levels of *S. mutans* in saliva
Method of analysis	MSB specific for *S. mutans* and determination by bioluminescence	Clinical periodontal parameters	Clinical and microbiological periodontal parameters	MSB specific for *S. mutans* and BHI, not specific for bacteria and fungus	Clinical periodontal parameters and PCR	MSB specific for *S. mutans*
Follow-up	5 w	18 m	7 d	21 d	18 w	2-3 m
Statistical analysis	T-tests (1-tailed, with $P < 0.05$). Chi-squared χ^2	χ^2 Wilcoxon Stata	ANOVA Tukey-Kramer	SPSS 13.0 Wilcoxon ($P < 0.05$)	T-tests Sidak post hoc Fisher's tests	ANOVA Minitab 14.20 χ^2
Outcome	SL favor reduced accumulation of *S. Mutans* and ATP by bioluminescence is useful in assessing plaque index	No advantages of SL over C with respect to the periodontal status of the mandibular anterior teeth	Bracket design can have a significant impact on bacterial load and on periodontal parameters	The hypothesis that self-ligating brackets favor greater aggregation of microorganisms was proved	Bracket design does not seem to have a strong influence on clinical parameters and periodontal pathogens in subgingival plaque.	The total levels of *S. mutans* do not seem to be significantly different between C and SL brackets

p = patients; y = years; m = months; w = weeks; d = days; h = hours; C = conventional brackets; SL = self-ligating brackets; S. = *Streptococcus*; SEM = scanning electron microscopy; ATP = adenosine triphosphate; MSB = Mitis Salivarius agar; BHI = brain heart infusion; PCR = polymerase chain reaction.

In the papers,[46,54] full alignment of the mandibular arch was necessary to eliminate crowding as a confounding factor, but the clinical variables were assessed by the same periodontist. The examiner in the study carried out by Pandis[46] was not blinded, which could have influenced the outcome of the research, making the results biased. The study conducted by Pithon[52] did not describe whether it had a blinded examiner, however, as a confounding factor, randomized participants were asked whether they had already received any kind of orthodontic treatment with fixed appliances, since this can have consequences for the smoothness of the tooth enamel and for microbial adhesion at the beginning of biofilm formation.[5,20,21] All six studies[33,46,48,52,54,55] used appropriate statistical methods. The examiner's calibration level was reported in one single study,[54] and only two papers[54,55] identified the sample calculation. Smoking or medical conditions were clearly identified in studies by van Gastel,[48] Pejda[54] and Pandis.[55] As for the other studies,[33,46,52] these conditions were declared only after the authors were requested to do so. The final score of the scientific relevance, in accordance with the Jadad scale,[44] was 10.0 for Pellegrini[33] and Pejda[54], 9.5 for van Gastel[48] and Pandis[55], and 9.0 for Pandis[46] and Pithon[52] (Table 4), which revealed high-quality researches and methodological soundness.

Assessment of the eligible studies outcomes

Among the selected studies, four[46,48,54,55] had their outcomes consistent in reporting that (a) SL brackets have no advantages over C in periodontal condition of anterior mandibular teeth;[46] (b) the design of the brackets can have significant impact on bacterial load and periodontal parameters;[48] and (c) in subgingival plaque and saliva, there seems to be no significant differences in the total levels of *S. Mutans* and periodontal pathogens between C and SL.[54,55] However, a study[52] confirmed the hypothesis that SL brackets favor the accumulation of micro-organisms, while another study[33] reported that SL brackets promote lower retention of *S. mutans* when compared to C (Table 3). The outcomes of the eligible studies[33,46,48,52,54,55] were not unanimous in reporting that there is evidence of a possible influence of bracket design (conventional or self-ligating) over adhesion and formation of *Streptococcus mutans* colonies.

DISCUSSION

A systematic review can confirm the quality of a research as well as the methodological soundness of works selected from the literature. Additionally, it can present them for consideration of the clinical and scientific communities. Evidence-based practice requires the construction of a research question and a literature review.

Conventionally, to attach the wire to the brackets, three methods are used: metal ligature, elastomeric ligatures, and the open-close devices of SL brackets. All these methods have advantages and disadvantages, but with regard to the accumulation of biofilm, the literature[8,33] suggests that elastomeric ligatures favor the retention of biofilm in comparison with the other two methods of ligatures. The question prepared for this review aimed to verify whether bracket design (conventional or self-ligating) influences the formation of *Streptococcus mutans* colonies. Micro-organisms exhibit significant adherence to brackets because there are favorable ecological niches in the porous (rough and irregular surfaces of these brackets).[39,47,49,51,56] Thus, the characteristics of the bracket surface can be considered as harboring favorable sites for the adhesion of biofilm.

Search strategy outcomes

This research was highly sensitive, addressing evidence of minimum bias. The study carried out by

Table 4 - Quality assessment of the six retrieved studies.

	Pellegrini et al[33] 2009 AJODO	Pandis et al[46] 2008 Orthod Craniofac Res	van Gastel et al[48] 2007 Journal of Clinical Periodontology	Pithon et al[52] 2011 Braz J Oral Sci.	Pejda et al[54] 2012 Angle Orthod	Pandis et al[55] 2010 Eur J Orthod
Type of study	2.0	2.0	2.0	2.0	2.0	2.0
Study description	1.0	1.0	1.0	1.0	1.0	1.0
Sample size	1.0	1.0	1.0	0.5	1.0	1.0
Sample selection description	1.0	1.0	1.0	1.0	1.0	1.0
Drop out description	1.0	0.5	0.5	1.0	1.0	0.5
Measurement method	0.5	0.5	0.5	0.5	0.5	0.5
Blind study	0.5	---	0.5	---	0.5	0.5
Statistics	1.0	1.0	1.0	1.0	1.0	1.0
Confounding factors	1.0	1.0	1.0	1.0	1.0	1.0
Clinical significance	1.0	1.0	1.0	1.0	1.0	1.0
Scale score (Jadad[44])	10.0	9.0	9.5	9.0	10.0	9.5
Quality standard assessed	high	high	high	high	high	high

Jordan and LeBlanc[50] was excluded due to: (a) having assessed one bracket system only, (b) having a not blinded examiner and (c) presenting unspecified statistical analyses. The *in vitro* studies that were excluded[47,49,51] did not have the inherent characteristics which contribute to the development of intraoral biofilm, and may provide bias results for clinical periodontal conditions.[22] The differences observed between the results of some papers[33,46,48-50,52] may be related to factors that include: variations in the shape, material and size between SL and C brackets, the individual level of oral hygiene, salivary flow, treatment variables, types of ligatures, bonding procedures and age of the individuals involved.[24,45,49,51,55] Thus, bracket type itself would not be a deciding factor for biofilm development, but its composition and material type should be included as factors behind *Streptococcus mutans* colonies formation.[56]

Assessment of the scientific relevance of the eligible studies

The statistical analysis of our results was not feasible, given that the methodological designs of the eligible articles were heterogeneous. However, the scientific relevance assessment revealed high-quality researches and methodological soundness of all six studies,[33,46,48,52,54,55] as shown in their final scores, according to the Jadad scale.[44]

Although SL brackets do not require ligatures, their opening and closing mechanism may provide sites for biofilm adhesion similarly to conventional brackets.[46] This mechanism of SL brackets is not renewed, as it occurs with elastomeric modules in conventional brackets. Moreover, plaque calcification in SL leads to a malfunction of the opening and closing mechanisms. Thus, the theoretical advantages of self-ligating over conventional brackets can be eliminated, as confirmed by other studies.[46,52] When using conventional brackets, neither the elastomeric rings nor the metal ligatures seem to affect the distribution of bacterial morphotypes in brackets or on the enamel surface.[3] Aged elastomeric surfaces can apparently favor plaque retention in comparison with polished stainless steel ligatures, but there are no differences between periodontal conditions of patients treated with these two types of ligatures.[8,57] Nevertheless, some studies[41,58] report that brackets with elastomeric rings favor damage to gingival conditions, with significant accumulation of biofilm, while the metal ligature had lower retention of biofilm in comparison with other brackets. Some reports[59,60] affirm that C brackets are directly related to the retention of biofilm, however, the study conducted by Pithon et al[52] suggests that cross-infection caused by replacement of elastomeric rings is controllable with the use of C brackets, because this type of brackets favors lower formation of *S. Mutans* colonies, which agrees with the study by van Gastel et al[48] that showed no difference between C and SL in gingival bleeding.

Assessment of the retrieved studies outcomes

The increase in oral microbiota attachment of *Streptococcus mutans* and *Lactobacillus* is associated with the use of orthodontic appliances,[6,8,9,33,45] with both C or SL brackets. This increase leads to higher cariogenic plaque, pH low enough to change the clinical periodontal parameters[46,48,54] and increased risk of enamel demineralization.[6,47]

Some eligible studies[52,54] evaluated not only the presence of *S. mutans*, but also of other microorganisms related to periodontal disease in patients with C or SL brackets. The study conducted by Pejda et al[54] found 23.8 times more chance of finding *Aggregatibacter actinomycetemcomitans* (AA) in subgingival plaque of patients with C brackets, but the increase in AA does not represent a risk factor for local periodontitis, as studies by Paolantonio et al[61,62] confirm. The differences found between the results of the study by Pithon et al[52] and the other studies assessed[33,46,48,54,55] may have been due to methodological differences in some of these studies[46,48,54,55] in which the CFU were counted from material collected from saliva; Pellegrini et al[33] collected it from tooth surfaces surrounding the bracket; and, in the study by Pithon,[52] it was directly collected from the surface of brackets (winglets, slot and cervical region). That was the reason why this latest study should have found statistically significant differences that reveal greater accumulation of biofilm in SL brackets.

Clinical implications

Some studies[8,33-39] report that SL brackets are less susceptible to bacterial colonization due to their shape and lack of metal or elastomeric ligatures. However, adequate control of biofilm is more strongly influenced by the correct orientation and cooperation of patients[24,55] than by simply choosing one system of brackets instead of another. The outcomes of the eligible studies[33,46,48,52,54,55] were not unanimous in reporting a possible influence of bracket design (conventional or self-ligating) over the adhesion and formation of *Streptococcus mutans* colonies.

The decision of orthodontists on prescribing the use of SL instead of C in their clinical routine, aiming at improving hygiene / plaque accumulation, cannot yet be applied due to lack of scientific evidence.[46,48,52,54,55] After this review, we presume that there is not enough evidence to support the use of fixed appliances with SL brackets in place of systems with C or vice versa, which agrees with the study by Fleming et al.[63]

Based on the limitations of some works,[64,66] further studies on other types of brackets, for example, esthetic self-ligating ones, must be performed to visualize the periodontal complications arising from different shapes, sizes and material types of brackets, and with that, guide the development of new systems of brackets design in order to reduce the formation of *Streptococcus mutans* colonies.

CONCLUSIONS

Within the limitations of this study, it was concluded that there is no evidence for a possible influence of bracket design (conventional or self-ligating) over colony formation and adhesion of *Streptococcus mutans*.

REFERENCES

1. O'Reilly MM, Featherstone JDB. Demineralization and remineralization around orthodontic appliances: an in vivo study. Am J Orthod Dentofacial Orthop. 1987;92(1):33-40.
2. Øgaard B, Rølla G, Arends J. Orthodontic appliances and enamel demineralization. Part 1. Lesion development. Am J Orthod Dentofacial Orthop. 1988;94(1):68-73.
3. Gwinnett JA, Ceen F. Plaque distribution on bonded brackets. Am J Orthod. 1979;75(6):667-77.
4. Mizrahi E. Surface distribution of enamel opacities following orthodontic treatment. Am J Orthod Dentofacial Orthop. 1983;84(4):323-31.
5. Alexander SA. Effects of orthodontic attachments on the gingival health of permanent second molars. Am J Orthod Dentofacial Orthop. 1991;100(4):337-40.
6. Balenseifen JW, Madonia JV. Study of dental plaque in orthodontic patients. J Dent Res. 1970;49(2):320-4.
7. Menzaghi N, Saletta M, Garattini G, Brambilla E, Strohmenger L. Changes in the yeast oral flora in patients in orthodontic treatment. Prev Assist Dent. 1991;17(4):26-30.
8. Forsberg CM, Brattström V, Malmberg E, Nord CE. Ligature wires and elastomeric rings: two methods of ligation, and their association with microbial colonization of Streptococcus mutans and lactobacilli. Eur J Orthod. 1991;13(5):416-20.
9. Rosenbloom RG, Tinanoff N. Salivary Streptococcus mutans levels in patients before, during, and after orthodontic treatment. Am J Orthod Dentofacial Orthop. 1991;100(1):35-7.
10. Saemundsson SR, Bergmann H, Magnusdottir MO, Holbrook WP. Dental caries and Streptococcus mutans in a rural child population in Iceland. Scand J Dent Res. 1992;100(5):299-303.
11. Sansone C, Van Houte J, Joshipura K, Kent R, Margolis HC. The association of mutans streptococci and non-mutans streptococci capable of acidogenesis at a low pH with dental caries on enamel and root surfaces. J Dent Res. 1993;72(2):508-16.
12. Mattousch TJ, van der Veen MH, Zentner A. Caries lesions after orthodontic treatment followed by quantitative light-induced fluorescence: a 2-year follow-up. Eur J Orthod. 2007;29(3):294-8.
13. Mizrahi E. Enamel demineralization following orthodontic treatment. Am J Orthod. 1982;82(1):62-7.
14. Benson PE, Parkin N, Millett DT, Dyer FE, Vine S, Shah A. Fluorides for the prevention of white spots on teeth during fixed brace treatment. Cochrane Database Syst Rev 2004;(3):CD003809.
15. Gorelick L, Geiger AM, Gwinnett AJ. Incidence of white spot formation after bonding and banding. Am J Orthod. 1982;81(2):93-8.
16. Øgaard B. Prevalence of white spot lesions in 19-year-olds: a study on untreated and orthodontically treated persons 5 years after treatment. Am J Orthod Dentofacial Orthop. 1989;96(5):423-7.
17. Anhoury P, Nathanson D, Hughes CV, Socransky S, Feres M, Chou LL. Microbial profile on metallic and ceramic bracket materials. Angle Orthod. 2002;72(4):338-43.
18. Loe H, Theilade E, Jensen SB. Experimental Gingivitis in Man. J Periodontol. 1965;36:177-87.
19. Zachrisson S, Zachrisson BU. Gingival condition associated with orthodontic treatment. Angle Orthod. 1972;42(1):26-34.
20. Shelley WB. Gingival hyperplasia from dental braces. Cutis. 1981;28:149-50.
21. Theilade E, Wright WH, Jensen SB, Loe H. Experimental gingivitis in man. II. A longitudinal clinical and bacteriological investigation. J Periodontal Res. 1966;1:1-13.
22. van Pelt AW, Weerkamp AH, Uyen MH, Busscher HJ, de Jong HP, Arends J. Adhesion of Streptococcus sanguis CH3 to polymers with different surface free energies. Appl Environ Microbiol. 1985;49(5):1270-5.
23. Socransky SS, Haffajee AD, Smith C, Dibart S. Relation of counts of microbial species to clinical status at the sampled site. J Clin Periodontol. 1991;18(10):766-75.
24. Quirynen M, Dekeyser C, van Steenberghe D. The influence of gingival inflammation, tooth type, and timing on the rate of plaque formation. J Periodontol. 1991;62(3):219-22.
25. Quirynen M, Dekeyser C, van Steenberghe D. Discriminating power of five plaque indices. J Periodontol. 1991;62(2):100-5.
26. Ramberg P, Axelsson P, Lindhe J. Plaque formation at healthy and inflamed gingival sites in young individuals. J Clin Periodontol. 1995;22(1):85-8.
27. Rowshani B, Timmerman MF, Van der Velden U. Plaque development in relation to the periodontal condition and bacterial load of the saliva. J Clin Periodontol. 2004;31(3):214-8.
28. Quirynen M, Marechal M, Busscher H, el-Abiad M, Arends J, Van Steenberghe D. The influence of surface characteristics on the early bacterial colonization of intra-oral hard surfaces. J Clin Dent. 1988;1 Suppl A:A14-9.
29. Bollen CM, Quirynen M. [Specimen collection in dental plaque and oral microbiology]. Rev Belge Med Dent. 1994;49(2):44-51.
30. Satou J, Fukunaga A, Satou N, Shintani H, Okuda K. Streptococcal adherence on various restorative materials. J Oral Rehabil. 2004;31(3):278-85.
31. Berger J. The engaging concept of self-ligation. Ont Dent. 1999;76(3):26-33.
32. Cacciafesta V, Sfondrini MF, Ricciardi A, Scribante A, Klersy C, Auricchio F. Evaluation of friction of stainless steel and esthetic self-ligating bráquetes in various bracket-archwire combinations. Am J Orthod Dentofacial Orthop. 2003;124(4):395-402.

33. Pellegrini P, Sauerwein R, Finlayson T, McLeod J, Covell DA Jr, Maier T, et al. Plaque retention by self-ligation vs elastomeric orthodontic brackets: quantitative comparison or oral bacteria detection with adenosine triphosphate-driven bioluminescence. Am J Orthod Dentofacial Orthop. 2009;135(4):426.e1-9.
34. Damon DH. The rationale, evolution and clinical application of the self-ligating bracket. Clin Orthod Res. 1998;1(1):52-61.
35. Shivapuja PK, Berger J. A comparative study of conventional ligation and self-ligation bracket systems. Am J Orthod Dentofacial Orthop. 1994;106(5):472-80.
36. Paduano S, Cioffi I, Iodice G, Rapuano A, Silva R. Time efficiency of self-ligating vs conventional brackets in orthodontics: effect of appliances and ligating systems. Prog Orthod. 2008;9(2):74-80.
37. Yu YL, Qian YF. The clinical implication of self-ligating brackets. Shanghai Kou Qiang Yi Xue. 2007;16(4):431-5.
38. Fernandes C, Almeida R. self-ligating appliances: evolution or revolution? Aust Orthod. 2008;24(1):97-103.
39. Türkkahraman H, Sayin MO, Bozkurt FY, Yetkin Z, Kaya S, Onal S. Archwire ligation techniques, microbial colonization, and periodontal status in orthodontically treated patients. Angle Orthod. 2005;75(2):231-6.
40. Polson AM, Subtelny JD, Meitner SW, Polson AP, Sommers EW, Iker HP. Long-term periodontal status after orthodontic treatment. Am J Orthod Dentofacial Orthop. 1988;93(1):51-8.
41. Garcez, AS, Suzuki SS, Ribeiro MS, Mada EY, Freitas AZ, Suzuki H. Biofilm retention by 3 methods of ligation on orthodontic brackets: a microbiologic and optical coherence tomography analysis. Am J Orthod Dentofacial Orthop. 2011;140(4):e93-8.
42. National Health Service (NHS) Centre for reviews and dissemination. Undertaking systematic reviews of research on effectiveness [report]. York (UK): York Publishing Services; 2001. Available from: www.york.ac.uk/inst/crd/crdrep.htm.
43. European Food Safety Authority. Application of systematic review methodology to food and feed safety assessments to support decision making. EFSA J. 2010;8(6):1637. Available from: http://www.efsa.europa.eu
44. Jadad AR, Moore RA, Carrol D, Reynolds DJ, Gavaghan DJ, McQuay HJ. Assessing the quality of reports of randomized clinical trials: is blinding necessary? Controlled Clin Trials 1996;17(1):1-12.
45. Sukontapatipark W, el-Agroudi MA, Selliseth NJ, Thunold K, Selvig KA. Bacterial colonization associated with fixed orthodontic appliances. A scanning electron microscopy study. Eur J Orthod. 2001;23(5):475-84.
46. Pandis N, Vlachopoulos K, Polychronopoulou A, Madianos P, Eliades T. Periodontal condition of the mandibular anterior dentition in patients with conventional and self-ligating brackets. Orthod Craniofac Res. 2008;11(4):211-5.
47. Faltermeier A, Burgers R, Rosentritt M. Bacterial adhesion of Streptococcus mutans to esthetic bracket materials. Am J Orthod Dentofacial Orthop. 2008;133(4 Suppl):S99-103.
48. van Gastel J, Quirynen M, Teughels W, Coucke W, Carels C. Influence of bracket design on microbial and periodontal parameters in vivo. J Clin Periodontol 2007;34(5):423-31.
49. Brusca MI, Chara O, Sterin-Borda L, Rosa AC. Influence of different orthodontic brackets on Adherence of microorganisms in vitro. Angle Orthod. 2007;77(2):331-6.
50. Jordan C, LeBlanc DJ. Influences of orthodontic appliances on oral populations of mutans streptococci. Oral Microbiol Immunol. 2002;17(2):65-71.
51. Fournier A, Payant L, Bouclin R. Adherence of Streptococcus mutans to orthodontic bráquetes. Am J Orthod Dentofacial Orthop. 1998;114(4):414-7.
52. Pithon MM, Santos RL, Nascimento LE, Ayres AO, Alviano D, Bolognese AM. Do self-ligating brackets favor greater bacterial aggregation? Braz J Oral Sci. 2011;10(3):208-12.
53. Ristic M, Vlahovic Svabic M, Sasic M, Zelic O. Clinical and microbiological effects of fixed orthodontic appliances on periodontal tissues in adolescents. Orthod Craniofac Res. 2007;10(4):187-95.
54. Pejda S, Varga ML, Milosevic SA, Mestrovic S, Slaj M, Repic d, Bosnjak A. Clinical and microbiological parameters in patients with self-ligating and conventional brackets during early phase of orthodontic treatment. Angle Orthod. 2013;83(1):133-9.
55. Pandis N, Papaioannou W, Kontou E, Nakou M, Makou M, Eliades T. Salivary Streptococcus mutans levels in patients with conventional and self-ligating brackets. Eur J Orthod. 2010;32(1):94-9.
56. Carneiro RC. Estudo da microbiota do biofilme supragengival de pacientes em tratamento ortodôntico com diferentes tipos de braquetes [tese]. Belo Horizonte (MG): Pontifícia Universidade Católica; 2008.
57. Gameiro GH, Nouer DF, Cenci MS, Cury JA. Enamel demineralization with two forms of archwire ligation investigated using an in situ caries model: a pilot study. Eur J Orthod. 2009;31(5):542-6.
58. Souza RA, Borges de Araújo Magnani MB, Nouer DF, Oliveira da Silva C, Klein MI, Sallum EA, et al. Periodontal and microbiologic evaluation of 2 methods of archwire ligation: Ligature wires and elastomeric rings. Am J Orthod Dentofacial Orthop. 2008;134(4):506-12.
59. Eliades T, Eliades G, Brantley WA. Microbial attachment on orthodontic appliances: I. Wettability and early pellicle formation on bracket materials. Am J Orthod Dentofacial Orthop. 1995;108(4):351-60.
60. Batoni G, Pardini M, Ota F, Guica MR, Gabriele M, Campa M, Senesi S. Effect of removable orthodontic appliances on oral colonization by mutans streptococci in children. Eur J Oral Sci. 2001;109(6):388-92.
61. Paolantonio M, Festa F, di Placido G, D'Attilio M, Catamo G, Piccolomini R. Site-specific subgingival colonization by Actinobacillus actinomycetemcomitans in orthodontic patients. Am J Orthod Dentofacial Orthop. 1999;115(4):423-8.
62. Paolantonio M, Pedrazzoli V, di Murro C, di Placido G, Picciani C, Catamo G, et al. Clinical significance of Actinobacillus actinomycetemcomitans in young individuals during orthodontic treatment. A 3-year longitudinal study. J Clin Periodontol. 1997;24(9 Pt 1):610-7
63. Fleming PS, Johal A. Self-ligating brackets in orthodontics. Angle Orthod. 2010;80:575-584.
64. Maza JL, Elguezabal N, Prado C, Ellacuria J, Soler I, Ponton J. Candida albicans adherence to resin–composite restorative dental material: influence of whole human saliva. Oral Surg Oral Med Oral Pathol Oral Radiol Endod. 2002;94(5):589-92.
65. Addy M, Shaw WC, Hansford P, Hopkins M. The effect of orthodontic appliances on the distribution of Candida and plaque in adolescents. Br J Orthod. 1982;9(3):158-63.
66. Park JH, Gakunga PT, Aemechi BT. Influence of self-ligating orthodontic brackets on plaque accumulation in vitro. J Dent Res. 2007;86(Spec Issue A), abstract 1937.

13

Does self-ligating brackets type influence the hysteresis, activation and deactivation forces of superelastic NiTi archwires?

José Rino Neto[1], Gilberto Vilanova Queiroz[2], João Batista de Paiva[3], Rafael Yagüe Ballester[4]

Objective: To compare hysteresis, activation and deactivation forces produced by first-order deformation of Contour 0.014-in NiTi wire (Aditek, Brazil) in four brands of self-ligating brackets: Damon MX, Easy Clip, Smart Clip and In-Ovation. **Methods:** Activation and deactivation forces were measured in an Instron universal tensile machine at 3 mm/minute speed to a total displacement of 4 mm. Tests were repeated eight times for each bracket/wire combination. Statistical analysis comprised ANOVA and Tukey's multiple comparisons test. **Results:** Using a 4-mm deformation, mean activation forces increased in the following order: Damon = 222 gf, Easy Clip = 228 gf, In-Ovation = 240 gf and Smart Clip = 306 gf. The same order was observed for mean hysteresis values, i.e., 128 gf, 140 gf, 150 gf and 206 gf, respectively. The respective values of deactivation forces for the Damon, Easy Clip, In-Ovation and Smart Clip brackets were 94 gf, 88 gf, 90 gf and 100 gf. **Conclusions:** Brackets with higher activation forces were accompanied by higher hysteresis values, which resulted in clinically similar deactivation forces, regardless of the type of self-ligating brackets used.

Keywords: Corrective orthodontics. Orthodontic brackets. Orthodontic wires.

[1] Associate Professor, Department of Orthodontics, School of Dentistry, University of São Paulo (FOUSP).
[2] MSc and PhD in Orthodontics, FOUSP.
[3] Full Professor, Department of Orthodontics, FOUSP.
[4] Full Professor, Department of Dental Materials, FOUSP.

» The author reports no commercial, proprietary or financial interest in the products or companies described in this article.

Gilberto Vilanova Queiroz
Via Piacenza, 144 – Jd. Paradiso – CEP: 13.331-545 – Indaiatuba/SP – Brazil
E-mail: gilbertovilanova@terra.com.br

INTRODUCTION

Activation force is defined as the force required to deform an archwire when it is inserted into a misaligned bracket slot,[8] whereas deactivation force is the force applied by the archwire on a misaligned bracket when it is reverting to its original shape. Friction in the contact region between wire and bracket is one of the factors affecting the magnitude of both activation and deactivation forces. The higher the friction, the greater the force required by an archwire to slide in the slots of brackets placed on anchorage teeth.[9,11]

Friction in orthodontic sliding mechanics can be divided into two key components: Classic friction and binding. Classic friction is caused by the elastomeric ligatures compressing the archwire against the bottom of the bracket slot,[9] which is controlled using self-ligating brackets, i.e., brackets that do not require the use of elastomeric ligatures given their own unique ligation devices.[1,2,3,5]

Binding, in turn, is a type of friction caused by archwire deformation (strain), with intensity depending on the force with which the archwire is pressed against the slots of the anchorage brackets.[9,11] The magnitude of binding produced by first order deformation in Contour NiTi 0.014-in wire (Aditek) varies according to the type of self-ligating brackets used.[14] Given that wire activation and deactivation forces are influenced by friction occurring between orthodontic wire and bracket[9,11] it is important to evaluate if different self-ligating brackets affect the forces produced by wire deformation in superelastic NiTi wires.

The aim of this study was to compare the forces of activation, deactivation and hysteresis produced by the deformation of Contour 0.014-in NiTi wire in four different self-ligating brackets, i.e., Damon, Easy Clip, Smart Clip and In-Ovation.

MATERIAL AND METHODS

A device attached to the Instron universal tensile machine comprising five 0.022 x 0.028-in brackets (central incisor, lateral incisor, canine, first and second premolars in the upper left quadrant) was used to compare the activation and deactivation forces produced by four types of self-ligating brackets: Damon MX (Ormco), Easy Clip (Aditek), In-Ovation (GAC) and Smart Clip (3M/Unitek).

The testing device consisted of four cylinders that could be moved vertically and two guiding slots with internal dimensions of 0.022 x 0.028-in positioned at the ends of the bracket area (Fig 1). In order to achieve parallelism and leveling between the bracket slots bonding was performed by simultaneously inserting a standard 0.022-in ruler into both the guiding slots and the bracket slots. Direct bonding of the brackets was performed individually and followed this sequence: Insertion of standard 0.022-in ruler into the guiding slots, application of cyanoacrylate (Superbonder, Henckel / Brazil) to the bracket base and positioning at the center of the cylinder, sliding of the cylinder until the bottom of the slot fit the 0.022-in standard ruler in its entire mesiodistal extension, determining the final bonding position (Fig 2). Direct bonding of the brackets with cyanoacrylate showed sufficient strength to stabilize the brackets during the mechanical tests, even in specimens without full contact between bonding surface and bracket base (Fig 2). The distance from bracket center to bracket center was 7.5 mm.

To obtain the forces produced by the 0.014-in SE NiTi archwire in the different types of self-ligating brackets a support was developed whose upper portion was inserted into the Instron tensile machine and bottom portion displayed a surface where the canine would be bonded.

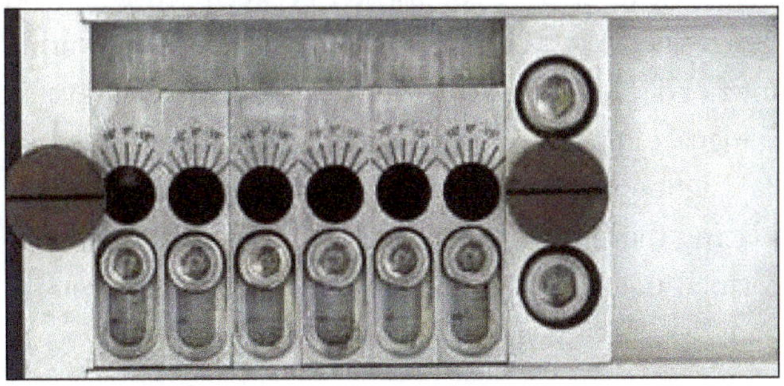

Figure 1 - Testing device.

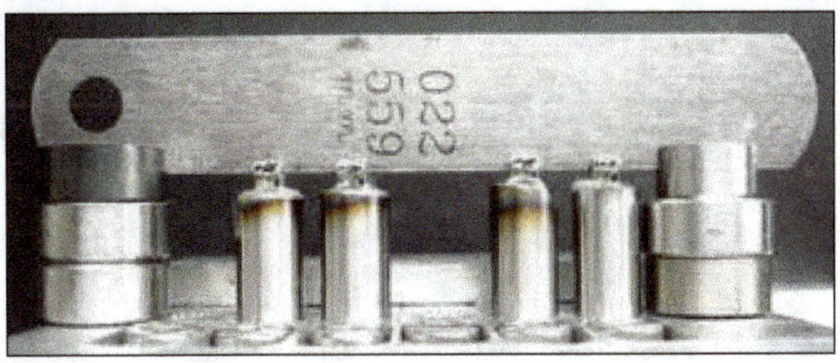

Figure 2 - Bracket positioning corresponding to incisors and premolars in a passive configuration.

The canine bracket was bonded with light-curing resin in the following order (Fig 3):

» Insertion of 0.021 x 0.025-in rectangular stainless-steel wire into the bracket slot and stabilization with conventional elastomeric ligatures.
» Insertion of the same rectangular wire into the previously bonded brackets with the canine bracket at an equidistant position to the adjacent brackets (Fig 3A).
» Application of composite resin to the support attached to the Instron machine (Fig 3B).
» The support was raised until it touched the bracket, proceeding with curing of composite resin (Fig 3C).

This procedure sequence ensured parallelism between the slot of the canine bracket, attached directly to the Instron machine, and the slots of the four brackets bonded to the cylinders.

A straight segment of Contour NiTi wire (Aditek) with round 0.014-in cross-section and 12 cm length was employed in all mechanical tests. The superelastic Contour NiTi wire, classified as active austenitic, was stabilized inside the slots by means of the lids or clips (ligation device) of the self-ligating brackets.

A model 5565 Instron universal mechanical testing machine was used with a load cell of 500 Newtons and crosshead speed of 0.05 mm/second. The forces were recorded every 0.1 mm during activation cycles until reaching the maximum displacement of 4.5 mm, and during deactivation back to zero. A comparison between activation and deactivation forces performed at 4 mm deformation during inferior displacement of the canine bracket, which simulated a lingual canine placement and a first order deformation.

Eight tests were performed for each bracket type replacing the archwires for each test. The tests were performed in a dry medium at a temperature between 24 and 26 Celsius degrees.

Statistical analysis

The values for means, standard deviations and amplitudes were calculated and normality tests applied for each orthodontic wire-bracket combination. The differences between the four self-ligating brackets were tested by comparing the mean values with ANOVA, and Tukey's multiple comparisons test was applied to verify between which bracket brands the differences occurred.

The analyses were performed with SAS (Statistical Analysis System) 8.0 software. All results for p values lower than 0.05 were considered statistically significant.

RESULTS

Figure 4 shows the average load-deflection curves for the four self-ligating brackets assessed. The Contour 0.014-in NiTi archwire exhibited activation and deactivation plateaus in all tests, confirming its superelastic properties.

Descriptive analysis of the activation, deactivation and hysteresis forces for the 0.014-in NiTi wire are displayed in Table 1. The lowest mean activation force was 228 gf, obtained using Damon brackets, while the highest was 312 gf, using Smart Clip brackets. Deactivation forces showed mean values between 88 and 100 gf while hysteresis exhibited greater fluctuations, with values between 134 gf (Damon) and 212 gf (Smart Clip). The reduced data scatter found in the standard deviations and amplitudes indicates adequate repeatability of the method used for the mechanical tests.[8]

Total results of Tukey's multiple comparisons test are shown in Table 2. Overall, the groups showed statistically significant differences in hysteresis and activation forces while deactivation forces were similar, except between Easy Clip and Smart Clip brackets.

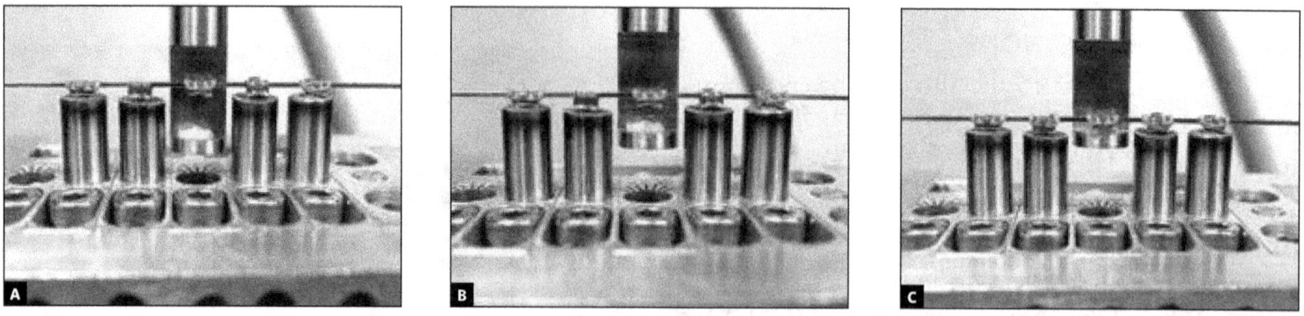

Figure 3 - A) Inferior displacement of the support and application of composite resin. **B)** Support rising. **C)** Placement of the canine bracket in a passive configuration.

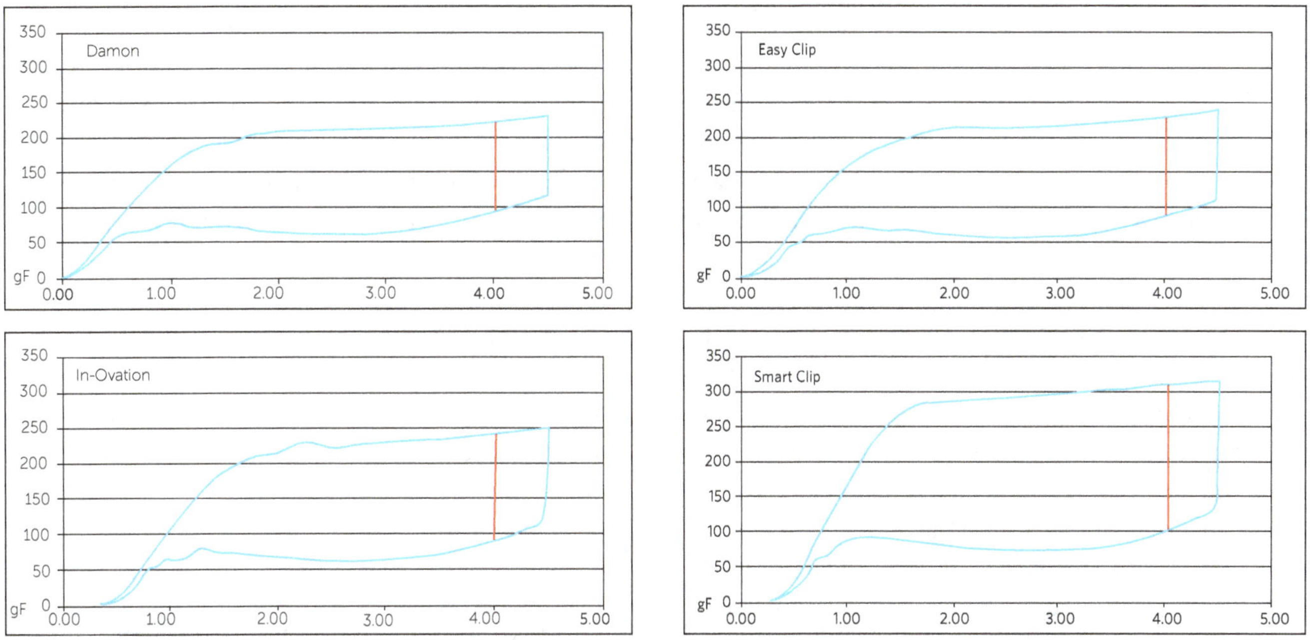

Figure 4 - Load/deflection curves for 0.014-in NiTi wire with Damon, Easy Clip, In-Ovation and Smart Clip brackets. The red line indicates hysteresis at a 4 mm deflection.

Table 1 - Mean, standard deviation (SD) and amplitude (A) in grams/force with 4 mm deflection.

	Activation		Deactivation		Hysteresis	
	Mean ± SD	A	Mean ± SD	A	Mean ± SD	A
Damon	228 ± 6	17	94 ± 4	13	134 ± 6	16
Easy Clip	235 ± 5	17	88 ± 2	6	147 ± 6	21
In-Ovation	247 ± 6	21	90 ± 2	7	157 ± 5	16
Smart Clip	312 ± 14	35	100 ± 4	13	212 ± 10	26

Table 2 - Results of Tukey's multiple comparisons test between self-ligating brackets ($p < 0.05$).

	Activation		Deactivation		Hysteresis	
	Mean	≠ Sig.	Mean	≠ Sig.	Mean	≠ Sig.
Damon (a)	228	c,d	94	--	134	b,c,d
Easy Clip (b)	235	d	88	d	147	a,d
In-Ovation (c)	247	a,d	90	--	156	a,d
Smart Clip (d)	312	a,b,c	100	b	211	a,b,c

DISCUSSION

Superelastic NiTi archwires exhibit plateaus of constant forces that allow orthodontists to select the ideal force according to the desired kind of movement.[10] To achieve this goal it is important to define whether the load-deflection curve of superelastic NiTi wire is constant or varies when different brands of self-ligating brackets are used.

Activation force is the force required to insert the archwire into the bracket slot. One of the factors influencing the magnitude of activation force is the friction force present in the wire-bracket interface. The higher the friction the greater the force required for the archwire to slide inside the slots of the brackets placed on the anchorage teeth, resulting in a higher activation force.[9,11] A previous study[14] found that a 4 mm horizontal deformation of the Contour 0.014-in NiTi wire produced significantly different friction forces between self-ligating brackets, with values increasing in the following order: Damon, Easy Clip, In-Ovation and Smart Clip. This outcome raised the hypothesis that the activation force might also vary depending on the use of different self-ligating brackets. The results of this study confirm this hypothesis. When subjected to 4 mm standardized horizontal deformations, the Contour 0.014-in NiTi archwire exhibited increasing activation forces in the same sequence found for friction forces between self-ligating brackets: Damon, Easy Clip, In-Ovation and Smart Clip.

Although increases in activation force may aggravate patient discomfort upon archwire insertion,[8] such fact bears limited importance since the actual forces delivered to the periodontium during orthodontic treatment are the deactivation forces.[13] Thus, within a strictly clinical perspective, comparisons between deactivation forces of self-ligating brackets are more relevant.

When comparing the deactivation forces produced by superelastic NiTi wires in different self-ligating brackets, Franchi et al[4] found no clinically relevant differences. This study found statistically significant differences between mean deactivation forces for the Easy Clip and Smart Clip brackets. However, since this difference only amounted to 12 gf, a value insufficient to produce clinically relevant differences, the deactivation forces found between Damon, Easy Clip, In-Ovation and Smart Clip brackets were considered similar. Therefore, from a clinical standpoint, the significant differences found for the activation forces between self-ligating brackets did not influence the magnitude of the deactivation forces.

Mechanical hysteresis — defined as the force difference between the archwires' activation and deactivation plateaus at identical deflection[6,7] — was significantly different between the self-ligating brackets, with lower values for the Damon bracket, intermediate values for Easy Clip and In-Ovation, and higher values for Smart Clip brackets. This indicates that the significant differences found in activation forces between the self-ligating brackets were absorbed by the NiTi SE wire, thereby rendering deactivation forces clinically similar. Such behavior may be explained by the special mechanical properties of superelastic nickel-titanium wires.

Superelastic NiTi wire conforms to Hooke's law in its initial deformation, when an increase in load results in proportional wire deformation. After this first phase, when deformation reaches a critical limit a second stage begins characterized by the transformation of the wire's crystal structure from austenite to martensite. During this transition wire stiffness collapses, causing progressive deformation of the archwire with almost constant force, a phenomenon evidenced by a plateau in the wire's activation force.[6,7,12] The martensitic phase is unstable in the absence of force. Therefore, as soon as wire compression ends, the process is reversed with a transformation from the martensitic phase into austenitic. Reversal of the crystal structure requires less energy, which justifies the presence of marked hysteresis in the early deactivation stage.

Although its participation in this process has not yet been clearly defined, the friction force that opposes the archwire sliding is one of the factors that influence the profile of the load-deflection curve and hysteresis magnitude.[6]

Considering that deactivation forces are of most relevance from a clinical point of view and that they proved similar between Damon, Easy Clip, In-Ovation and Smart Clip brackets, the results suggest that the self-ligating brackets assessed in this study are equivalent, regardless of the activation forces. It should be noted however that wire deformation produces moments of force both in the misaligned tooth and in the adjacent anchorage teeth. These factors were not addressed in this research.

CONCLUSIONS

High activation force values of the Contour 0.014-in NiTi wire were accompanied by higher hysteresis values, which resulted in clinically similar deactivation forces, regardless of type of self-ligating brackets used.

REFERENCES

1. Baccetti T, Franchi L. Friction produced by types of elastomeric ligatures in treatment mechanics with the preadjusted appliance. Angle Orthod. 2006;76(2):211-6.
2. Cacciafesta V, Sfondrini MF, Ricciardi A, Scribante A, Klersy C, Auricchio F. Evaluation of friction of stainless steel and esthetic self-ligating brackets in various bracket-archwire combinations. Am J Orthod Dentofacial Orthop. 2003;124:395-402.
3. Demicheli M, Migliorati MV, Balboni C, Biavati AS. Confronto tra differenti sistemi bracket/filo/legatura - Misurazione in vitro dell'attrito su un'intera arcata. Mondo Ortod. 2006;4:273-89.
4. Franchi L, Baccetti T, Giuntini V. Forces released by nonconventional bracket or ligature systems during alignment of buccally displaced teeth. Am J Orthod Dentofacial Orthop. 2009;136:316.e1–e6.
5. Gandini P, Orsi L, Bertoncini C, Massironi S, Franchi L. In vitro frictional forces generated by three different ligation methods. Angle Orthod. 2008;78:917-21.
6. Garrec P, Jordan L. Stiffness in bending of a superelastic Ni-Ti orthodontic wire as a function of cross-sectional dimension. Angle Orthod. 2004;74:691-6.
7. Garrec P, Tavernier B, Jordan L. Evolution of flexural rigidity according to the cross-sectional dimension of a superelastic nickel titanium orthodontic wire. Eur J Orthod. 2005;27:402-7.
8. Kasuya S, Nagasaka S, Hanyuda A, Ishimura S, Hirashita A. The effect of ligation on the load-deflection characteristics of nickel-titanium orthodontic wire. Eur J Orthod. 2007;29(6):578-82.
9. Kusy R, Whitley, JQ. Influence of archwire and bracket dimensions on sliding mechanics: Derivations and determinations of the critical contact angles for binding. Eur J Orthod. 1999;21:199-208.
10. Mallory DC, English JD, Powers JM, Brantley WA, Bussa HI. Force-deflection comparison of superelastic nickel-titanium archwires. Am J Orthod Dentofacial Orthop. 2004;126:110-2.
11. Meling TR, Odegaard J, Holthe K, Segner D. The effect of friction on the bending stiffness of orthodontic beams: A theoretical and in vitro study. Am J Orthod Dentofacial Orthop. 1997;112:41-9.
12. Miura F, Mogi M, Ohura Y, Hamanaka H. The super-elastic property of the Japanese NiTi alloy wire for use in orthodontics. Am J Orthod Dentofacial Orthop. 1986;90:1-10.
13. Nakano H, Satoh K, Norris R, Jin T, Kamegai T, Ishikawa F, et al. Mechanical properties of several nickel-titanium alloy wires in three-point bending tests. Am J Orthod Dentofacial Orthop. 1999;115:390-5.
14. Queiroz G, Rino JN, Paiva JB, Ballester RY. Estudo comparativo da força de atrito produzida pela deformação de arco NiTi em diferentes braquetes ortodônticos. Avaliação in vitro. Dental Press J Orthod. 2012;17(4):45-50.

14

Shear bond resistance and enamel surface comparison after the bonding and debonding of ceramic and metallic brackets

José Maurício da Rocha[1], Marco Abdo Gravina[2], Marcio José da Silva Campos[3], Cátia Cardoso Abdo Quintão[4], Carlos Nelson Elias[5], Robert Willer Farinazzo Vitral[6]

Objective: To evaluate, *in vitro*, the shear bond strength presented by three brands of polycrystalline ceramic brackets and one brand of metallic bracket; verify the adhesive remnant index (ARI) after the tests, and analyze, through scanning electron microscopy (SEM) the enamel surface topography after debonding, detecting the release of mineral particles. **Methods:** Sixty bovine lower incisors were used. Three ceramic brackets (Allure®, InVu®, and Clarity®) and one metallic bracket (Geneus®) were bonded with Transbond XT®. Kruskal-Wallis's test (significance level set at 5%) was applied to the results of share bond and ARI. Mann Whitney's test was performed to compare the pairs of brackets in relation to their ARI. Brown-Forsythe's test (significance level set at 5%) was applied to the results of enamel chemical composition. Comparisons between groups were made with Games-Howell's and the Post-hoc tests. **Results:** No statistically significant difference was observed in relation to the shear bond strength loads. Clarity® brackets were the most affected in relation to the surface topography and to the release of mineral particles of enamel (calcium ions). **Conclusion:** With regard to the ARI, there was a prevalence of score 4 (40.4%). As for enamel surface topography, the Geneus® bracket was the only one which did not show superficial tissue loss. The InVu® and Clarity® ones showed cohesive fractures in 33.3% and the Allure® in 50%, the latter being the one that presented most fractures during removal.

Keywords: Shear bond strength. Tooth enamel. Orthodontic brackets. Scanning electron microscopy.

[1] MSc in Orthodontics, Adjunct professor, Department of Orthodontics - School of Dentistry — Federal University of Juiz de Fora (FO/UFJF).
[2] PhD in Dentistry, State University of Rio de Janeiro (UERJ). Adjunct professor, Department of Orthodontics, FO/UFJF.
[3] Postdoc in Orthodontics and professor, FO/UFJF.
[4] PhD in Orthodontics and Adjunct professor of Orthodontic, UERJ.
[5] Adjunct professor of Biomaterials, Fluminense Federal University (UFF).
[6] Associate professor, Department of Orthodontics, FO/UFJF.

» The authors report no commercial, proprietary or financial interest in the products or companies described in this article.

Marco Abdo Gravina
Av. Barão do Rio Branco, 2595 – Salas 1203 e 1204 – Centro
Juiz de Fora/MG – Brazil — CEP: 36010-011
E-mail: marcoabdogravina@yahoo.com.br

INTRODUCTION

The need for esthetic orthodontic treatment, especially by adults, culminated in the development of the first ceramic brackets in the late 1980's. Since then, new technologies for manufacturing esthetic brackets have been developed.[10] Ceramic brackets may be monocrystalline or polycrystalline, according to the manufacturing process. Polycrystalline brackets are produced by precipitation of aluminum oxide particles blended with a binder, and then textured and fired to remove surface imperfections and stress, caused by the cutting process. This manufacturing process may produce structural failures in the accessories. Monocrystalline brackets are produced by a completely different process. Single sapphire crystals involve the combination of aluminum oxide particles at 2,100°C.[13,19] The crystalline structure of monocrystalline brackets has higher purity than that of polycrystalline ones, with fewer structural failures but higher manufacturing costs.[3]

Bracket bonding became a routine in orthodontic treatment with fixed appliances after Buonocore[4] introduced the technique of acid-etching the enamel surface. Buonocore[4] proposed that the enamel surface could be modified by acids in order to become more receptive to bonding. The technique consisted in enamel prophylaxis, in which the enamel is cleaned, dried and freed from saliva, followed by application of acid on its surface. Several materials have been developed for this purpose. Due to presenting adhesive properties,[4] composite resins have become the main bonding material.

When a bracket is removed, bond failure may occur in the bracket/adhesive interface (adhesive), in the adhesive/enamel interface (adhesive), in the adhesive layer (cohesive), or both (adhesive and cohesive). Failures in the adhesive/enamel interface lead to a higher risk of having enamel fragments removed along with the bracket base resin. Therefore, many authors suggest that the orthodontist use a technique that promotes failure in the bracket/adhesive interface in order to prevent damage to the tooth structure.[2,4,11,12,14,24]

Due to a great difficulty in obtaining extracted human teeth for dental research, a substitute, with similar physical characteristics, has become necessary. Human teeth are morphologically and histologically similar to the teeth of other mammals. Thus, bovine incisors have become a good option in dental research, as they are adequate in size and easily available.[5]

The shear bond test is one of the most simple and widely used tests for determining adhesion resistance of bonded orthodontic brackets.[8] In this test, the bond is fractured with the application of a force parallel to the adhesive interface. The test may be conducted with a metallic blade or a steel wire loop, as close as possible to the adhesive interface.[8] Failure starts at the point where the blade applies a normal force, therefore, failure does not always happen at the weakest point.[23]

Scanning electron microscopy (SEM) has a wide range of applications in different fields of knowledge, and provides detailed structural information with a wide magnification range (up to 300,000X). SEM may be coupled to an X-ray energy dispersive spectroscopy (X-EDS) system, which allows the qualitative and semi-quantitative composition of the samples to be determined through emission of characteristic X-rays.[7]

In vivo studies may have several variables which can be minimized by *in vitro* research protocols performed with standard procedures and variables as limited as possible, thus yielding more representative and amenable-to-comparison results. The purpose of this study was to perform *in vitro* assessments of the shear resistance of three commercial brands of polycrystalline ceramic orthodontic brackets, using SEM to analyze the superficial enamel topography after bracket debonding and detect the release of mineral particles.

Proposition

1. Assess, *in vitro*, the shear resistance of three commercial brands of polycrystalline ceramic orthodontic brackets and of one metallic orthodontic bracket, all with mechanical retention.
2. Assess, by means of light microscopy, the adhesive remnant index (ARI) after bracket removal;
3. Assess, with SEM, the enamel superficial topography after bracket debonding.
4. Detect, by means of SEM adapted with an X-EDS microanalysis system, the release of mineral particles from the enamel after removal of ceramic and metallic brackets.
5. Observe and calculate bracket fracture during removal.

MATERIAL AND METHODS

Sixty recently extracted bovine lower incisors were obtained from the Municipal Abattoir of Juiz de Fora. The inclusion criteria demanded that the teeth had intact buccal surfaces, and no cavities, fractures, stains or enamel lesions.

All teeth were examined under light microscopy with a stereomicroscope (Stemi 2000C, Zeiss), at the Department of Physics of the Federal University of Juiz de Fora. After selection, the teeth were immersed for seven days into a 0.1% thymol-water solution[17] at room temperature, for asepsis and dehydration prevention. After this period, the remaining soft tissues, calculi and root-adhered bone fragments were removed.[17]

All teeth were subsequently kept at distilled water at 4°C, which was replaced every seven days, for a period not greater than three months before inclusion in the molded samples. Before inclusion, the teeth had their radicular tips sectioned so as to have the same radicular length.[16] Prior to plaster casting, carboril disk retentions were performed in the roots in order to increase their retention.

Three commercial brands of polycrystalline ceramic orthodontic brackets (Allure /GAC; InVu /TP and Clarity/3M-Unitek) and a metallic orthodontic bracket brand (Geneus/ GAC), all with mechanical retention, were used. They were divided into four groups with 15 brackets each. The study was conducted in two parts: 1) shear test; 2) SEM with X-EDS microanalysis.

To build the molded samples, 26 mm high PVC pipes with a 25 mm internal diameter were used. The molded samples were filled with type IV pink stone plaster[16] (Vigodent, Bonsucesso, Rio de Janeiro, Brazil). For bracket bonding, the teeth underwent prophylaxis of their buccal surfaces, with pumice stone and water, and were brushed with a Robinson's brush in low-rotation. The teeth were then washed with water for 10 seconds, and dried with an oil-free and humidity-free air spray.

All brackets were bonded with the Transbond XT adhesive (3M Unitek Orthodontics Products, Mowrovia, USA), according to the manufacturer's instructions. The teeth were initially immersed into a 37% phosphoric acid solution (Condac 3M, FGN, Joinvile, Santa Catarina, Brazil) for 15 seconds, sprayed with water for 10 seconds, and dried with an air spray. By the end of the process, they acquired a chalk-white color.

The adhesive (Primer Transbond XT, 3M Unitek Orthodontics Products, Monrovia, USA) was applied and light-cured for 10 seconds.[4] At last, the brackets were positioned at the center of the buccal surfaces, excess resin was removed and a light-curing process was performed for 20 seconds (ceramic brackets) and 40 seconds (metallic brackets). The Opti Light digital light curing device (Gnatus, São Paulo, Brazil) was used. After bonding, the teeth remained immersed in distilled water at 37°C, for 24 hours.

In order to standardize the molded samples for the shear test, a 0.021 x 0.025-in rectangular steel wire guide, inserted into the bracket slots and fixed with elastomeric ligatures, was used for positioning the teeth in the PVC pipes. This device allowed the brackets to remain at the same distance from the molded sample bases, and the buccal surfaces of the teeth to lie on a vertical plane parallel to the blade of the testing machine. Thus, all the molded samples were positioned at the base of the testing machine in such a way that the cleaver would be placed between the base and the occlusal tying-wings of the brackets, directing the force to an axis that was parallel to the bonding surface.

The mechanical shear tests were performed in a universal testing machine (EMIC DL 2000) adapted with a microprocessor, at the Post-Graduation Laboratory of the School of Dentistry — Federal University of Juiz de Fora. A 50 Kgf load cell was used at a 0.5 mm/min testing speed. For bracket debonding, the shear load values applied were gradually increased. The data obtained from these tests were stored in a computer directly linked to the mechanical testing device.

In order to analyze the morphology of the enamel debonding surfaces, the secondary electron analysis technique, through SEM (JEOL, JSM5800 LV), was performed at the Military Engineering Institute of Rio de Janeiro. All the images were under magnification of 200X for observation of the entire surface from which photographs were obtained. To detect enamel mineral chemical elements in the debonding surfaces, SEM with X-EDS microanalysis was employed. This test assessed the damage inflicted to the enamel after debonding, being performed in only five teeth of each group (the ones with the smallest ARI).

In addition, two other variables were assessed: 1) ARI after debonding and; 2) frequency of cohesive bracket fractures during the shear tests.

Therefore, all dental elements were analyzed and classified taking into account their ARI[1,6] after bracket removal. The scores ranged from zero to five, as follows: (0) no resin remained adhered to the tooth after debonding; (1) less than 25% of resin remained adhered to the tooth after debonding; (2) between 25 and 50% of resin remained adhered to the tooth after debonding; (3) between 50 and 75% of resin remained adhered to the tooth after debonding; (4) more than 75% of resin remained adhered to the tooth after debonding and; (5) all resin remained adhered to the tooth after debonding.[1,6]

The results were statistically analyzed and the Shapiro-Wilk's test did not show normal distribution in the sample. Levene's test demonstrated the homoscedasticity of the sample, while Kruskal-Wallis's test was used, with a significance level set at 5%, to obtain the shear test results and calculate the adhesive remnant index (ARI) in the enamel. Furthermore, Mann-Whitney's test, with a significance level set at 1.25% (equivalent to 0.05/4), was used to compare pairs of brackets with regard to their ARI.

To analyze the chemical composition of the enamel (X-EDSD), Brown-Forsythe's test, with a statistical significance of 5%, was used. Comparisons between groups were made with the Post-hoc and Games-Hoewell's tests.

RESULTS

Table 1 presents the results (in MPa) of the mechanical shear tests. The mean shear resistance values were as follows: GI (9.97 ± 5.29); GII (11.74 ± 4.52), GIII (10.91 ± 4.37); GIV (12.71 ± 5.81). Kruskal-Wallis's test (5% significance) had P = 0.43, showing that no group differed from one another with regard to the central tendency.

GI (Geneus®) was the only group that did not show bracket fracture during the mechanical testing. On the other hand, GII (Allure®) had 50% of its brackets with cohesive fractures, while GIII (InVu®) and GIV (Clarity®) had fractures of five brackets each, corresponding to 33.3% of the sample in each group. Out of the total number of ceramic brackets used (n = 44), 17 fractured, which represents 38.63% of the sample.

As for the ARI results, some teeth could not be analyzed, as the whole bracket base remained adhered to the crown after removal. The results of this analysis are shown in Table 2. Kruskal-Wallis's Test (5% significance) had P = 0.03, showing statistically significant differences between groups with regard to the central tendency.

Table 3 shows the differences between pairs with regard to ARI (Mann-Whitney'ss Test). The pairs were analyzed with a general significance level (P = 0.003), and with specific significance levels not greater than 0.0125 (0.05/4). Statistically significant differences were observed between the following brackets: Clarity® and InVu® (P = 0.002); Allure® and InVu® (P = 0.006) and Clarity® and Geneus® (P = 0.002). The other comparisons yielded no statistically significant differences.

Five teeth from each group were selected for enamel analysis with SEM. The choice was based on the molded samples with the smallest ARI value in each group. Since these samples would supposedly have suffered the greatest enamel damage after the shear test, they would probably allow better visualization of the enamel surface. After individual analysis of the 20 teeth (5 from each group) under SEM, all molded samples were found to have microscopic enamel topographic characteristics that were similar within groups. These characteristics are shown in Figures 1 to 4.

All molded samples selected for SEM analysis were also submitted to X-EDS for analysis of the enamel chemical composition.

Table 1 - Means, standard deviation, minimum and maximum values and number of teeth regarding the mechanical shear tests (MPa).

Group	Mean ± SD	Minimum	Maximum	Number of teeth
I) Geneus	9.97 ± 5.29	4.05	17.71	15
II) Allure	11.74 ± 4.52	5.72	22.00	15
III) InVu	10.91 ± 4.37	4.93	17.34	15
IV) Clarity	12.71 ± 5.81	6.16	23.22	15
Total	11.33 ± 5.01	4.05	23.22	60

Kruskal-Wallis' test. p = 0.43.

Table 4 presents the data referring to the chemical composition, described by means and intra-group standard deviations of the percentages of the chemical elements found. Because most chemical elements found were not present in all groups of brackets, statistical analysis was precluded for most of them.

Only comparative analysis of calcium could be performed, at it was the only chemical element present in all groups of brackets. To this end, Brown-Forsythe's test was used, given that neither Kolmogorov-Smirnov's and Shapiro-Wilk's normality tests nor Levene's equality of variance test found variance normality and similarity between groups.

It is important to point out that, out of all chemical elements found with X-EDS, calcium percentages should be the most noteworthy in the enamel, as higher values would indicate minor damage to the enamel after bracket removal, whereas lower values would suggest severe damage. This is the reason why only the data referring to calcium were presented in this study. The Brown-Forsythe's test reached 5% statistical significance for calcium.

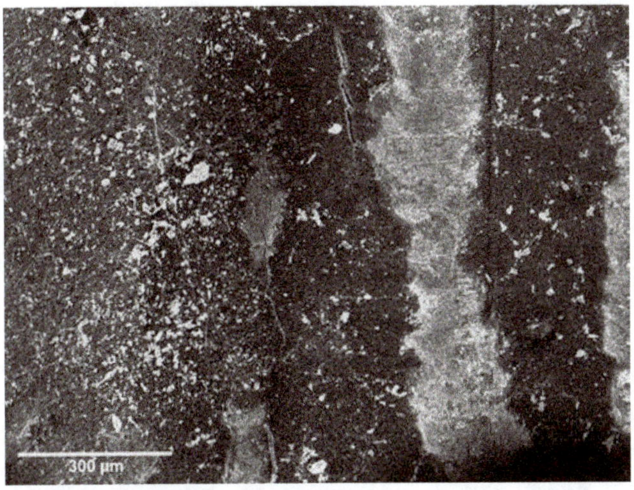

Figure 1 - Enamel sample from the Geneus® group, with no superficial tissue loss, showing only small fissures, probably due to the debonding technique.

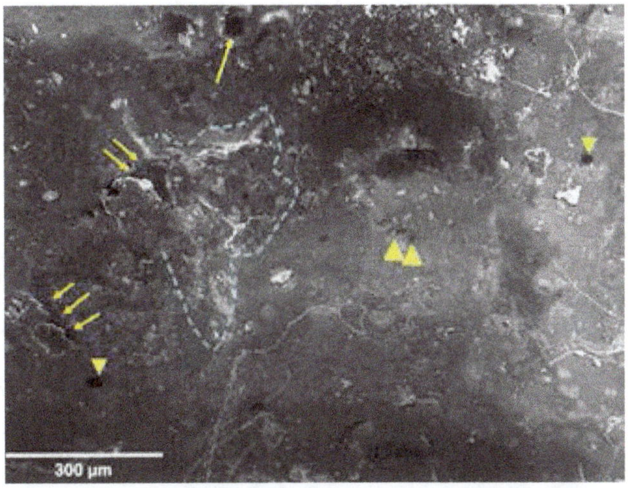

Figure 2 - Enamel sample from the Allure® group, showing erosions (yellow arrow) and well-established pores (green arrow point), depressions (orange arrow) and slight loss of the aprismatic enamel layer (blue dotting).

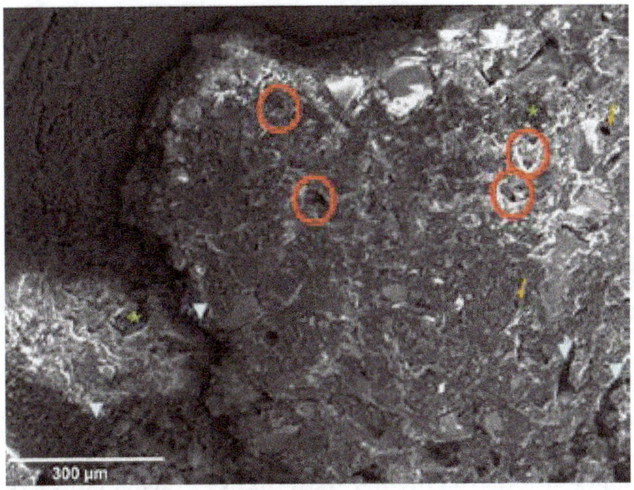

Figure 3 - Enamel sample from the InVu® group, showing small craters (green asterisk) surrounded by areas of loss of the aprismatic enamel layer, pores (orange arrow), erosions (red circle) and depressions (blue arrow heads).

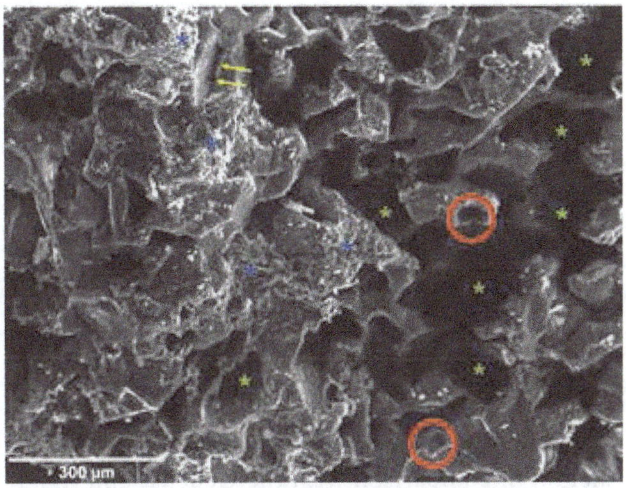

Figure 4 - Enamel sample of the Clarity® group, showing significant alterations of the enamel microstructure, with electron-lucent areas, corresponding to craters characteristic of "erosion deepening" (green asterisk), surrounded by extensive loss of the aprismatic enamel layer (blue asterisk) and depressions (yellow arrows) and some erosions (red circle).

Table 2 - Scores for ARI assessment in the study groups.

ARI groups	Scores						Total
	0	1	2	3	4	5	
I) Geneus	0 (0%)	5 (33.3%)	4 (26.7%)	0 (0%)	2 (13.3%)	4 (26.7%)	15
II) Allure	0 (0%)	0 (0%)	1(7.1%)	0 (0%)	9 (64.3%)	4 (28.6%)	14
III) InVu	2 (20%)	1(10%)	2 (20%)	1(10%)	4 (40%)	0 (0%)	10
IV) Clarity	0 (0%)	0 (0%)	0 (0%)	1(7.7%)	6 (46.2%)	6 (46.2%)	13
Total	2	6	7	2	21	14	52

Table 3 - Differences between bracket pairs, according to the ARI.

	Geneus (I)	Allure (II)	InVu (III)	Clarity (IV)
I) Geneus		0.057	0.605	0.002*
II) Allure	0.057		0.006*	0.488
III) InVu	0.605	0.006*		0.002*
IV) Clarity	0.002*	0.488	0.002*	

Table 4 - X-ESD results referring to the mean percentages of calcium present in tooth enamel and their statistical analysis.

Group	Mean	Bracket	Bracket	Mean difference	Mean standard error	p-value
Geneus	52.77	Geneus	Allure	19.10800	13.90868	0.564
			InVu	-7.54000	4.50529	0.421
			Clarity	45.56600 (*)	4.94396	0.000
Allure	33.66	Allure	Geneus	-19.10800	13.90868	0.564
			InVu	-26.64800	13.34571	0.320
			Clarity	26.45800	13.50011	0.327
InVu	60.31	InVu	Geneus	7.54000	4.50529	0.421
			Allure	26.64800	13.34571	0.320
			Clarity	53.10600 (*)	3.01652	0.000
Clarity	7.20	Clarity	Geneus	-45.56600 (*)	4.94396	0.000
			Allure	-26.45800	13.50011	0.327
			InVu	-53.10600 (*)	3.01652	0.000

The Post-hoc and Game-Hoewel's tests were used for comparison between groups, with the Clarity® group showing statistically lower percentages of calcium in comparison with the Geneus® and InVu® groups. As for the Allure® group, no statistically significant difference was found between the former and the other groups (Table 4).

DISCUSSION

Santos et al[17] and Vicente et al[21] demonstrated the superiority of Transbond XT® in comparison with glass ionomer cements, with higher bracket adhesive resistance to enamel and higher percentage of fractures in the bracket-adhesive interface. This is the reason why this was the material chosen in this study.

All brackets were conventionally bonded as proposed by Buonocore[4] in 1955, that is: prophylaxis of the bonding dental surfaces, acid etching, application and light-curing of the Transbond XT® adhesive and bonding with the Transbond XT® resin. Romano[15] reported the need for acid etching of the enamel to reach shear resistance values that were compatible with clinical use. Savaris and Menezes,[18] on the other hand, did not observe statistically significant differences in the shear loads between samples in which the Transbond XT adhesive (primer) was light-cured and samples in which no light-curing process was performed. We chose to proceed with acid etching of the enamel and light-curing of the adhesive, as this is a traditional protocol used in shear and enamel surface analysis research.

The mechanical shear tests were performed 24 hours after bracket bonding, with the molded samples being kept in distilled water during this period. We chose this time interval in accordance with Hajrassie and Khier[9] who did not observe significant differences, *in vitro* or *in vivo*, in the debonding loads of metallic brackets bonded to premolars with Transbond XT® after four different bonding times: 10 minutes, 24 hours, 1 week and 4 weeks.

As for the values obtained with the mechanical shear tests (loads between 9.97 and 12.71 MPa), we concluded that all brackets studied could be successfully used in a clinical scenario, given that the minimum shear resistance loads necessary to tooth movement range from 5.9 to 7.9 MPa, according to Vasques et al.[20]

Cohesive fractures were observed in the three commercial brands of ceramic brackets, with 33.3% for Invu® and Clarity®, and 50% for Allure®. No fractures were observed in the group of metallic brackets. As for SEM, the samples of the Clarity® group had significant alterations in the enamel microstructure in comparison with the other groups, with electron-lucent areas corresponding to craters, erosion deepening and extensive loss of the aprismatic enamel layer. This was confirmed by X-EDS, in which the Clarity® group had a significantly lower percentage of calcium in the enamel after bracket removal. Likewise, Chen et al[6] observed cohesive fractures in 25% of the Clarity® brackets after machine-driven debonding. On the other hand, in the same study, Chen et al[6] observed by means of SEM that most fractures occurred in the bracket/adhesive interface, with no significant enamel damage after bracket removal. However, it is noteworthy that Chen et al[6] submitted their total sample to SEM with X-EDS microanalysis, whereas in the present study only the teeth with smaller ARI were analyzed, which might have contributed to less favorable results concerning the superficial topography of the enamel.

Savaris and Menezes[18] as well as Chen et al[6] did not observe damage or important fractures in the enamel surface after removal of the Clarity® brackets bonded to bovine teeth, reporting that debonding predominantly occurred in the resin layer (cohesive failure, ARI 3), with enamel fracture in just one of the 60 teeth analyzed. Similarly to the study conducted by Chen et al,[6] the whole sample was submitted to SEM.

Substantial enamel loss and significant enamel damage were observed under SEM analysis for all groups of ceramic brackets. Vilchis, Hotta and Yamamoto[22] used SEM to observe the superficial enamel topography of premolars submitted to bracket bonding according to two methods: (1) etching with 37% phosphoric acid for 30 seconds + Transbond XT® adhesive + Transbond XT® resin cement; and (2) Transbond Plus Self Etching Primer® (SEP) + Transbond XT® resin cement. Based on the yielded results, they demonstrated that the phosphoric acid etching group had greater enamel loss in comparison to the Transbond Plus Self Etching Primer® group. Additionally, the enamel-adhesive interfaces had more irregularities with phosphoric acid etching. The differences between our findings and some literature reports may be related to such etching, as phosphoric acid was used in our study.

In a search for a more conservative orthodontic bonding, we suggest that further studies comparing Transbond Plus Self Etching Primer®, 37% phosphoric acid and other etching materials be undertaken to identify the orthodontic material causing the least enamel damage after bracket removal. This study demonstrated that enamel damage after bracket removal can occur in teeth conditioned with 37% phosphoric acid, with this damage being more frequent and extensive when ceramic brackets are used.

CONCLUSION

1. There were no statistically significant differences between groups with regard to the shear loads necessary to promote bracket debonding.
2. As for the adhesive remnant index, there were statistically significant differences between the following groups: Clarity® and Invu®; Allure® and InVu®; Clarity® and Geneus®. No statistically significant differences were found between other pairs. In a general context, score 4 prevailed, with 40.4%.
3. Analysis of the enamel superficial topography showed that the Geneus® group was the only one with no superficial tissue loss, having suffered only small fissures, probably due to the debonding technique. All ceramic bracket groups had erosions, pores, depressions and loss of the aprismatic enamel layer, with the Clarity® group being most affected, with significant alterations in enamel microstructure.
4. As for the X-EDSD, the Clarity® group had a significantly lower percentage of calcium in the enamel after bracket removal.
5. Metallic brackets did not fracture during removal. The InVu® and Clarity® groups had fractures in 33.3% of their samples, while the Allure® group had fractures in 50%.

REFERENCES

1. Artun J, Bergland S. Clinical trials with crystal growth conditioning as an alternative to acid-etch enamel pretreatment. Am J Orthod. 1984;85(4):333-40.
2. Bennett CG, Shen C, Waldron JM. The effects of debonding on the enamel surface. J Clin Orthod. 1984;18(5):330-4.
3. Bigarella CA. Avaliação in vitro da resistência friccional entre bráquetes cerâmicos e metálico [dissertação]. São Paulo (SP): Universidade de Marília; 2005.
4. Buonocore MGA. A simple method of increase the adhesion of acrylic filling materials to enamel surfaces. J Dent Res. 1955;34(6):849-53.
5. Campos MIC, Campos CN, Vitral RWF. O Uso de dentes bovinos como substitutos de dentes humanos em pesquisas odontológicas: uma revisão da literatura. Pesq Bras Odontoped Clin Integr. 2008;8(1):127-32.
6. Chen HY, Su MZ, Chang HF, Chen YJ, Lan WH, Lin CP. Effects of different debonding techniques on the bonding forces and failure modes of ceramic brackets in simulated clinical set-ups. Am J Orthod Dentofacial Orthop. 2007;132(5):680-6.
7. Duarte LC, Juchem PL, Pulz GM, Brum TMM, Chodur N, Liccardo A, et al. Aplicações de microscopia eletrônica de varredura (MEV) e sistema de energia dispersiva (EDS) no estudo de gemas: exemplos brasileiros. Pesq Geociências. 2003;30(2):3-15.
8. Garcia FCP , D'Alpino PHP, Terada RSS, Carvalho RM. Testes mecânicos para a avaliação laboratorial da união resina/dentina. Rev Fac Odontol. 2002;10(3):118-27.
9. Hajrassie MK, Khier SE. In-vivo and in vitro comparison of bond strengths of orthodontic brackets bonded to enamel and debonded at various times. Am J Orthod Dentofacial Orthop. 2007;131(3):384-90.
10. Karamouzos A, Athanasiou AE, Apadopoulos MA. Clinical characteristics and properties of ceramic brackets: a comprehensive review. Am J Orthod Dentofacial Orthop. 1997;112(1):34-40.
11. Katona TR. Stresses developed during clinical debonding of stainless steel orthodontic brackets. Angle Orthod. 1997;67(1):39-46.
12. Newman GV. A posttreatment surgery of directed bonding of metal brackets. Am J Orthod. 1971;60(6):600-10.
13. Omana HM, Moore RN, Bagby MD. Frictional properties of metal and ceramic brackets. J Clin Orthod. 1992;26(7):425-32.
14. Redd TB, Shivapuja PK. Deboning ceramic brackets: effects on enamel. J Clin Orthod. 1991;25(8):475-81.
15. Romano FL. Análise in vitro da resistência ao cisalhamento de bráquetes metálicos colados em várias condições de esmalte [dissertação]. Piracicaba (SP): Universidade Estadual de Campinas; 2003.
16. Rosa CB, Pinto RAC, Habib FAL. Colagem ortodôntica em esmalte com presença ou ausência de contaminação salivar: é necessário o uso de adesivo autocondicionante ou de adesivo hidrofílico? Rev Dental Press Ortod Ortop Facial. 2008;13(3):34-42.
17. Santos PCF, Santos JFF, Chaves Júnior CM, Campos BGP, Santos HMG. Colagem em ambiente úmido: avaliação da capacidade de resistência à tração de bráquetes metálicos. Rev Dental Press Ortod Ortop Facial. 2000;5(6):33-43.
18. Savaris FL, Menezes LM. Avaliação in vitro de diferentes tempos de fotoativação na colagem de bráquetes cerâmicos. Rev Odonto Ciênc. 2004;19(44):139-44.
19. Swartz ML. Ceramic brackets. J Clin Orthod. 1988;22(2):82-8.
20. Vasques WO, Ciruffo PSD, Tubel CAM, Miyamura ZY, Vedovello Filho M. Resistência ao cisalhamento de diferentes bráquetes metálicos: colados com resina composta fotoativada (Transbond). Estudo comparativo "in vitro". Rev Goiana Odontol. 2005;53(3):186-90.
21. Vicente A, Bravo LA, Romero M, Ortíz AJ, Canteras M. Effects of 3 adhesion promoters on the shear bond strength of orthodontic brackets: an in-vitro study. Am J Orthod Dentofacial Orthop. 2006;129(3):390-5.
22. Vilchis RJ, Hotta Y, Yamamoto K. Examination of enamel-adhesive interface with focused ion beam and scanning electron microscopy. Am J Orthod Dentofacial Orthop. 2007;131(5):646-50.
23. Watanabe I, Nakabayashi N. Measurement methods for adhesion to dentine: the current status in Japan. J Dent. 1994;22(2):67-72.
24. Zachrisson BU. Colagem em Ortodontia. In: Graber TM, Vanarsdall Júnior RL. Ortodontia princípios e técnicas atuais. Rio de Janeiro: Guanabara Koogan; 1996. cap. 12, p. 524-35.

15

Differences in the force system delivered by different beta-titanium wires in elaborate designs

Renato Parsekian Martins[1], Sergei Godeiro Fernandes Rabelo Caldas[2], Alexandre Antonio Ribeiro[3], Luís Geraldo Vaz[4], Roberto Hideo Shimizu[5], Lídia Parsekian Martins[6]

Objective: Evaluation of the force system produced by four brands of β-Ti wires bent into an elaborate design. **Methods:** A total of 40 T-loop springs (TLS) hand-bent from 0.017 x 0.025-in β-Ti were randomly divided into four groups according to wire brand: TMA™ (G1), BETA FLEXY™ (G2), BETA III WIRE™ (G3) and BETA CNA™ (G4). Forces and moments were recorded by a moment transducer, coupled to a digital extensometer indicator adapted to a testing machine, every 0.5 mm of deactivation from 5 mm of the initial activation. The moment-to-force (MF) ratio, the overlapping of the vertical extensions of the TLSs and the load-deflection (LD) ratio were also calculated. To complement the results, the Young's module (YM) of each wire was determined by the slope of the load-deflection graph of a tensile test. The surface chemical composition was also evaluated by an energy dispersive X-ray fluorescence spectrometer. **Results:** All groups, except for G2, produced similar force levels initially. G3 produced the highest LD rates and G1 and G4 had similar amounts of overlap of the vertical extensions of the TLSs in "neutral position". G1 and G3 delivered the highest levels of moments, and G2 and G3 produced the highest MF ratios. β-Ti wires from G3 produced the highest YM and all groups showed similar composition, except for G2. **Conclusion:** The four beta-titanium wires analyzed produced different force systems when used in a more elaborate design due to the fact that each wire responds differently to bends.
Keywords: Orthodontics. Tooth movement. Orthodontic wires.

[1] Adjunct professor, Universidade Estadual Paulista Julio de Mesquita Filho (UNESP), School of Dentistry, Department of Orthodontics, Araraquara, São Paulo, Brazil.
[2] Adjunct Professor, Universidade Federal do Rio Grande do Norte (UFRN), Department of Dentistry, Natal, Rio Grande do Norte, Brazil.
[3] Professor, Universidade Potiguar (UnP) and Associação Brasileira de Odontologia (ABO), Specialization course in Orthodontics, Natal, Rio Grande do Norte, Brazil.
[4] Professor, Universidade Estadual Paulista Julio de Mesquita Filho (UNESP), School of Dentistry, Department of Prosthesis and Dental Material, Araraquara, São Paulo, Brazil.
[5] Professor, Universidade Tuiuti do Paraná (UTP), School of Dentistry, Curitiba, Paraná, Brazil.
[6] Professor, Universidade Estadual Paulista Julio de Mesquita Filho (UNESP), School of Dentistry, Department of Orthodontics and Pediatric Dentistry, Araraquara, São Paulo, Brazil.

» The authors report no commercial, proprietary or financial interest in the products or companies described in this article.

Renato Parsekian Martins.
Rua Carlos Gomes, 2158, Araraquara, São Paulo - Brazil. CEP: 14801-320.
E-mail: dr_renatopmartins@hotmail.com

INTRODUCTION

Beta-titanium (β-Ti) was introduced in Dentistry in the late 70's;[1] since then it has been widely used in Orthodontics due to its excellent mechanical properties, such as high spring-back, low stiffness, high formability, and good weldability.[2-6] After expiration of the patent[2] on the first commercial brand of β-Ti (TMA™, Ormco Co., Glendora, USA), the use of this alloy expanded drastically with a wide range of prices and quality. Even though there are several brands available to the clinician, only a few studies[2,7,8] have been conducted in order to compare different β-Ti commercial brands. These studies, however, compare mechanical properties of β-Ti alloys either through tensile[2,8] or through 3-point bending tests[7] on straight pieces of wire. This might not represent the true behavior of the different β-Ti alloys when bends are placed in the wire or when more elaborate designs, such as loops, are used.

It has been established that the T-loop spring (TLS) has the greatest ability to produce high moment-to-force (MF) ratios in order to control tooth movement when compared to other designs of springs. Several parameters of TLS have already been studied, such as spring's height,[9-13] the location of the spring within inter bracket distance,[9,12-15] the intensity and type of pre-activation,[11,12,13,16,17,18] horizontal activation,[11,13] alloy wire type,[3,19,20] and stress relaxation;[21] all of which can alter the MF ratio and force produced. However, differences between TLS manufactured with different β-Ti have not yet been systematically studied and are not completely understood. Thus, it is suggested that these alloys may present different biomechanical behavior, thereby affecting the force system released by the springs.

The objective of this study was to evaluate whether the behavior of four different brands of beta-titanium bent into an elaborate design (T-loop spring) are similar when forces, moments and MF ratios produced are compared.

MATERIAL AND METHODS

Force system

Sixty 6 x 10-mm T-loop springs (TLSs) were blindly bent out of four different commercial brands of 0.017 x 0.025-in β-Ti, using a Marcotte plier (Hu-Friedy dental instruments, Chicago, USA), a custom template (Fig 1). They were divided into four groups of 15 springs made of the same wire brand. The groups were previously labeled to assure impartiality of results. The wires used in the groups were TMA (Ormco Co., Glendora, USA) (G1), BETA FLEXY (Orthometric Imp.Exp.Ltda, Marília, Brazil) (G2), BETA III WIRE (Morelli Ortodontia, Sorocaba, Brazil) (G3) and BETA CNA (Ortho Organizers, INC., San Marcos, USA) (G4) (Table 1) TLSs were hand-bent in a random order; and out of the 15 TLSs bent, ten were randomly selected for testing.

A universal testing machine (EMIC, São José dos Pinhais, Brazil), set up with a load cell of 0.1 kN, was coupled to a moment transducer and a digital extensometer indicator (Transdutec, São Paulo, Brazil) for the tests. The test speed was 5 mm/min and the digital extensometer excitation and sensitivity was 5 V and 0.5 mV/V, respectively (Fig 2).

Prior to the test, concentrated bends were used to pre-activate the TLSs[22] which were positioned symmetrically in an inter bracket distance (IBD) of 23 mm. At this distance, they were checked with a digital caliper and the testing device was zeroed. To assure the correct activation and the centralization of the TLSs, 9 mm were measured from the center of the loop towards each extremity of the horizontal extensions, and marked with a permanent marker (Fig 3). Those markings would allow the TLS to be correctly secured in place and centralized with the correct horizontal activation. The TLS was rigidly clamped to the test apparatus in one extremity and tied to a bracket on the other one with an elastomeric ligature.

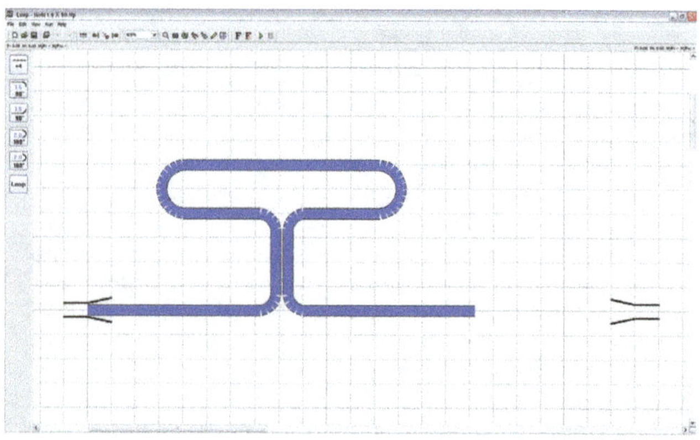

Figure 1 - Template developed in the Loop software (dHAL Orthodontic Software, Athens, Greece) used for the design of the TLS. The software allows the template to be printed in 1:1 ratio. Each square measures 1 mm².

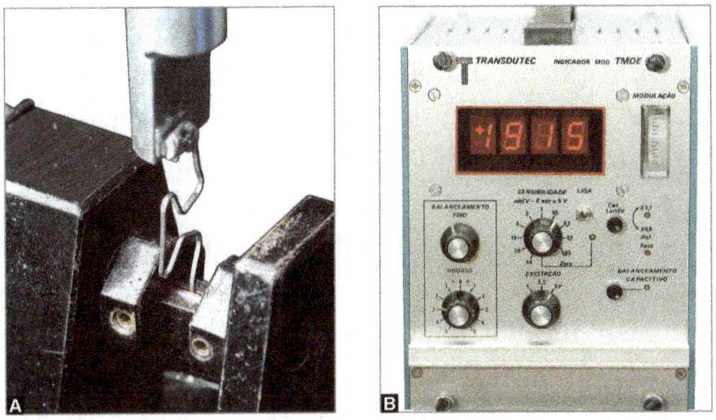

Figure 2 - A) Detail of the device used for the measurements: the bottom extremity of the TLS is firmly clamped by the moment transducer, while the top part of the TLS is tied to a bracket soldered to the universal testing machine, which records the horizontal force; B) Moment transducer used.

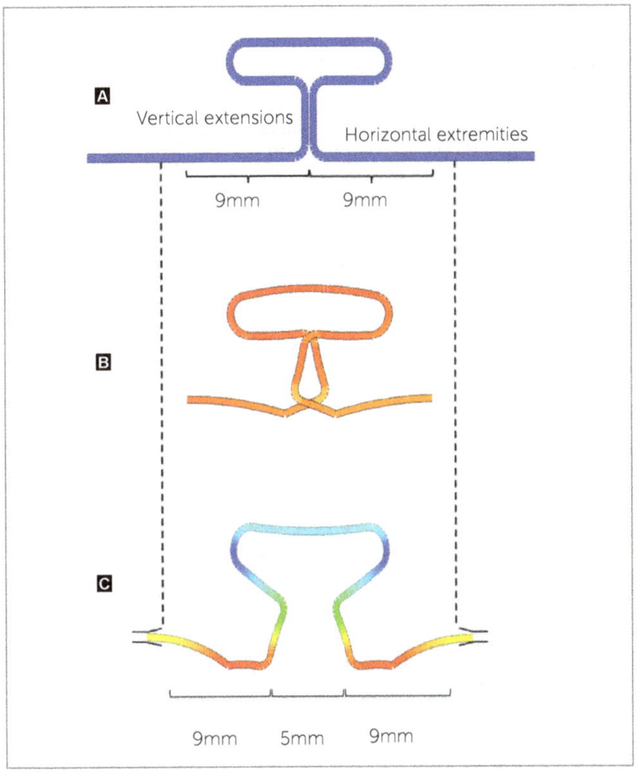

Figure 3 - A) Loop horizontal dimensions were marked to assure correct activation and TLS centralization; B) Neutral position of the TLS simulated by the Loop Software; C) TLS shape simulated by the Loop Software when positioned symmetrically in an IBD of 23 mm and activated 5 mm. Colored areas reflect stress distribution over the wire, going from red, being high stress areas; to dark blue, being low stress areas.

After a horizontal activation of 5 mm, the horizontal force and moment developed were recorded for every 0.5 mm of deactivation at the extremity of the TLSs attached to the testing machine, and the MF ratios were calculated. Furthermore, the amount of overlap of the vertical extensions of the TLSs in neutral position (deformation assumed when the loop's extremities are placed parallel to the position that they will be once installed, producing only moments) was calculated by linear interpolation. The load-deflection (LD) ratio of each TLS was obtained by calculating the slope of the respective deactivation graph (Fig 4).

Wire dimensions

The height and width of each wire were measured to the nearest 0.001 mm with a digital micrometer accurate to ± 1 µm (Mitutoyo, Kyoto, Japan). Five wires were taken from each group, totaling 20 readings, and the mean value was used in the subsequent calculations (Table 1).

Mechanical properties

The sample comprised five 30-cm segments of each wire and was divided as presented in Table 1. The tensile test was performed on a universal testing machine (EMIC, São José dos Pinhais, Brazil) set up with a load cell of 5 kN and speed of 2 mm/min until rupture of the wire. Young's module (YM) was determined by the slope of the LD graph of the tensile test.[23]

Chemical composition

An energy dispersive X-ray fluorescence spectrometer machine, model EDX-800, (Shimadzu Corporation, Kyoto, Japan), was used to determine the surface chemical composition of the wires in each group, using different wires from the same batch. Based on this analysis, it was assumed that the bulk composition was similar to surface compositions within the limits of accuracy. A fractographic image was obtained and the chemical composition was determined automatically in percentages.

Statistical analysis

SPSS v.16.0 (SPSS Inc., Chicago, USA) statistical analysis software was used in this study. Kolmogorov-Smirnov test indicated normal distribution of data and one-way ANOVA test was used to identify differences among groups. Tukey post hoc test, at a significance level of 5%, was used to compare differences among groups.

RESULTS

Force system

The TLSs measured produced horizontal forces ranging from 116.7 gf to 498.9 gf (G1), -15.9 gf to 311.4 gf (G2), 35.8 gf to 452.6 gf (G3) and 121.9 gf to 463.7 gf (G4) between 0.5 and 5 mm of activation. TLSs from G2 produced the lowest initial forces of deactivation compared to the other three groups. (Table 2 and Fig 4) The TLSs from G3 showed the highest LD rates (93.7 gf/mm), followed by G1 (85.5 gf/mm), and by G2 and G4 (72.7 and 76.0 gf/mm, respectively), which showed similar LD rates.

The amount of overlap of the vertical extensions of TLSs (in neutral position) was different between G2 (0.72 mm) and G3 (0.13 mm), which, on the other hand, were different from the similar overlap that occurred between G1 and G4 (-0.86 mm and -1.13 mm, respectively) (Table 2 and Fig 5).

TLSs delivered moments that ranged from 1452.0 gf.mm to 2030.7 gf.mm (G1), 919.0 gf.mm to 1482.0 gf.mm (G2), 1366.1 gf.mm to 1992.1 gf.mm (G3) and 1276.9 gf.mm to 1721.3 gf.mm (G4) between 0.5 and 5 mm of activation. G1 and G3 produced the highest levels of moments initially, while G4 produced lower moments than G1, but the values were similar to G3 and G2. G2 was different from all other groups. (Table 3 and Fig 6)

G2 and G3 showed the highest MF ratios initially (4.9 and 4.4 mm, respectively), followed by G1 (4,1 mm) which was similar to G3 and G4 (3.7 mm). From 1.5 mm of deactivation on, there was no difference among groups. (Table 4 and Fig 7).

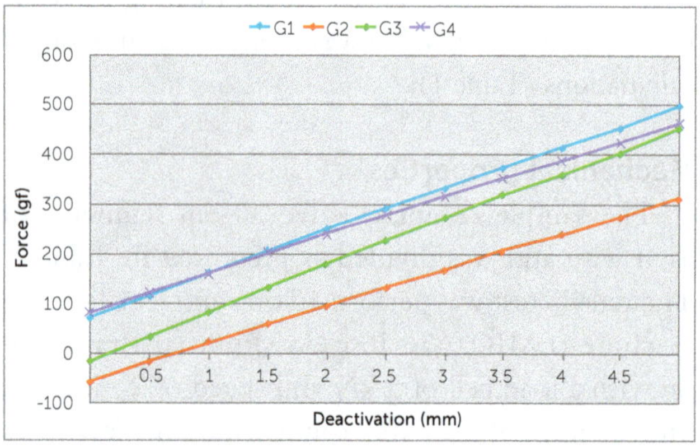

Figure 4 - Horizontal force (in grams-force) produced on deactivation by the four groups of β-Ti TLSs over a range of 5 mm.

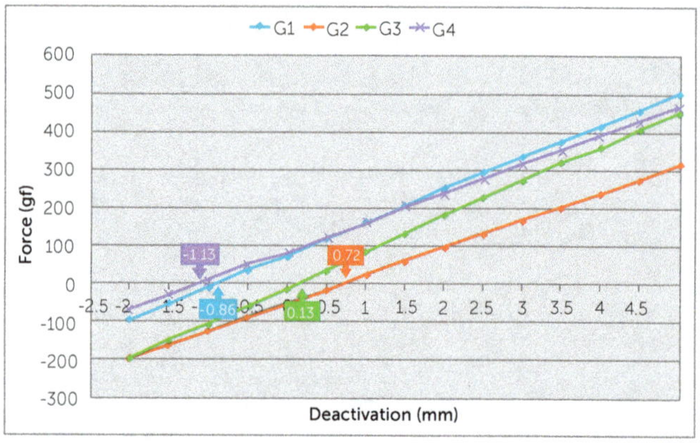

Figure 5 - Figure 4 slightly modified. The x- intercepts, pointed by the arrows, depict the amount of horizontal overlap of the vertical extensions of the TLSs in "neutral position" and were calculated by linear interpolation.

Table 1 - β-Ti wires used in the study.

Group	Wire	Manufacturer	Batch	Measured dimensions (inches) Height Mean	SD		Range	p (95%)	Width Mean	SD		Range	p (95%)
1	TMA	Ormco Corporation	03F2F	0.0165	0.00	A	0.0	<0.001	0.024	0.00	B	0.0	0.007
2	BETA FLEXY	Orthometric Imp. Exp.	148	0.0161	0.00	B	0.0005		0.024	0.00	B	0.0	
3	BETA III TiMo	Morelli Ortodontia	1072448 100004	0.0165	0.00	A	0.0		0.0244	0.00	A	0.0005	
4	CNA	Ortho Organizers	401682D06	0.0165	0.00	A	0.0		0.0242	0.00	AB	0.0005	

Table 2 - Means and standard deviations for forces (gf), neutral position (mm), LD ratio (gf.mm) and ANOVA results over a range of 5 mm of deactivation.

	1			2			3			4			*p* (95%)
	Mean	SD		Mean	SD		Mean	SD		Mean	SD		
5 mm	498.9	18.7	B	311.4	79.92	A	452.58	26.73	B	463.65	13.8	B	< 0.001
4.5 mm	453.74	18.78	B	273.67	72.85	A	406.47	24.43	B	424.35	13.91	B	< 0.001
4 mm	414.1	18.41	C	238.37	68.59	A	362.21	24.27	B	388.57	14.05	BC	< 0.001
3.5 mm	373.93	18.3	C	203.04	64.58	A	317.58	24.1	B	352.48	14.22	BC	< 0.001
3 mm	333.22	18.18	C	167.3	60.78	A	272.42	24.29	B	315.85	14.48	C	< 0.001
2.5 mm	291.66	18.16	C	131.48	57.3	A	226.65	24.4	B	278.65	14.92	C	< 0.001
2 mm	249.29	18.29	C	95.34	54.15	A	180.0	24.58	B	240.77	15.5	C	< 0.001
1.5 mm	206.05	18.51	C	58.55	51.22	A	132.61	24.82	B	201.93	15.94	C	< 0.001
1 mm	161.89	18.86	C	21.53	48.83	A	84.48	25.06	B	162.28	16.4	C	< 0.001
0.5 mm	116.66	19.42	C	-15.87	47.1	A	35.77	25.31	B	121.94	17.29	C	< 0.001
Neutral position	-0.86	0.22	A	0.72	0.62	C	0.13	0.29	B	-1.13	0.27	A	< 0.001
LD	85.5	3.04	B	72.7	12.51	A	93.71	2.59	C	75.96	3.01	A	< 0.001

Different letters indicate group differences.

Table 3 - Means and standard deviations for moments (gf.mm) and ANOVA results over a range of 5 mm of deactivation.

	1			2			3			4			*p* (95%)
	Mean	SD		Mean	SD		Mean	SD		Mean	SD		
5 mm	2030.7	290.16	C	1482.0	278.8	A	1992.1	179.27	BC	1721.3	110.65	AB	< 0.001
4.5 mm	1977.8	282.51	C	1430.7	272.23	A	1941.5	177.57	BC	1677.7	113.48	AB	< 0.001
4 mm	1934.9	276.38	C	1382.3	269.75	A	1891.9	170.27	BC	1641.3	116.98	AB	< 0.001
3.5 mm	1874.7	265.35	C	1329.43	268.39	A	1837.9	169.29	BC	1601.4	117.46	B	< 0.001
3 mm	1812.1	253.31	C	1271.4	267.33	A	1761.0	148.82	BC	1557.1	119.2	B	< 0.001
2.5 mm	1745.3	236.17	B	1211.3	268.41	A	1687.6	125.73	B	1507.7	117.62	B	< 0.001
2 mm	1683.3	224.98	B	1149.1	269.11	A	1615.6	124.93	B	1455.7	114.46	B	< 0.001
1.5 mm	1597.2	180.45	B	1075.8	267.83	A	1538.2	126.97	B	1402.0	112.18	B	< 0.001
1 mm	1527.8	174.18	B	1000.2	265.97	A	1459.4	131.14	B	1339.2	106.87	B	< 0.001
0.5 mm	1452.0	169.17	B	919.0	265.91	A	1366.1	132.17	B	1276.9	106.35	B	< 0.001

Different letters indicate group differences.

Table 4 - Means and standard deviations for MF ratios (mm) and ANOVA results over a range of 5 mm of deactivation.

	1			2			3			4			p (95%)
	Mean	SD		Mean	SD		Mean	SD		Mean	SD		
5 mm	4.07	0.55	AB	4.86	0.72	C	4.4	0.33	BC	3.72	0.28	A	< 0.001
4.5 mm	4.36	0.59	AB	5.35	0.86	C	4.78	0.37	BC	3.96	0.33	A	< 0.001
4 mm	4.67	0.64	AB	5.98	1.06	C	5.23	0.41	BC	4.23	0.37	A	< 0.001
3.5 mm	5.02	0.69	AB	6.83	1.43	C	5.8	0.49	B	4.55	0.42	A	< 0.001
3 mm	5.44	0.73	AB	8.12	2.16	C	6.48	0.5	B	4.94	0.49	A	< 0.001
2.5 mm	5.99	0.77	A	10.4	4.02	B	7.48	0.74	A	5.43	0.58	A	< 0.001
2 mm	6.77	0.89	A	17.25	13.64	B	9.09	1.15	A	6.08	0.7	A	0.003
1.5 mm	7.79	1.01		-3.03	49.35		11.91	2.18		6.99	0.9		0.537
1 mm	9.53	1.42		13.76	29.44		18.74	6.21		8.35	1.26		0.425
0.5 mm	12.71	2.35		3.09	71.76		23.65	131.14		10.71	2.1		0.927

Different letters indicate group differences.

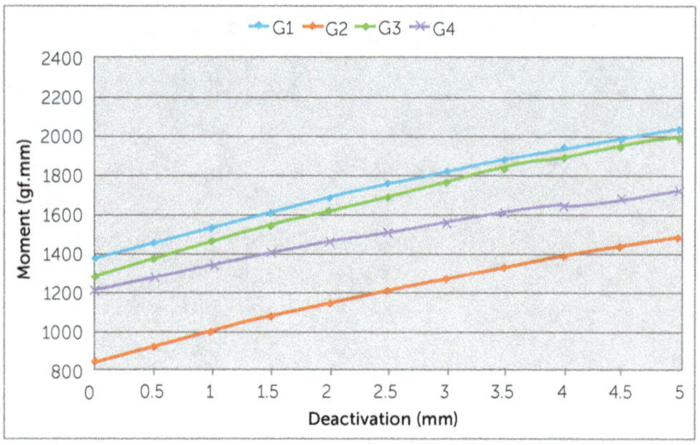

Figure 6 - Moments produced by the β-Ti TLSs over a range of 5 mm of deactivation.

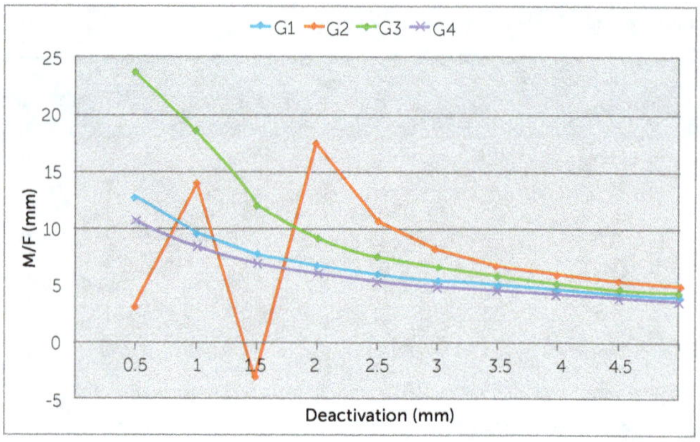

Figure 7 - MF ratio produced by the β-Ti TLSs over a range of 5 mm of deactivation.

Table 5 - Means and standard deviations for YM and ANOVA results over a range of 5 mm of deactivation.

Group	Mean Young's test Modulus (GPa)		SD	Range	p (95%)
1	51.0	ab	1.7	3.9	0.012
2	50.3	ab	2.9	7.3	
3	56.5	b	6.2	14.6	
4	48.1	a	0.7	1.6	

Different letters indicate group differences.

Table 6 - Composition of β-Ti wires used in the study (in % of total composition).

Group	Ti	Mo	Zr	S	Sn	p	Sum (%)
1	68.4	13.6	6.1	4.7	3.4	3.2	99.4
2	72.6	11.3	6.2	4.0	2.9	2.5	99.6
3	68.1	13.0	5.5	5.8	4.0	3.6	100.0
4	69.7	13.3	5.9	4.2	4.0	2.8	100.0

Wire dimensions

Significant differences were found among the sizes of wires (Table 1). Groups 1, 3 and 4 had the same height (0.0165-in) which was larger than the dimension of G2 (0.0161-in). Regarding the width of the wires, G1, G2 and G4 had the same dimensions (0.024-in; 0.024-in; 0.0242-in, respectively), while G3 (0.0244-in) was different from all of them, except for G4.

Mechanical properties

β-Ti wires from G3 showed the highest YM at 56.5 GPa, which was similar to G1 (51.0 GPa) and G2 (50.3 GPa). G4 showed the lowest YM (48.1 GPa), which was different from G3, but similar to G1 and G2 (Table 5).

Chemical composition

The wires from all groups showed similar composition regarding Titanium (Ti), Molybdenum (Mo), Zirconium (Zn), Sulfur (S), Tin (Sn) and Phosphorus (P), except for the wires from G2 which had a higher concentration of Ti and a lower concentration of Mo (Table 6).

DISCUSSION

All groups produced similar force levels at 5 mm of deactivation, except for G2 which showed lower forces. Even though there were differences found in the dimensions of the wires, these differences were small (ranging from 0.0004 to 0.0002) and probably unable to influence the results significantly. The neutral position of the loops is probably the factor that can best explain these differences. The amount of overlap of the vertical extensions of the loops, when in neutral position, may create an over or underactivation of the loop initially, which is the consequence of the shape of pre-activation of the loop.[17,18,21] In this study, however, the groups tested had the same pre-activation shapes, which does not explain the differences found in neutral position. Chemical differences among wires, on the other hand, could influence how each particular brand of β-Ti responds to the bends made to the design of the loop, and could, therefore, play a major role in causing these differences.[3]

All groups had similar composition, except for G2 which showed a higher percentage of Ti and a lower percentage of Mo. Even though this could explain only partially the differences found (G2 produced lower forces initially), it cannot explain why all groups, but G1 and G4, were different among themselves regarding the neutral position. The differences might finally be explained by other factors, such as the manufacturing process, which can alter the wires properties.[3]

Throughout deactivation, the TLSs from all groups acted differently, except for G1 and G4. This result can be substantiated by the differences found in LD rate. These differences can be explained by the design,[9-13] method of pre-activation,[11,12,13,16-18] and chemical composition of the wire[3,19,20] and, finally, by the method of manufacture of the wires.[3] In this study, the design, method of pre-activation and size of the wire were controlled. The similar chemical composition among groups, except for G2, could only partially explain the differences because it does not explain the different behavior of G3. The physical properties of the wires due to the manufacturing process might play a role on the subject, as well as how each beta-titanium wire brand responds to bends in the wire and stress relief, since the tensile test made found similar LD rates (Young's modulus) among all groups.[21,22,24]

The differences found in the moments among groups were similar, as the ones found in the force levels. In this study, the differences among groups were probably due to neutral position and stress relief differences.[21,22,24] This was expected, since the residual moment, or the moment produced by the concentrated bends, is related to the way each wire will behave to those particular bends.[11,12,13,16-18] The effect of bends in the behavior of the wires can be confirmed if data are mathematically adjusted to neutral position, as already shown in the literature, because it can subtract the effect of how the wires respond to bends (Figs 8 and 9).[17,18] This can be done by transposing the x-intercept of each line of the graph to the origin of the graph, along with every point of the line, isolating the effects of horizontal overlapping of the vertical extensions of the TLSs. It can be seen on the charts that the relation of force among groups is very similar to the relation of moments among them, if neutral position is not taken into consideration, and that TLSs behavior is pretty similar among groups.

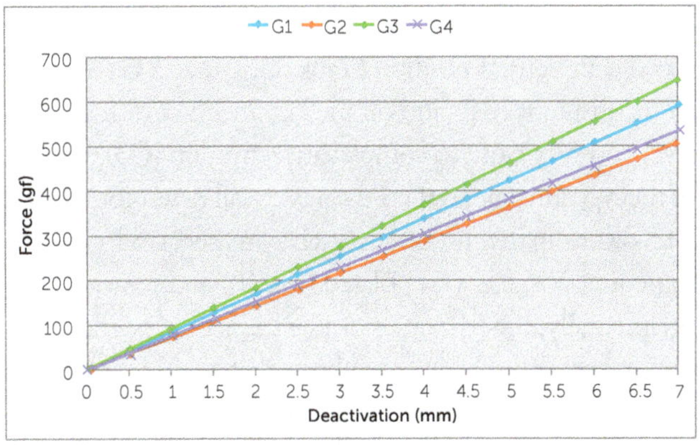

Figure 8 - Figure 4 mathematically adjusted in order to isolate the effect of the overactivation on the force produced by the groups caused by the overlapping of the vertical extensions.

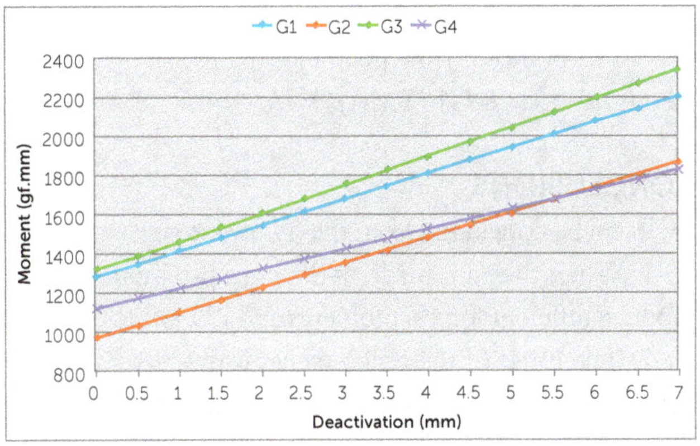

Figure 9 - Figure 6 mathematically adjusted in order to isolate the effect of the overactivation on the moments produced by the groups caused by the overlapping of the vertical extensions.

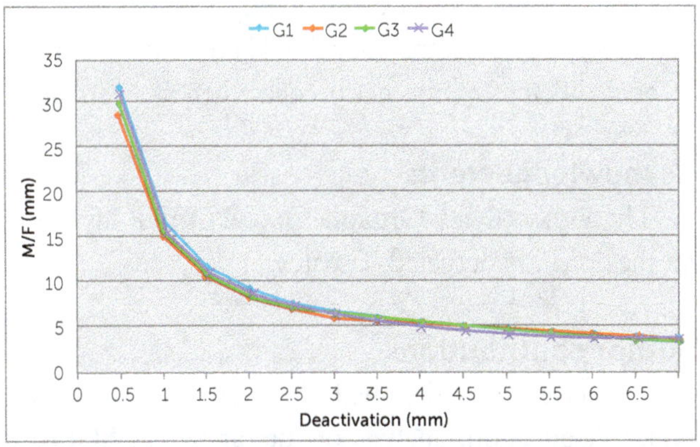

Figure 10 - Figure 7 mathematically adjusted in order to isolate the effect of the overactivation on the MF ratios produced by the groups caused by the overlapping of the vertical extensions The force systems developed by the groups was quite similar.

MF rate significantly varied among groups, since it is a proportion between the already variable force levels and moment levels. The fact that G1 and G4 produced similar

MF rates is consistent with the similar behavior that they showed in neutral position (Table 2). G2 and G3 showed an inconsistent MF ratio on the last 2 mm of deactivation (G2) and very close to complete deactivation (G3) because of their positive neutral position (vertical extensions of the TLSs were apart). If the way each wire behaves in regards to neutral position was isolated (Fig 10) and removed experimentally, the MF ratios of all wires would be the same. Unfortunately, that is something that would not occur clinically. This, however, does not mean that the wires from G2 and G3 should not be used clinically. They can be used, but a different approach is needed when those wires are used in loops. If a TLS is to be used, the clinician should compensate the differences in the overlapping of the vertical extensions of the loop by opening less the inner "ears" of those two wire brands than what is normally recommended for G1 (TMA).[9,22]

CONCLUSIONS

It can be concluded from the TLSs tested:

1. When they are made of different β-Ti wires, TLSs produce different forces, moments and LD ratios.

2. The cause of these differences is the way each wire behaves in relation to bends, thereby producing different shapes in neutral position.

3. Groups 1 (TMA) and 4 (CNA) showed a more consistent MF ratio throughout deactivation.

4. Even though groups 2 (BETA-FLEXY) and 3 (BETA III TIMO) behaved differently from groups 1 and 4, this does not mean that they should not be used clinically, but a different approach is needed when loops are used.

Acknowledgements

The authors thank Orthometric and OrthoOrganizers for the donation of their β-Ti wires for this study.

Author contributions

Conceived and designed the study: RPM, LGV, RHS; Acquisition, analysis or interpretation: SGFRC; Data collection: AAR; Wrote the article: SGFRC, AAR; Critical revision of the article: RPM, LPM; Final approval of the article: LPM; Statistical analysis: SGFRC.

REFERENCES

1. Goldberg J, Burstone CJ. An evaluation of beta titanium alloys for use in orthodontic appliances. J Dent Res. 1979 Feb;58(2):593-99.
2. Verstrynge A, Van Humbeeck J, Willems G. In-vitro evaluation of the material characteristics of stainless steel and beta-titanium orthodontic wires. Am J Orthod Dentofacial Orthop. 2006 Oct;130(4):460-70.
3. Burstone CJ, Goldberg AJ. Beta titanium: a new orthodontic alloy. Am J Orthod. 1980 Feb;77(2):121-32.
4. Goldberg AJ, Burstone CJ. Status report on beta titanium orthodontic wires. Council on Dental Materials, Instruments, and Equipment. J Am Dent Assoc. 1982 Oct;105(4):684-5.
5. Donovan MT, Lin JJ, Brantley WA, Conover JP. Weldability of beta titanium arch wires. Am J Orthod. 1984 Mar;85(3):207-16.
6. Kapila S, Sachdeva R. Mechanical properties and clinical applications of orthodontic wires. Am J Orthod Dentofacial Orthop. 1989 Aug;96(2):100-9.
7. Johnson E. Relative stiffness of beta titanium archwires. Angle Orthod. 2003 Jun;73(3):259-69.
8. Juvvadi SR, Kailasam V, Padmanabhan S, Chitharanjan AB. Physical, mechanical, and flexural properties of 3 orthodontic wires: an in-vitro study. Am J Orthod Dentofacial Orthop. 2010 Nov;138(5):623-30.
9. Burstone CJ, Koenig HA. Optimizing anterior and canine retraction. Am J Orthod. 1976 Jul;70(1):1-19.
10. Chen J, Markham DL, Katona TR. Effects of T-loop geometry on its forces and moments. Angle Orthod. 2000 Feb;70(1):48-51.
11. Faulkner MG, Fuchshuber P, Haberstock D, Mioduchowski A. A parametric study of the force/moment systems produced by T-loop retraction springs. J Biomech. 1989;22(6-7):637-47.
12. Martins RP, Buschang PH, Martins LP, Gandini LG Jr. Optimizing the design of preactivated titanium T-loop springs with Loop software. Am J Orthod Dentofacial Orthop. 2008 Jul;134(1):161-6.
13. Viecilli RF. Self-corrective T-loop design for differential space closure. Am J Orthod Dentofacial Orthop. 2006 Jan;129(1):48-53.
14. Hoenigl KD, Freudenthaler J, Marcotte MR, Bantleon HP. The centered T-loop: a new way of preactivation. Am J Orthod Dentofacial Orthop. 1995 Aug;108(2):149-53.
15. Kuhlberg AJ, Burstone CJ. T-loop position and anchorage control. Am J Orthod Dentofacial Orthop. 1997 Jul;112(1):12-8.
16. Manhartsberger C, Morton JY, Burstone CJ. Space closure in adult patients using the segmented arch technique. Angle Orthod. 1989 Fall;59(3):205-10.
17. Martins RP, Buschang PH, Viecilli R, dos Santos-Pinto A. Curvature versus v-bends in a group B titanium T-loop spring. Angle Orthod. 2008 May;78(3):517-23.
18. Caldas SG, Martins RP, Galvão MR, Vieira CI, Martins LP. Force system evaluation of symmetrical beta-titanium T-loop springs preactivated by curvature and concentrated bends. Am J Orthod Dentofacial Orthop. 2011 Aug;140(2):e53-8.
19. Lim Y, Quick A, Swain M, Herbison P. Temperature effects on the forces, moments and moment to force ratio of nickel-titanium and TMA symmetrical T-loops. Angle Orthod. 2008 Nov;78(6):1035-42.
20. Rose D, Quick A, Swain M, Herbison P. Moment-to-force characteristics of preactivated nickel-titanium and titanium-molybdenum alloy symmetrical T-loops. Am J Orthod Dentofacial Orthop. 2009 Jun;135(6):757-63.
21. Caldas SG, Martins RP, Viecilli RF, Galvão MR, Martins LP. Effects of stress relaxation in beta-titanium orthodontic loops. Am J Orthod Dentofacial Orthop. 2011 Aug;140(2):e85-92.
22. Marcotte M. Biomechanics in Orthodontics. Philadelphia: BC Decker; 1990.
23. World Health Organization. International Organization for Standardization, ISO 15841 dentistry-wires for use in orthodontics. Geneva, Switzerland: World Health Organization; 2006. p. 1-9.
24. Burstone CJ, van Steenbergen E, Hanley KJ. Modern Edgewise Mechanics & the segmented arch technique. Glendora: Ormco; 1995.

16

Does the CO_2 laser reduce bond strength in different types of ceramic brackets?

Fábio Lourenço Romano[1], Giovanna Pessoti[2], Rodrigo Galo[3], Jaciara Miranda Gomes-Silva[4], Marília Pacífico Lucisano[4], Maria Cristina Borsatto[5], Paulo Nelson-Filho[5]

Objective: The aim of this study was to assess *in vitro* the influence of the CO_2 laser and of the type of ceramic bracket on the shear bond strength (SBS) to enamel. **Methods:** A total of 60 enamel test surfaces were obtained from bovine incisors and randomly assigned to two groups, according to the ceramic bracket used: Allure (A); Transcend (T). Each group was divided into 2 subgroups (n = 15): L, laser (10W, 3s); C, no laser, or control. Twenty-four hours after the bonding protocol using Transbond XT, SBS was tested at a crosshead speed of 0.5 mm/min in a universal testing machine. After debonding, the Adhesive Remnant Index (ARI) was evaluated at 10x magnification and compared among the groups. Data were analyzed by one-way ANOVA, Tukey's, Mann-Whitney's and Kruskal-Wallis tests (α = 0.05). **Results:** Mean SBS in MPa were: AL = 0.88 ± 0.84; AC = 12.22 ± 3.45; TL = 12.10 ± 5.11; TC = 17.71 ± 6.16. ARI analysis showed that 73% of the specimens presented the entire adhesive remaining on the tooth surfaces (score 3). TC group presented significantly higher SBS than the other groups. The lased specimens showed significantly lower bond strength than the non-lased groups for both tested brackets. **Conclusion:** CO_2 laser irradiation decreased SBS values of the polycrystalline ceramic brackets, mainly Allure.

Keywords: Carbon dioxide. Dental debonding. Lasers. Orthodontic brackets. Shear strength.

[1] Professor, Universidade de São Paulo, Ribeirão Preto Dental School, Department of Pediatric Clinics, Ribeirão Preto/SP, Brazil.
[2] Dental surgeon, Universidade de São Paulo, Ribeirão Preto Dental School, Ribeirão Preto/SP, Brazil.
[3] Professor, Universidade Federal dos Vales do Jequitinhonha e Mucuri, School of Biological and Health Sciences, Department of Dentistry, Diamantina/MG, Brazil.
[4] Dental surgeon, Universidade de São Paulo, Ribeirão Preto Dental School, Department of Pediatric Clinics, Ribeirão Preto/SP, Brazil.
[5] Full professor, Universidade de São Paulo, Ribeirão Preto Dental School, Department of Pediatric Clinics, Ribeirão Preto/SP, Brazil.

» The authors report no commercial, proprietary or financial interest in the products or companies described in this article.

Fábio Lourenço Romano
Avenida do Café s/n, Monte Alegre, CEP: 14.040-904
Ribeirão Preto/SP, Brasil – E-mail: fabioromano@forp.usp.br

INTRODUCTION

The use of ceramic brackets has become widespread in orthodontic treatments due to the increased number of adult patients seeking care and esthetic appliances.[1] However, compared to conventional metallic brackets, ceramic brackets are more costly, with a questionable clinical performance, since their rigid properties may cause antagonist tooth contact wear. Also, conventional methods for debonding ceramic brackets (pliers and drills) can cause injuries and fractures to the enamel.[2-5] The difficulties for debonding ceramic brackets can be attributed to the high bond strength and to the low fracture strength of ceramics,[5,6] which can lead to iatrogenic enamel damages, bracket fractures and longer clinical chairtime.[1-6]

Therefore, several techniques were suggested for debonding of ceramic brackets, such as electrothermal devices,[7] ultrasound,[8] solvents[9] and recently the lasers.[5,10-17] The use of electrothermal devices has been an effective method in debonding ceramic brackets, however, due to irreversible heating damages to the pulp, this device lost popularity among the clinicians.[7]

The laser debonding technique is based on controlled thermal softening of the adhesive resin that leads to adhesion strength degradation. Studies have shown no pulp damage when debonding brackets with a laser device.[5,10,11,18]

In this way, despite the good results obtained with different types of lasers, carbon dioxide (CO_2) laser has been considered the best choice for removing ceramic brackets, due to the high absorption of its wavelength in ceramic surfaces.[14,15]

There are several variables in the studies concerning ceramic bracket removal by lasers, such as: laser settings, type of brackets and bonding agents, as well as the employed methodology. Therefore, in view of the increased use of ceramic brackets in orthodontic patients and the improvements in laser technology and adhesive dentistry in dental practice, the aim of the current investigation was to assess *in vitro* the influence of CO_2 laser use and of the type of ceramic bracket on the shear bond strength (SBS) to enamel. The null hypothesis tested was that the CO_2 laser irradiation does not decrease SBS values of the evaluated polycrystalline ceramic brackets.

MATERIAL AND METHODS

This study had no need to be submitted to an ethics committee in animal experimentation, since the samples were product of commercial slaughter of animal.

Recently extracted sound bovine permanent mandibular incisors were immersed in 0.1% thymol solution at 4 °C for 1 week. Prior to use, the teeth were hand scaled, cleaned with pumice-water slurry using Robinson bristle brushes in a low-speed handpiece and examined with a stereomicroscope (Nikon Inc. Instrument Group, Melville, NY, USA) at 10x magnification to discard those with cracks, fractures or structural abnormalities that could interfere in the results. Sixty bovine teeth were selected, thoroughly washed in running water to eliminate storage solution traces, and maintained in distilled water at 4°C. The samples followed the ISO TR11405[19] instructions, that recommend 15 teeth per group for shear bond strength tests.

The crowns were embedded in chemically activated acrylic resin (Jet Clássico, São Paulo/SP, Brazil) and after resin polymerization, the buccal enamel surfaces were flattened with #400- to #1200-grit silicon carbide (SiC) papers (Buehler Ltd., Lake Bluff, IL, USA) in a low-speed polishing machine (Politriz DP-9U2; Struers, A/S, Copenhagen, Denmark) in order to obtain the test sites that, for standardization, were demarcated by attaching a piece of insulating tape with a central square (5 x 5 mm) on each surface. Next, the roots were embedded in chemically activated acrylic resin (Jet Clássico, São Paulo/SP, Brazil) using polyvinyl chloride rings (2.1 cm diameter and 1.1 cm high) in order to facilitate the laser irradiation and the SBS test immediately after.

The 60 enamel test surfaces were randomly assigned to two groups (n = 30), according to the used polycrystalline ceramic bracket: A) Allure (GAC, New York, NY, USA), and T) Transcend (3M Unitek, Monrovia, CA, USA).

Prior to the bracket bonding protocol, the test surfaces were cleaned by rubber cup/pumice prophylaxis for 10 s, rinsed and dried for the same time with an oil-free air stream. Next, the enamel surfaces were etched with 37% phosphoric acid gel (ScotchBond etchant, 3M/ESPE, St. Paul, MN, USA) for 15 s, rinsed thoroughly for 15 s, dried with a mild, oil-free air stream to obtain a uniformly white, opaque, chalk-like appearance. Transbond XT primer (3M Unitek, Monrovia,

CA, USA) was applied to the acid etched enamel bonding site in a uniform layer, slightly thinned with a mild, oil-free air stream.

The ceramic brackets for lower central incisor were bonded to the center of the specimens using Transbond XT composite (3M Unitek, Monrovia, CA, USA) according to the manufacturer's recommendations. All bonding procedures were performed by the same operator, who used a pair of pliers (Ortoply, Philadelphia, PA, USA), and the excess of material was removed with a sharp explorer (Duflex, Juiz de Fora/MG, Brazil). Each bracket bonding was photoactivated at a 1 mm distance between the bracket base and the light-curing device for 40 s (10 s for each side of the bracket) with a visible light curing unit (XL 1500; 3M/ESPE, St. Paul, MN, USA) with a 450 mW/cm^2 output power. Light intensity of each device was measured prior to each photo-activation cycle using a curing radiometer (Demetron, Danbury, CT, USA). Then the specimens were randomly divided into two subgroups (n = 15): Laser (L) and No Laser, or control (C). The specimens were stored in distilled water at 37 °C for 24 h.

Immediately before the SBS test, the samples in the laser group were irradiated. The equipment used for CO_2 laser irradiation was a UM-L30 device (Shangai-Jue Hua Technology Development Shangai, PR China) emitting at 10.6 μm wavelength. The laser beam was delivered in non-contact mode. The laser tip was held perpendicularly at a 4-mm distance from the bracket surface and the light was delivered in focused mode. The parameter settings were 10 W for 3s. The laser operated at ultra-pulse mode with pulse duration of 100 μs (interval time: 0,01s). The time delay between laser irradiation and force application was up to 3s[17].

The SBS was tested to failure using a knife-edge blade in a universal testing machine (Model DL 500, EMIC Ltda., São José dos Pinhais/PR, Brazil) running at a crosshead speed of 0.5 mm/min with a 50 kgf load cell (Fig 1).

Mean SBS values (in MPa) and standard deviations were calculated and data were analyzed statistically by one-way ANOVA. Tukey's test was used for multiple comparisons at 5% significance level.

The debonded specimens were observed with a 10x stereomicroscope (Carl Zeiss, Goettingen, Germany) by an calibrated and experienced examiner, in order to assess the amount of resin material adhered to enamel after bracket removal, which were classified according to the Adhesive Remnant Index (ARI) scores established by Artun and Bergland:[20] 0 = no adhesive remaining adhered to enamel; 1 = less than half of the adhesive remaining adhered to enamel; 2 = more than half of the adhesive remaining adhered to enamel; 3 = all the adhesive remaining adhered to enamel. All examinations were done by a single examiner blinded to the groups to which the specimens belonged. The ARI scores data were statistically analyzed by the Kruskal-Wallis test and Mann-Whitney complementary test, at a significance level of 5%.

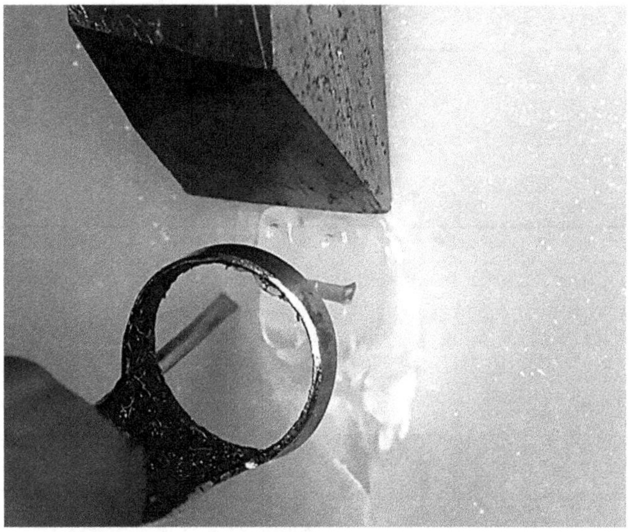

Figure 1 - Specimen with the active chisel tip acting on the upper part of the bracket base during the shear bond strength test.

RESULTS

SBS means (in MPa), standard deviation, and statistical analysis are presented in Table 1. Group TC presented the highest and group AL present the lowest SBS values of all groups ($p < 0.05$), respectively. There was no statistically significant difference between groups AC and TL. Nevertheless, the SBS values were statistically lower in the CO_2 laser irradiated specimens for both Allure and Transcend tested ceramic brackets.

Statistically significant difference ($p < 0.05$) was found in the ARI scores among the four groups. ARI scores are illustrated in Figure 2. According to the results, 73% of the specimens presented ARI score 3, indicating that bond failure occurred predominantly at the bracket–adhesive interface, leaving most of the adhesive on the enamel surface. ARI score 0 was only observed in one specimen of TL group.

Table 1 - Comparison of shear bond strength means values (MPa).

Groups	n	Mean (SD)	Tukey's test*
AC	15	12.22 (3.45)	a
AL	15	0.88 (0.84)	b
TC	15	17.71 (6.16)	c
TL	15	12.10 (5.11)	a

* Same letters indicate no statistically significant difference.
AC = Allure Control; AL = Allure Laser; TC = Transcend Control; TL = Transcend Laser.

Table 2 - Comparison of ARI scores by p values (Mann-Whitney test).

Groups	AC	AL	TC	TL
AC	--------------	0.029*	0.011*	0.000*
AL	0.029*	----------------	0.000*	0.000*
TC	0.011*	0.000*	----------------	0.000*
TL	0.000*	0.000*	0.000*	----------------

*Changes are significant at $p < 0.05$.

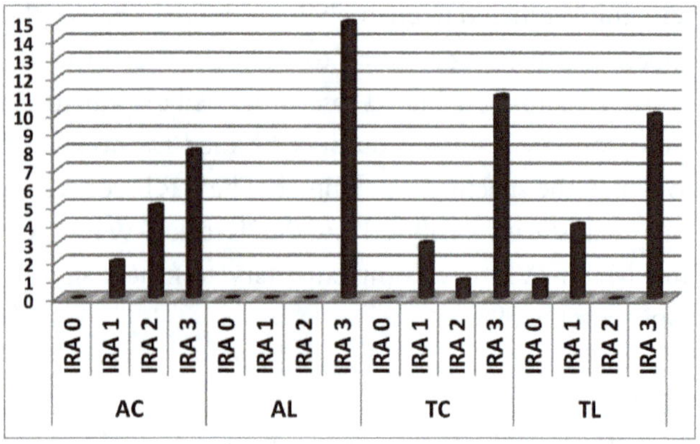

Figure 2 - ARI scores after bracket debonding.

DISCUSSION

Recently, Orthodontics experienced a great scientific advance regarding the improvement of materials and techniques, allowing more esthetic treatments. Ceramic brackets offer esthetics, durability and better color stability. Nevertheless, enamel cracks and fractures or bracket breakage due to the brittleness, low ductility, high elastic modulus and high adhesion strength to teeth of ceramics have been observed in the conventional debonding of these appliances.[1,3]

According to some authors, laser debonding of ceramic brackets eliminates damages to enamel by reducing the required force to remove it.[13,14,18,21] The lasers act softening the adhesive bonding agent by heat conductivity.[11,21] Saito et al.[22] concluded that ceramic bracket debonding with CO_2 laser, when adhesives containing thermal expansion microcapsules are used, can be an effective and safe method. CO_2 laser has been considered the favorite laser device for debonding ceramic brackets since its wavelength is more easily absorbed by these brackets.[14,15] In the present research, the CO_2 laser irradiation decreased the force required to remove the polycrystalline ceramic brackets.

Studies have reported no pulp or enamel tissue injuries and also a decreased debonding force and operation time with CO_2 laser.[11,15] Lijima et al.[10] have observed that the hardness and elastic modulus of enamel are not affected by CO_2 laser irradiation. Nevertheless, the workable laser parameters are directly related to the lasers' ability to soften the adhesive resin without adversely affecting tooth tissues.

The laser settings applied (10W/3s) in this study were based on the findings of a previous investigation done by this research group, in which these CO_2 laser parameters did not increase the intrapulpal temperature above the pulp physiologic tolerance.[17] The employed ultra-pulse CO_2 laser can provide short pulses with sufficient time to permit tooth tissues to cool down between pulses.[15] Obata et al.[11] have shown that CO_2 laser at 3W/3s are safe settings when debonding brackets, while other authors[23] reported that CO_2 laser irradiation at 50w for 2s increased 0.70°C in pulp chamber temperatures. Yassaeiet al.[5] found a 1.46°C increase in intrapulpal temperature after diode laser irradiation at 2.5 W for 10 s.

As regards as the type of bracket, ceramic brackets are constituted by alumina and are monocrystalline (sapphire) or polycrystalline structures. The monocrystalline ceramic brackets show greater strength, but the fracture resistance is generally below that of the polycrystalline brackets.[24,25] Also, monocrystalline brackets require lower laser energy for debonding than the polycrystalline brackets[21] since polycrystalline units do not allow high transmissibility, thus increasing energy loss.[26] Thus, in the present study, polycrystalline brackets were used and higher values of SBS were observed for the Transcend ceramic brackets, which might be attributed to differences in the base design, structure, and composition of the tested brackets. Perhaps if other laser parameters were used, different SBS values would be reported.

Under clinical conditions, adequate bracket bond strength values might be between 6 to 8 MPa in order to prevent risk of tooth damages at debonding.[27] However, the force required to remove ceramic brackets can reach values of 20MPa, which might cause tooth or bracket fractures by exceeding the cohesive strength of the enamel or the bracket.[2,3,27] Confirming these facts, in this study, Transcend ceramic bracket reached a SBS mean of 17.71 MPa, which is much higher than the ideal bracket bond strength value.

Additionally, even though the laser decreased the ceramic brackets bond strength, only for the Allure group this reduction (93%) reached clinically applicable values for debonding (0.88 MPa). The Transcend lased group showed a reduction in 68%, but SBS values (12.10 MPa) were still near the limit of force (11.1 MPa) that can cause tooth fractures at debonding.[28] In the different treatments (with laser or without laser), the adhesion of Transcend ceramic brackets were higher than Allure. However, significant reduction in the adhesion with both brackets was observed when laser was applied.

Ma et al.[18] have observed that specimens debonded with CO_2 laser (18W/2s) were only 25% (1.48 MPa) of the mean of the non-lased group. Other authors[10] reported that CO_2 laser irradiated specimens showed a 31% decrease in SBS, if they were bonded with a conventional etch and rinse adhesive system, and a 25% decrease with a self-etching adhesive system, compared with control (non-irradiated) specimens. However, these studies tested other materials and techniques.

Concerning ARI scores, the fractures after bracket debonding occurred predominantly at the bracket/resin interface (73%, score 3), which reduces the risk of bracket or tooth damages.[29] ARI scores 1 and 2 occurred as the SBS increased and score 0 was observed only in one TL group specimen, situation in which cracking of the enamel is more probable.[28] These findings suggest that, in addition to softening, the adhesive resin might have undergone thermal ablation and photoablation, resulting in vaporization and decomposition of the material.[1] The high percentage of score 3 (all composite remain after debonding) indicated that laser irradiation didn't cause injuries or fractures in the enamel surface, preserving the dental structure (Fig 2). In groups 1, 3 and 4, this score was predominant and in group 2, all sample obtained this same result. These results are promising, and probably during laser irradiation procedure a slight softening of the composite occurred, without heating the tooth.

In view of the above considerations and based on findings of the current investigation, the CO_2 laser has been noted as a promising technology in debonding ceramic brackets, mainly for the Allure, since it was observed a greater adhesive remnant index on the tooth surface together with decreased SBS values.

There is still much to be investigated concerning specific laser parameters for the adhesive resins and ceramic brackets available for orthodontic treatment, in order to justify the use of such protocols in clinical orthodontic practice. As regards time saving, lower complexity of treatment, decreased damages to tooth structures and discomfort, the use of lasers for debonding esthetic ceramic brackets has a significant advantage over the traditional method. The lack of reported studies testing the same methodology and materials used in the present study did not allow a reliable comparison with the outcomes of previous researches.

CONCLUSION

The null hypothesis was rejected. The CO_2 laser irradiation decreased the adhesion of the ceramic brackets and enhanced brackets debonding.

Acknowledgements

The authors would like to thank the National Council for Research - CNPq (#11.1.754.58.0) for the research grant and financial support.

Authors contribution

Conception or design of the study: FLR, MCB, PNF. Data acquisition, analysis or interpretation: GP, MPL, RG. Writing the article: FLR, JMGS. Critical revision of the article: FLR, PNF. Final approval of the article: FLR. Obtained funding: GP.

REFERENCES

1. Azzeh E, Feldon PJ. Laser debonding of ceramic brackets: a comprehensive review. Am J Orthod Dentofacial Orthop. 2003 Jan;123(1):79-83.
2. Jena AK, Duggal R, Mehrotra AK. Physical properties and clinical characteristics of ceramic brackets: a comprehensive review. Trends Biomater Artif Organs. 2007;20:201-19.
3. Jeiroudi MT. Enamel fracture caused by ceramic brackets. Am J Orthod Dentofacial Orthop. 1991 Feb;99(2):97-9.
4. Bishara SE, Fonseca JM, Boyer DB. The use of debonding pliers in the removal of ceramic brackets: force levels and enamel cracks. Am J Orthod Dentofacial Orthop. 1995 Sept;108(3):242-8.
5. Yassaei S, Soleimanian A, Nik ZE. Effects of diode laser debonding of ceramic brackets on enamel surface and pulpal temperature. J Contemp Dent Pract. 2015 Apr 1;16(4):270-4.
6. Scott GE Jr. Fracture toughness and surface cracks--the key to understanding ceramic brackets. Angle Orthod. 1988 Jan;58(1):5-8.
7. Dovgan JS, Walton RE, Bishara SE. Electrothermal debracketing: patient acceptance and effects on the dental pulp. Am J Orthod Dentofacial Orthop. 1995 Sept;108(3):249-55.
8. Boyer DB, Engelhardt G, Bishara SE. Debonding orthodontic ceramic brackets by ultrasonic instrumentation. Am J Orthod Dentofacial Orthop. 1995 Sept;108(3):262-6.
9. Larmour CJ, McCabe JF, Gordon PH. An ex vivo investigation into the effects of chemical solvents on the debond behaviour of ceramic orthodontic brackets. Br J Orthod. 1998 Feb;25(1):35-9.
10. Iijima M, Yasuda Y, Muguruma T, Mizoguchi I. Effects of CO(2) laser debonding of a ceramic bracket on the mechanical properties of enamel. Angle Orthod. 2010 Nov;80(6):1029-35.
11. Obata A, Tsumura T, Niwa K, Ashizawa Y, Deguchi T, Ito M. Super pulse CO2 laser for bracket bonding and debonding. Eur J Orthod. 1999 Apr;21(2):193-8.
12. Sarp AS, Gülsoy M. Ceramic bracket debonding with ytterbium fiber laser. Lasers Med Sci. 2011 Sept;26(5):577-84.
13. Oztoprak MO, Nalbantgil D, Erdem AS, Tozlu M, Arun T. Debonding of ceramic brackets by a new scanning laser method. Am J Orthod Dentofacial Orthop. 2010 Aug;138(2):195-200.
14. Tehranchi A, Fekrazad R, Zafar M, Eslami B, Kalhori KA, Gutknecht N. Evaluation of the effects of CO2 laser on debonding of orthodontics porcelain brackets vs. the conventional method. Lasers Med Sci. 2011 Sept;26(5):563-7.
15. Ahrari F, Heravi F, Fekrazad R, Farzanegan F, Nakhaei S. Does ultra-pulse CO(2) laser reduce the risk of enamel damage during debonding of ceramic brackets? Lasers Med Sci. 2012 May;27(3):567-74.
16. Tozlu M, Ostoprak MO, Arun T. Comparison of shear bond strengths of ceramic brackets aftediferente times lags between lasing and debonding. Lasers Med Sci. 2012 Nov;27(6):1151-5.
17. Macri RT, Lima FA, Bachmann L, Galo R, Romano FL, Borsatto MC, et al. CO2 laser as auxiliary in the debonding of ceramic brackets. Lasers Med Sci. 2015 Sept;30(7):1835-41.
18. Ma T, Marangoni RD, Flint W. In vitro comparison of debonding force and intrapulpal temperature changes during ceramic orthodontic bracket removal using a carbon dioxide laser. Am J Orthod Dentofacial Orthop. 1997 Feb;111(2):203-10.
19. International Organization for Standardization. Guidance on testing of adhesion to tooth structure. ISSO/TC106/SC 1 N236, Resolution 61. CD TR 11405, Trieste, Oct 1994.
20. Artun J, Bergland S. Clinical trials with crystal growth conditioning as an alternative to acid-etch enamel pretreatment. Am J Orthod. 1984 Apr;85(4):333-40.
21. Strobl K, Bahns TL, Willham L, Bishara SE, Stwalley WC. Laser-aided debonding of orthodontic ceramic brackets. Am J Orthod Dentofacial Orthop. 1992 Feb;101(2):152-8.
22. Saito A, Namura Y, Isokawa K, Shimizu N. CO2 laser debonding of a ceramic bracket bonded with orthodontic adhesive containing thermal expansion microcapsules. Lasers Med Sci. 2015 Feb;30(2):869-74.
23. Abdul-Kader HM, Ibrahim AS. A comparative study of CO2 laser debonding of three types of ceramic brackets. J Dent Sci. 1999;2:79-84.
24. Mimura H, Deguchi T, Obata A, Yamagishi T, Ito M. Comparison of different bonding materials for laser debonding. Am J Orthod Dentofacial Orthop. 1995 Sept;108(3):267-73.
25. Flores DA, Caruso JM, Scott GE, Jeiroudi MT. The fracture strength of ceramic brackets: a comparative study. Angle Orthod. 1990 Winter;60(4):269-76.
26. Eliades T, Johnston WM, Eliades G. Direct light transmittance through ceramic brackets. Am J Orthod Dentofacial Orthop. 1995 Jan;107(1):11-9.
27. Reynolds I. A review of direct orthodontic bonding. Br J Orthod. 1975;2(3):71-8.
28. Bishara SE, Fehr DE, Jakobsen JR. A comparative study of the debonding strengths of different ceramic brackets, enamel conditioners, and adhesives. Am J Orthod Dentofacial Orthop. 1993 Aug;104(2):170-9.
29. Nalbantgil D, Oztoprak MO, Tozlu M, Arun T. Effects of different application durations of ER:YAG laser on intrapulpal temperature change during debonding. Lasers Med Sci. 2011 Nov;26(6):735-40.

17

A comparative clinical study of the failure rate of orthodontic brackets bonded with two adhesive systems: Conventional and Self-Etching Primer (SEP)

Gladys Cristina Dominguez[1], André Tortamano[2], Luiz Vicente de Moura Lopes[3], Priscilla Campanatti Chibebe Catharino[4], Camillo Morea[5]

Objective: This study compared the clinical performance of orthodontic brackets bonded with Transbond adhesive paste after two priming systems: a two-stage conventional system (acid etching + Transbond XT adhesive primer) and a single-stage self-etching primer (SEP) (Transbond Plus). **Methods:** The sample comprised 480 metal brackets bonded to the teeth of 24 consecutive patients treated for 36 to 48 months. A split-mouth design was used for bonding, and both systems were used in each patient. Bracket failure rates for each system were analyzed; and failure causes as reported by the patients and the quadrant of teeth for which brackets failed were recorded. **Results:** The conventional system group had a failure rate of 5.41%, whereas the rate for SEP was 4.58%. In this group, there were 5 failures (38.4%) in the right maxillary quadrant, 2 (15.4%) in the left maxillary quadrant, 4 (30.8%) in the right mandibular quadrant, and 2 (15.4%) in the left mandibular quadrant. In the SEP group, there were 4 (36.4%) failures in the right maxillary quadrant, 1 (9%) in the left maxillary quadrant, 3 (27.3%) in the right mandibular quadrant, and 3 (27.3%) in the left mandibular quadrant. Results of descriptive statistical analysis and odds ratio did not show any significant differences between rates (p = 0.67). **Conclusion:** The clinical efficiency of SEP was similar to that of the conventional system.

Keywords: Orthodontic brackets. Bonding. Dental adhesive.

[1] Associate Professor, Department of Orthodontics and Pediatric Dentistry, School of Dentistry, São Paulo University (FOUSP), São Paulo, Brazil.
[2] Professor, PhD, Department of Orthodontics and Pediatric Dentistry, FOUSP, São Paulo, Brazil.
[3] PhD student, Department of Orthodontics, FOUSP, São Paulo, Brazil.
[4] MSc student, Department of Orthodontics, FOUSP, São Paulo, Brazil.
[5] Post-doctor in Orthodontics, USP.

» The author reports no commercial, proprietary or financial interest in the products or companies described in this article.

Luiz Vicente de Moura Lopes
Av. Prof. Lineu Prestes, 2227 – Cidade Universitária – São Paulo/SP, Brazil
CEP: 05.508-000 – E-mail: luizvicentelopes@me.com

INTRODUCTION

The sixth generation of adhesive systems, called self-etching primers (SEP), reduced the number of bonding stages because it eliminated the need to apply phosphoric acid and, consequently, reduced clinical time and the risk of contamination. However, Transbond Plus SEP (3M Unitek, Monrovia, CA) has a more conservative pattern and produces a smaller amount of demineralization and less penetration into the enamel surface than phosphoric acid (37%).[1]

Dominguez-Rodriguez et al conducted a series of studies from 2002 to 2004 to evaluate the reliability of this SEP system. In an *in vitro* study to evaluate resistance to traction,[2] brackets were bonded to human premolars extracted for orthodontic reasons. Mean resistance to traction was 6.25 ± 1.61 MPa, practically the same optimal values recommended in the literature[3,4] (6 MPa).Their next *in vitro* study of bonding to extracted human premolars compared SEP resistance to traction with that of a conventional system using Victory (3M Unitek, Monrovia, CA) metal brackets and the adhesive pre-coated (APC) system.[5] Mean values were 8.1 ± 2.7 MPa in the SEP group, and 10.3 ± 3.2 MPa for the conventional system, similar to those found by Grubisa et al[6] in another comparative study: 7.7 ± 4.2 MPa for SEP and 9.8 ± 4.2 MPa for the conventional system.

These findings suggested that the clinical applicability of SEP should be confirmed in clinical trials. A study to measure the frequency of metal bracket failure during orthodontic treatment included 278 teeth of 17 patients.[7] All brackets were bonded using a SEP system. Patients were followed up for 30 months, and results showed a bracket failure rate of 5.8% for all the teeth included in the analysis. Failure causes were associated with excessive application of force and with biting food that should have been excluded from regular diet according to initial instructions, such as candy and lollypops.

Reis et al,[8] who followed up 30 patients for 18 months, found a failure rate of 15.6% for SEP and 17.6% for the conventional system, a difference that was not statistically significant. Pandis et al[9] conducted a study to compare SEP with the Orthosolo and Enlight conventional systems in 62 patients for 12 months and found that the risk of failure in the SEP group was not any greater than in the conventional system group.

Elekdag-Turk et al,[10] in 2008, compared failure rates between SEP and the conventional adhesive systems. They followed up patients for 6 months and reported that there were no significant differences between the adhesive systems under study and that both had a failure rate of 0.6%. In another study, the same authors[11] compared the failure rates of self-ligating brackets bonded with either SEP or a conventional adhesive system. They followed up patients for 12 months and reported that there was a significant difference between the two systems, as the SEP group had a rate of 4.7%, whereas the rate for the conventional system was 1.7%.

Santos et al[12] conducted a study with a 6-month follow-up; they found that failures were associated with the adhesive-enamel interface, and that failure rates for SEP and the conventional system were 10.6% and 7.4%. In the same way, Murfitt et al[13] recorded bracket failure rates for 12 months and found a significantly greater rate for teeth to which brackets had been bonded with SEP (11.2%) rather than the conventional adhesive system (3.9%).

In a recent study, Paschos et al[14] compared different SEP adhesive systems: Transbond Plus (3M Unitek, Germany) and Clearfil Protect Bond (Kuraray Medical, Japan). They included 480 brackets in their study and, after a 12-month follow-up, found a failure rate of 5.4% (26 brackets), which was significantly greater than that found for brackets bonded with Clearfil Protect Bond (4.4%).

This clinical study used the split-mouth bonding design to evaluate bracket failure rates in individuals that underwent full orthodontic treatment for 36 to 48 months using the conventional system with acid etching (37% phosphoric acid) together with the Transbond XT adhesive (3M Unitek, Monrovia, CA) and the Transbond Plus SEP (3M Unitek, Monrovia, CA).

MATERIAL AND METHODS

The sample comprised 480 metal brackets (Victory) bonded to the teeth of 24 consecutive patients that were treated in the MBT Orthodontic Treatment Clinic of São Paulo University. No patient had received previous orthodontic treatment. After diagnosis and treatment plan, patients were treated with extraction of the four first premolars.

The split-mouth design was used for bracket bonding, and was divided into groups randomly. Patient dentition was divided into four quadrants, and one adhesive system was used in the right maxillary and left mandibular quadrants, and the other, in the left maxillary and right mandibular quadrants. In one group, 240 teeth underwent etching and priming using the two-stage conventional method: Acid etching with 37% phosphoric acid and bonding with Transbond XT adhesive paste. The other 240 teeth were primed using the Transbond Plus SEP (3M Unitek, Monrovia, CA). After that, all brackets were bonded using the Transbond XT resin.

The same bracket bonding protocol was strictly followed for each patient. First, prophylaxis was performed with rubber cup, pumice and water spray using a low-speed handpiece, and then teeth were rinsed with water. The place where to bond the brackets was defined according to the tables of the MBT treatment system and marked with a lead pencil on the buccal surface of the teeth. After that, the field was isolated using cheek retractors, and the actual process of bonding the brackets started.

In the quadrants chosen for the Transbond Plus SEP system, application followed the manufacturer's instructions: 1) contents of the first two reservoirs were squeezed into the third; 2) a micro brush was used to mix and apply the liquid to the enamel surface in circular movements while applying some pressure for three seconds; 3) excessive liquid was removed with a gentle air burst to leave a thinner liquid layer on the enamel. After that, direct bonding was performed. A thin layer of Transbond XT resin was applied to the base of each bracket. After removing excess resin, a halogen light was used for curing for 40 seconds (10 s for each surface).

In the contralateral quadrants chosen for conventional bonding, the field was isolated, teeth underwent acid etching (37% phosphoric acid; Dentsply) for 20 seconds, rinsing for 5 seconds per tooth, and drying for 10 seconds. A thin layer of Transbond XT adhesive primer was then applied to the surface of the tooth using a micro brush. The procedures to dispense resin onto the bracket base and directly bond the brackets were the same as those for bonding in the contralateral quadrant, which used the SEP system.

The leveling phase started on the same day. Patients received routine instructions about appliance cleaning and care, particularly about foods and habits that may damage the appliance.

Bracket failures were controlled and their causes and corresponding tooth were recorded during all treatments, which ranged from 36 to 48 months.

Statistical analysis

Descriptive statistics was used to analyze the number of bracket failures per individual, what bonding system was used in maxilla and mandible, failure causes and their percentages, and mean time between bonding and failure in months. The values obtained for bracket failure were compared (odds ratio – 0.839; $p = 0.676$).

RESULTS

The results are presented in Table 1 to 5.

DISCUSSION

Bracket failure rates were compared for the conventional and the SEP bonding systems. Orthodontic treatments with extraction of the maxillary and mandibular first premolars in 24 consecutive patients were evaluated during the different treatment phases: Leveling, alignment, space closure and finishing. Several factors were taken into consideration: Whether the tooth was in the maxilla or mandible; the quadrant (right and left); the type of tooth (incisor, canine, premolar and molar); failure causes; and mean time between bonding and failure.

Efficient bracket bonding and low failure rates are important factors in orthodontic treatments. As a complete orthodontic treatment may last from 24 to 48 months, bonding efficiency of the two systems under study was evaluated during all the treatments, which ranged from 36 to 48 months.

A split-mouth design for bonding was used to compare the two systems in each patient. This randomized method ensures that, of each 10 brackets bonded consecutively, 5 will be bonded using the conventional system in the maxillary right quadrant and 5 will use the SEP in the maxillary left quadrant. The same bonding system is used in contralateral quadrants so that, together with different bonding systems, analyses may include eating habits and individual mastication forces for each patient.[12,13]

Tables 1 and 2 show that the distribution of failure was similar in the maxilla and mandible for both

Table 1 - Number of failures according to tooth and bonding system in the upper arch.

Tooth	Right quadrant		Left quadrant	
	SEP	Conventional	SEP	Conventional
Incisors	0	2	0	0
Canines	1	0	0	0
Premolars	2	2	0	2
2nd molars	1	1	1	0
Total	4	5	1	2

Table 2 - Number of failures according to tooth and bonding system in the lower arch.

Tooth	Right quadrant		Left quadrant	
	SEP	Conventional	SEP	Conventional
Incisors	0	2	0	0
Canines	1	1	0	1
Premolars	0	1	1	1
2nd molars	2	0	2	0
Total	3	4	3	2

Table 3 - Total number of bracket failures according to bonding system.

Quadrant	SEP	Conventional
Right maxillary	4	5
Left maxillary	1	2
Right mandibular	3	4
Left mandibular	3	2
Total	11	13
% of failures	4.58	5.41

Table 4 - Cause of bracket failure (number and percentage of failures).

Failure cause	SEP	Conventional
Biting candy	3 (27.3%)	4 (30.7%)
Biting olive	1 (9%)	1 (7.7%)
Trauma	2 (18.2%)	0
Diet in general	5 (45.5%)	8 (61.6%)

Table 5 - Mean time between bonding and failure (months).

Teeth	Upper arch				Lower arch			
	Right quadrant		Left quadrant		Right quadrant		Left quadrant	
	SEP	Conventional	SEP	Conventional	SEP	Conventional	SEP	Conventional
Incisors	0	9.5	0	0	0	5	0	0
Canines	1	0	0	0	24	2	0	6
Premolars	1	1	0	2	0	2	36	2
2nd molars	3	1	11	0	1	0	1.5	0

SEP (maxilla = 5; mandible = 6) and conventional (maxilla = 7; mandible = 6) systems. Studies in the literature, as well as this study, found a nonsignificant difference in bracket failure rates between the two arches. There were 12 failures in the maxilla and 12 in the mandible, which confirmed equal rates.

The comparison of right and left quadrants in the maxilla and in the mandible revealed that there were 16 failures in the right quadrant (SEP = 7; conventional = 9) and 8 in the left quadrant (SEP = 4; conventional = 4). One possible explanation for that might be the patients' masticatory habits.[9] *In vivo* studies should take into consideration factors that might be associated with failure rates, such as patient socioeconomic status, malocclusion classification and type of mechanics used during treatment. Moreover, masticatory forces vary according to facial patterns, and diet is associated with cultural factors.[8,11]

The number of times the bracket is handled during bonding should also be evaluated in the analysis of bracket failures. Brackets handled more than three times when a SEP system is used have twice as many chances of failure than those bonded with a conventional bonding system.[13]

Several authors conducted shorter studies to compare SEP and conventional systems, from 6 to 12 or 18 months.[8-14] Our follow-up lasted longer, from 36 to 48 months.

Some authors found that the failure rate for SEP ranged from 0.6%10 to 15.6%[8] and that the SEP performance was equal to or better than that of conventional systems. Of the 240 brackets bonded with each of the two bonding systems, 11 in the SEP group and 13 in the conventional system group failed, which indicates failure rates of 4.58% and 5.41% (Table 3). Odds ratio results showed that there were no significant differences between these values, in agreement with most reports in the literature,[9,10,11,12] but different from studies that found greater failure rates for brackets bonded with SEP than for those bonded with conventional systems.[13,15] The fact that numbers and percentages are very close suggests that both the SEP and the conventional systems are equally efficacious.

Most failures occurred in premolars, at 9 failures, followed by molars, with 7, and the least failures were seen in incisors and canines, at 4 failures each (Tables 1 and 2). These findings are in agreement with studies that reported a three times greater rate for posterior teeth than for anterior teeth.[11,13,16,17] The fact that premolars are the teeth with the highest rate may be explained as a result of several factors: Lower risk of contamination by humidity in the anterior region during bonding; occlusal forces that exceed the limits of adhesive resistance of the brackets; greater amount of prismless enamel, which may affect the quality of micromechanical bonding and result in poor adhesion; and the difficulty to isolate the posterior region.[7]

Mean time between bonding and bracket failure (Table 5) showed great variation and ranged from 1 to 36 months. Despite that, most failures occurred in the first 6 months of treatment, and only four means indicated longer times. Two of these four cases were assigned to the sum of one failure in the beginning of the treatment and one at the end of it. The other two high means represented failures at the end of the treatment. The fact that most failures occurred in the first 6 months may be assigned to one of three causes. First, any problem during bonding becomes evident in the beginning of the treatment. Second, the initial period of the treatment is a time for adaptation of the patient to the diet. Finally, there may be excessive occlusal forces during the initial stage of treatment.[8,11] Some authors have reported a failure rate of up to 82% during this time.[10]

Other studies confirmed the efficacy of SEP systems during the first 6 months of treatment when compared with conventional systems.[8] After a longer treatment time, the difference between failure rates for the two bonding systems may become imperceptible. This is explained by the hydrophilic component of the monomer, which leads to increased water absorption and may weaken the adhesive-bracket interface along time. This was confirmed in our study, because mean time between bonding and bracket failure was greater when the SEP system was used (Table 5).

Regardless of time, failures were assigned to either patient diet in general, because patients did not follow initial diet recommendations, or to trauma (Table 4).

CONCLUSIONS

The efficacy of the SEP bonding system was similar to that of the conventional system, and its use in orthodontics seems to be reliable.

REFERENCES

1. Cal-Neto JP, Miguel JA. Scanning electron microscopy evaluation of the bonding mechanism of a sel-etching primer on enamel. Angle Orthod. 2006;76(1):132-6.
2. Dominguez-Rodriguez GC, Carvalho PAL, Horliana R, Bomfim RA, Vigortio, JW. Avaliação in vitro da resistência à tração de braquetes metálicos colados com o novo sistema adesivo self etching primer (SEP). Ortodontia. 2002;35(2):28-34.
3. Reynolds IA. A review of direct orthodontic bonding. Br J Orthod. 1975;2(3):171-8.
4. Whitlock BO, Eick JD, Ackerman RJ, Glaros AG, Chappell RP. Shear strength of ceramic brackets to porcelain. Am J Orthod Dentofacial Orthop. 1994;106(4):358-64.
5. Dominguez-Rodriguez GC, Horliana R, Carvalho PAL, Vigorito JW. Avaliação in vitro da resistência à tração de dois sistemas adesivos usados na colagem de braquetes metálicos com resina pré-incorporada à base. Ortodontia. 2003;36(3):8-14.
6. Grubisa HS, Heo G, Raboud D, Glover KE, Major PW. An evaluation and comparison of orthodontic bracket bond strengths achieved with self-etching primer. Am J Orthod Dentofacial Ortop. 2004;126(2):213-9.
7. Dominguez GC, Tortamano A, Carvalho PAL, Bonfim RA, Horliana R, Vigortio JW. Self-etching primer - resistência confiável na colagem de acessórios ortodônticos? Estudo clínico. Ortodontia. 2004;38(1):10-5.
8. Reis A, Santos JE, Loguercio AD, Bauer JRO. Eighteen-month bracket survival rate: conventional versus self-etch adhesive. Eur J Orthod. 2008;30(1):94-9.
9. Pandis N, Polychronopoulou A, Eliades T. Failure rate of self-ligating and edgewise brackets bonded with conventional acid etching and a self-etching primer. Angle Orthod. 2006;76(1):119-22.
10. Elekdag-Turk S, Isci D, Turk T, Cakmak F. Six-month bracket failure rate evaluation of self-etching primer. Eur J Orthod. 2008;30(2):211-6.
11. Elekdag-Turk S, Cakmak F, Isci D, Turk T. 12-month self-ligating bracket failure rate with a self-etching primer. Angle Orthod. 2008;78(6):1095-100.
12. Santos JE, Quioca J, Loguercio AD, Reis A. Six-month bracket survival with self-etch adhesive. Angle Orthod. 2006;76(5):863-8.
13. Murfitt PG, Quick AN, Swain MV, Herbison GP. A randomized clinical trial to investigate bond failure rates using a self-etching primer. Eur J Orthod. 2006;28(5):444-9.
14. Paschos E, Kurochkina N, Huth KC, Hansson CS, Rudzki-Janson I. Failure rate of brackets bonded with antimicrobial and fluoride-releasing, self-etching primer and the effect on prevention of enamel demineralization. Am J Orthod Dentofacial Orthop. 2009;135(5):613-20.
15. Ireland AJ, Knight H, Sherrif M. An in vivo investigation into bond failure rates with a new self-etching primer system. Am J Orthod Dentofacial Orthop. 2003;124(3):323-6.
16. Barry GRP. A clinical investigation of the effects of omission of pumice prophylaxis on band and bond failure. J Orthod. 1995;22(3):245-8.
17. Sunn S, Rock W. Clinical performance of orthodontic brackets and adhesive system: a randomized clinical trial. J Orthod. 1998;25(4):283-7.

18

Evaluation of stiffness and plastic deformation of active ceramic self-ligating bracket clips after repetitive opening and closure movements

Grace Kelly Martins Carneiro[1], Juliano Alves Roque[2], Aguinaldo Silva Garcez Segundo[3], Hideo Suzuki[4]

Objective: The aim of this study was to assess whether repetitive opening and closure of self-ligating bracket clips can cause plastic deformation of the clip. **Methods:** Three types of active/interactive ceramic self-ligating brackets (n = 20) were tested: In-Ovation C, Quicklear and WOW. A standardized controlled device performed 500 cycles of opening and closure movements of the bracket clip with proper instruments and techniques adapted as recommended by the manufacturer of each bracket type. Two tensile tests, one before and one after the repetitive cycles, were performed to assess the stiffness of the clips. To this end, a custom-made stainless steel 0.40 x 0.40 mm wire was inserted into the bracket slot and adapted to the universal testing machine (EMIC DL2000), after which measurements were recorded. On the loading portion of the loading-unloading curve of clips, the slope fitted a first-degree equation curve to determine the stiffness/deflection rate of the clip. **Results:** The results of plastic deformation showed no significant difference among bracket types before and after the 500 cycles of opening and closure ($p = 0.811$). There were significant differences on stiffness among the three types of brackets ($p = 0.005$). The WOW bracket had higher mean values, whereas Quicklear bracket had lower values, regardless of the opening/closure cycle. **Conclusion:** Repetitive controlled opening and closure movements of the clip did not alter stiffness or cause plastic deformation.

Keywords: Orthodontic brackets. Biomechanics. Fatigue. Laboratory automation.

[1] Master's student in Orthodontics, Faculdade e Centro de Pesquisas São Leopoldo Mandic, Campinas, São Paulo, Brazil.
[2] Assistant professor, Faculdade e Centro de Pesquisas São Leopoldo Mandic, Department of Orthodontics, Campinas, São Paulo, Brazil.
[3] Professor, Faculdade e Centro de Pesquisas São Leopoldo Mandic, Department of Orthodontics, Campinas, São Paulo, Brazil.
[4] Head of the Master's program in Orthodontics, Faculdade e Centro de Pesquisas São Leopoldo Mandic, Department of Orthodontics, Campinas, São Paulo, Brazil.

» The authors report no commercial, proprietary or financial interest in the products or companies described in this article.

Grace Kelly Martins Carneiro
E-mail: carneirogkm@yahoo.com.br

INTRODUCTION

Self-ligating brackets are not a new concept, they were first developed in the 1930s. Since then, several types of self-ligating brackets have been commercially available. In general, the self-ligating system is intended to replace elastomeric and stainless steel ligatures and has proved to have many advantages over conventional appliance systems. Most of them are related to reduced frictional resistance.

Advantages of metal ligatures are as follows: they do not deteriorate in oral environments, have their shape and strength unchanged, provide less retention of bacterial plaque and are easier to clean in comparison to elastomeric ligatures.[1] Conversely, the disadvantages are: they are time-consuming and tiresome in terms of placement,[2,3] produce variable effects depending on tension, and might occasionally cause discomfort and lesions on soft tissues.[4,5] On the other hand, elastomeric ligatures may not provide and maintain full archwire engagement and, in addition, they might increase biofilm retention, thereby hindering good oral hygiene.[6,7,8] They also undergo permanent deformation and, thus, force decays with time.[9] Most important, elastomeric ligatures have shown increased friction in sliding mechanics.[4,10]

Self-ligating brackets were developed with promises of eliminating ligatures by producing a continuous light force, thereby avoiding frequent appointments for replacement and creating a low friction environment at the bracket-archwire interface, which allows better sliding mechanics and, as a consequence, decreases overall treatment duration.[11,12] Nevertheless, whether self-ligating brackets low friction have a clinical effect on faster alignment or space closure, remains under discussion.[13,14]

For didactic proposes, self-ligating brackets may be divided into two groups, according to the type of ligation: active clip (also known as interactive clip) and passive clip. In an active system, the ligation clip exerts pressure on the archwire against the slot base. The passive self-ligating design uses a closing mechanism that transforms the open slot into a tube.[15]

Different self-ligating brackets showed opening and closure forces that varied among brands as well as among maxillary and mandibular designs of the same brand.[16] However, all benefits provided by self-ligating brackets can be hindered by a damaged clip, which may affect elasticity and the magnitude of force applied on the archwire, specially regarding active/interactive self-ligating bracket systems. Few studies have been conducted in order to assess clip resistance of self-ligating brackets. Some types of material are more prone to aging due to exposure into the oral cavity by calcification of the adsorbed complexes of ions and proteinaceous matter, which might alter the morphologic, structural and compositional characteristics as well as the mechanical properties of orthodontic alloys and polymers.[15]

In addition to the effects of intraoral aging, another concern might derive from the potential effect of repeated opening and closing movements of self-ligating brackets during the overall term of treatment, in particular for those containing an active/interactive mechanism.

The hypothesis tested in this study was whether an active/interactive self-ligating bracket clip, designed to be flexible and to produce a certain amount of seating force against the archwire, could present changes in stiffness, breakage or permanent deformation during repetitive opening and closure maneuvers.

MATERIAL AND METHODS

Twenty maxillary incisor ceramic self-ligating In-Ovation C active/interactive brackets (Dentsply GAC International, Bohemia, NY, USA), twenty maxillary incisor Quicklear active/interactive self-ligating brackets (Forestadent, St. Louis, MO, USA), and twenty maxillary incisor WOW active/interactive self-ligating brackets (Hubit, Uiwang-si, Gyeonggy-do, Korea) were used in this study. These specific bracket brands were chosen due to being among the ceramic brackets most used within the Brazilian market, including those that have an active clip and are not made with alloys that present with shape memory.

To assess initial clip stiffness, each bracket clip was assessed by a tensile test performed in an universal testing machine (Emic model DL2000) with a TRD 20 cell (20 Kgf) and 1 mm/min speed. For the tensile test, each sample was fixed to an iron support (Fig 1) 12° inclined (according to the bracket prescription) so that the bracket slot was parallel to the machine test cell, and pulled by a stainless steel 0.40 x 0.40 mm wire. Measurements were performed twice and an average was calculate in order to minimize the possibility of interference or position errors.

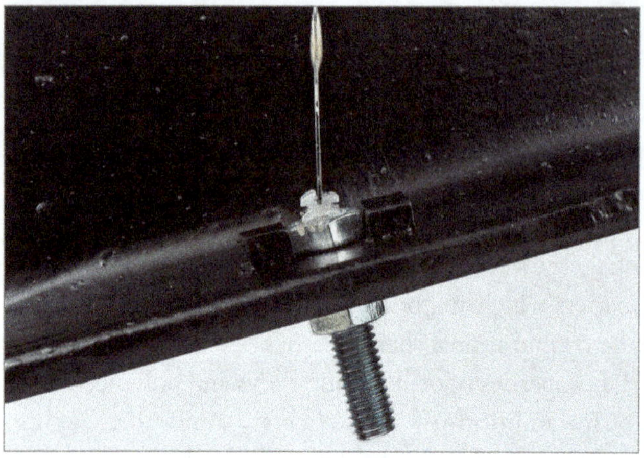

Figure 1 - Iron support customized for the tensile test with 12° inclination, so that the bracket slot was parallel to the machine test cell and the stainless steel 0.40 x 0.40 mm wire was engaged.

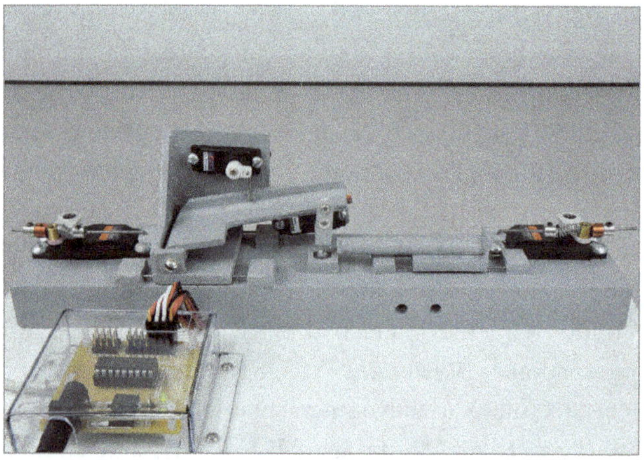

Figure 2 - Experiment device configuration. Note the four servo motors at the end of the gray support and the controlling plate for the computer interface.

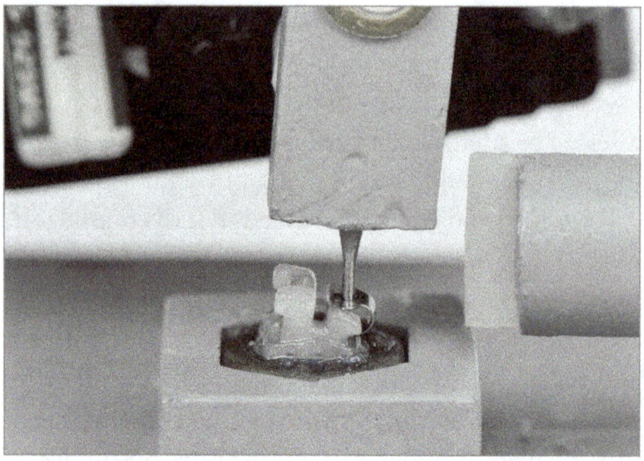

Figure 3 - Adapted devices recommended by the manufactures for clip opening and closure.

Since the universal testing machine is capable of performing various measurements during the tensile test, the resultant force-deflection curves were recorded and divided into three portions. The initial portion, which is parallel to the x axis, corresponds to the sliding of the wire attached to the clip (with no interaction between the clip and the stainless steel wire positioned into the bracket slot); the intermediate portion corresponds to the elastic deformation of the clip (wire-clip interaction); and the final portion corresponds to the locking mechanism of the clip inside the clip notch. In the present study, the line corresponding to the elastic deformation of the clip is defined by the first-order equation $y = ax + b$, and identified by an appropriate software. In this equation, "y" stands for force, "x" for deformation, "b" for the projection of the line in the y axis, and "a" for the slope of the line (stiffness). The software uses the coordinates of points on the loading curve to mathematically deduce the stiffness of the clip and compare the initial and final tensile results in order to calculate the plastic deformation of the clip.

After the initial tensile test, the bracket clip was submitted to an opening and closure test of 500 cycles in an automatic device specially designed for this experiment. The automatic device for the opening and closure cycles was constructed over an acrylic table on which four digital servo motors model DS821 (Spektrum, Champaign, IL, USA)were fixed and connected to a controller board and then to a computer interface.

Two additional components sliding onto 1.25-mm carbon steel rails were tied to the servos on the acrylic table; one containing the active end of the bracket opening instrument, and the other containing the closure device (Fig 2). Both instruments are recommended by the manufacturer (Fig 3) and the force applied was the minimum necessary for the opening and closing of the clip. Speed was calculated and controlled by the software.

To replicate the oral environment, the automatic device and each one of the tested brackets were kept under an acrylic chamber with controlled temperature (37 °C) for 5 minutes before the experiment and during the time necessary to perform the 500 cycles (Fig 3). Additionally, a drop of artificial saliva was placed on top of the clip, so as to mimic the natural lubrication of the oral cavity on the opening/closure bracket mechanism.

Tensile test results reveal that the stiffness of the clip was mathematically deduced throughout the slope of the elastic deformation line. The plastic deformation of the clip was calculated by comparing the displacement of this line between the initial and final tests.

Data of clip stiffness of ceramic orthodontic brackets were subjected to analysis of variance with two criteria for repeated measures and Tukey's test. In order to establish deformation values, considering non-normal distribution, we used the non parametric Kruskal-Wallis test. Significance level was set at 5% and all statistical calculations were conducted by means of SPSS 20 (SPSS Inc., Chicago, IL, USA).

RESULTS

There were significant differences on stiffness among the three types of brackets (p = 0.005). The WOW bracket had the highest mean values; whereas the In-Ovation C bracket had intermediate values and the Quicklear bracket had the lowest values, regardless of the 500 opening and closure cycles, as identified by Tukey's test and shown in Figure 4 and Table 1.

Regarding the slope of the force-deflection curve (clip stiffness), data revealed no significant difference among brackets before or after the 500 cycles of opening and closure (p = 0.811), as shown in Figure 4 and Table 1.

The Kruskal-Wallis test showed no significant difference among the values of plastic deformation observed for Quicklear, In-Ovation C and WOW brackets (p = 0.205), as shown in Figure 5.

DISCUSSION

The results yielded herein support the capability of an active/interactive clip, represented in this study by In-Ovation C, Quicklear and WOW brackets,

Table 1 - Mean values of elastic constant (standard deviation) of clips, expressed in N/mm, according to bracket brand and time of analysis.

Bracket	Elastic constant		Total mean
	Initial	Final	
Quicklear®	14.92 (0.95)	14.91 (0.95)	14.91 (0.92)[A]
In-Ovation C®	18.63 (2.29)	18.15 (1.62)	18.39 (1.95)[B]
WOW®	20.40 (1.44)	20.71 (1.85)	20.56 (1.62)[C]

* Elastic constant of bracket clips regardless of time. Total mean values followed by different letters suggest significant difference.

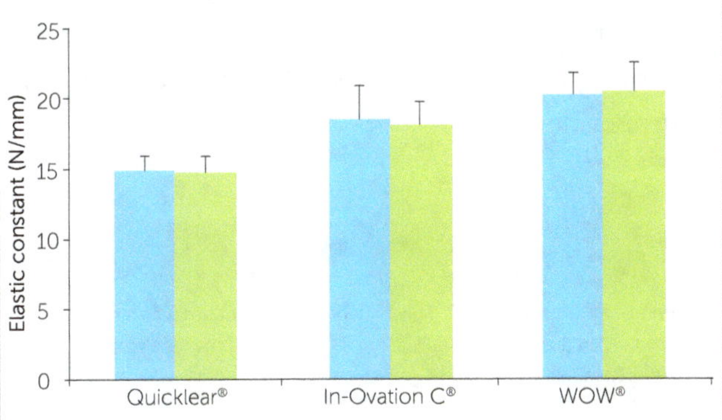

Figure 4 - Box plots of measured slope (N/mm) according to the bracket tested and period.

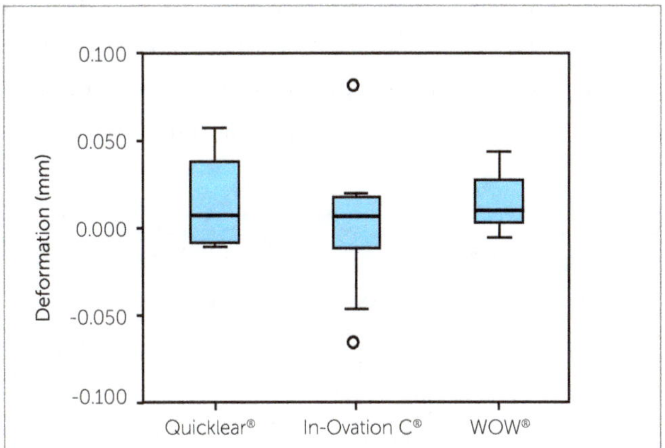

Figure 5 - Box plots of plastic deformation range (mm) according to the bracket tested.

to resist consecutive opening and closure cycles, maintaining the clip integrity with no loss of seating force or clip elasticity and, therefore, keeping ligation secure, fully archwire engagement and resistant to inadvertent loss of ligation.[17]

The benefits of an active clip include early buccolingual alignment, even in smaller archwire dimensions; and achievement of more significant alignment than a passive clip with the same dimension wire, since the existing freedom of the archwire within the bracket slot is lower in active/interactive self-ligating brackets.[18]

The literature about self-ligating bracket clips stiffness and deformation is scarce. Ideally, a clip must be rigid enough so as not to undergo permanent deformation, and flexible enough so as to store, together with the archwire, part of orthodontic forces applied.

In a similar study, Pandis et al[19] assessed changes in stiffness of retrieved self-ligating brackets, and did not find difference in the force exerted by the clip in SPEED brackets (Speed System Orthodontics, Cambridge, Ontario, Canada) after 15 months of use. Nevertheless, they found extensive relaxation (reduction of nearly 50%) on this force over In-Ovation R brackets (Dentsply GAC International, Bohemia, USA). In our study, absence of permanent deformation or change in stiffness of the clip, for both self-ligating bracket systems used during the tests, may be associated with the use of a standardized instrument, following the manufacturer's instructions, in controlled and ideal conditions regarding the amount and direction of opening and closing forces. Thus, during orthodontic practice, clinicians might manipulate the clip in different conditions, such as archwire/clip interaction in severe crowding with archwire deflection or a more rigid archwire, manipulation of different instruments causing damage to the clip, application of greater force during the opening procedure, presence of masticatory forces in deep bite cases, calculus and plaque formation around the bracket, making the mechanism difficult to open. These factors might contribute to clip breakage and deformation.

Other changes in the self-ligating clip may not only be caused by oxidation of material exposed to the oral environment for a long time, but also by chewing forces and friction due to oral hygiene. The literature is scarce regarding the degradation of the clip during orthodontic treatment; thus, further studies should be conducted on this subject.

The difference in clip stiffness between the two self-ligating bracket systems, in this study and according to results found by Pandis et al,[19] could be likely due to differences in alloy composition and the manufacturing process of these clips. In order to determine the number of cycles to be applied to this study, a pilot study was performed using 50 cycles and assessment of stiffness and deformation every five cycles. Nevertheless, no significant alteration was found even after 500 cycles of opening and closure movements. Further research should be conducted to test other clinical factors that might compromise clip integrity.

CONCLUSION

There was no significant change in stiffness or plastic deformation of the clip for both bracket systems used during the standardized controlled test, even after up to 500 cycles of opening and closure movements. There was significant difference on stiffness among the three bracket types: WOW bracket had the highest mean values, In-Ovation C bracket had intermediate values and Quicklear bracket had the lowest values, regardless of the 500 opening and closure cycles.

REFERENCES

1. Ridley J, Garret S, Moon, P. Frictional forces of ligated plastic and metal edgewise brackets. J Dent Res. 1979;21:98.
2. Maijer R, Smith, DC. Time saving with self-ligating brackets. J Clin Orthod. 1990;24(1):29-31.
3. Shivapuja PK, Berger J. A comparative study of conventional ligation and self- ligation bracket systems. Am J Orthod Dentofacial Orthop. 1994;106(5):472-80.
4. Sims AP, Waters NE, Birnie DJ, Pethybridge RJ. A comparison of the forces required to produce tooth movement in vitro using two self-ligating brackets and a pre-adjusted bracket employing two types of ligation. Eur J Orthod. 1993;15(5):377-85.
5. Bendar D, Gruendeman G. The influence of bracket design on moment production during axial rotation. Am J Orthod Dentofacial Orthop. 1993;104(3):254-61.
6. Kuster R, Ingervall B, Burgin W. Laboratory and intra-oral tests of the degradation of elastic chains. Eur J Orthod. 1986;8:202-8.
7. Eliades T, Eliades G, Watts DC. Structural conformation of in vitro and in vivo aged orthodontic elastomeric modules. Eur J Orthod. 1999;21:649-58.
8. Garcez AS, Suzuki SS, Ribeiro MS, Mada EY, Freitas AZ, Suzuki H. Biofilm retention by 3 methods of ligation on orthodontic brackets: a microbiologic and optical coherence tomography analysis. Am J Orthod Dentofacial Orthop. 2011;140:193-8.

9. Wong AK. Orthodontic elastic materials. Angle Orthod. 1976;46(2):196-205.
10. Thomas S, Sherriff M, Birnie D. A comparative in vitro study of the frictional characteristics of two types of self-ligating brackets and two types of pre-adjusted edgewise brackets tied with elastomeric ligatures. Eur J Orthod. 1998;20:589-96.
11. Eberting JJ, Straja SR, Tuncay OC. Treatment time, outcome, and patient satisfaction comparisons of Damon and conventional brackets. Clin Orthod Res. 2001;4:228-34.
12. Voudouris JC. Seven clinical principles of interactive twin mechanisms. J Clin Orthod. 1997;31(1):55-65.
13. Chen SS, Greenlee GM, Kim JE, Smith CL, Huang GJ. Systematic review of self-ligating brackets. Am J Orthod Dentofacial Orthop. 2010;137(6): 726.e1-726.e18; discussion 726-7
14. Fleming PS, Johal, A. Self-ligating brackets in orthodontics. A systematic review. Angle Orthod. 2010;80(3):575-84.
15. Harradine NWT. Self-ligating brackets: where are we now? J Orthod. 2003;30:262-73.
16. Gandini P, Orsi L, Sfondrini MF, Scribante A. Opening and closure forces of sliding mechanisms of different self-ligating brackets. J Appl Oral Sci. 2013;21(3):231-4.
17. Eliades T, Bourauel C. Intraoral aging of orthodontic materials: the picture we miss and its clinical relevance. Am J Orthod Dentofacial Orthop. 2005;127(4):403-12.
18. Harradine NWT. The History and Development of Self-Ligating Brackets, Semin Orthod. 2008;14(1):5-18.
19. Pandis N, Bourauel C, Eliades T. Changes in the stiffness of the ligating mechanism in retrieved active self-ligating brackets. Am J Orthod Dentofacial Orthop. 2007;132(6):834-7.

19

Shear bond strength of metallic and ceramic brackets using color change adhesives

Aisha de Souza Gomes Stumpf[1], Carlos Bergmann[2], José Renato Prietsch[3], Juliane Vicenzi[4]

Objective: To determine the shear bond strength of orthodontic brackets using color change adhesives that are supposed to aid in removing excess of bonding material and compare them to a traditional adhesive. **Methods:** Ninety metallic and ninety ceramic brackets were bonded to bovine incisors using two color change adhesives and a regular one. A tensile stress was applied by a universal testing machine. The teeth were observed in a microscope after debonding in order to determine the Adhesive Remnant Index (ARI). **Results:** The statistical analysis (ANOVA, Tukey, and Kruskall-Wallis tests) demonstrated that the mean bond strength presented no difference when metallic and ceramic brackets were compared but the bond resistance values were significantly different for the three adhesives used. The most common ARI outcome was the entire adhesive remaining on the enamel. **Conclusions:** The bond strength was similar for metallic and ceramic brackets when the same adhesive system was used. ARI scores demonstrated that bonding with these adhesives is safe even when ceramic brackets were used. On the other hand, bond strength was too low for orthodontic purposes when Ortho Lite Cure was used.

Keywords: Orthodontic brackets. Dental materials. Adhesives.

[1] Assistant Professor, UFRGS.
[2] Professor of Materials Science, School of Engineering, UFRGS.
[3] Professor of Orthodontics, Dental School, UFRGS.
[4] Assistant Professor, School of Engineering, UFRGS.

» The authors report no commercial, proprietary or financial interest in the products or companies described in this article.

Aisha de Souza Gomes Stumpf
Rua Oswaldo Aranha, 99 – sala 705c – Centro – Porto Alegre/RS, Brazil
CEP: 90.035-190 – Email: aishastumpf@terra.com.br

INTRODUCTION

Brackets bonding on tooth enamel is one of the most important procedures in orthodontic practice. The adhesive force should be enough to keep the bracket in position throughout the orthodontic treatment, but not strong enough to cause damage on its debonding. Lopez,[14] as well as Reynolds,[21] suggests that shear strength should be 6-8 MPa. Equivalent traction would be about 5 MPa.[1] This adhesive force would be clinically effective and would minimize the risk of enamel fracture. Unions stronger than 14 MPa can be disastrous to human enamel.[20]

Bonding strength depends on the design of the bracket base, the adhesive used, the bonding technique, the adhesive thickness, the bracket geometry and experience of the professional.[2,6,8,23] Experimental procedures used in the test brackets may affect the results.[12] Bonding force may vary according to the material used in manufacturing the bracket. Currently, the use of ceramic brackets is becoming increasingly common as more patients seek esthetic appearance.[5] Unfortunately, the bond strength between ceramic brackets and enamel can be very high, causing damage to the enamel during debonding.[4]

Besides the adhesive strength, while fixing orthodontic appliances, it is important to consider that they may increase the accumulation of dental plaque, enabling the development of gingival inflammation and carious lesions.[10,16] In a short period of 3 months, orthodontic appliances can alter the subgingival microbiota.[16] Thus, removal of any excess of adhesive material around the bracket is highly recommended. It is sometimes difficult to remove all material since the color of resins is very similar to enamel. Recently, colored resins that aid in the removal of excess material were introduced in the orthodontic market. These adhesives lose their color after polymerization.

The objective of this study is to evaluate the tensile strength of metal and ceramic brackets when two colored resins and a traditional one are used.

MATERIAL AND METHODS

Ninety metallic brackets (Morelli, Sorocaba, SP, Brazil) and 90 ceramic brackets (Virage, American Orthodontics, Sheboygan, WI, USA) were bonded in the center of the buccal surface of the lower incisors of healthy bovines, according to the manufacturer's instructions. Next, the teeth were placed in plastic tubes which were filled with acrylic resin.

The teeth were randomly divided into 6 groups: Group 1 (G1) = metallic brackets bonded with Ortho Lite Cure (Orthosource, N. Hollywood, CA, USA); Group 2 (G2) = ceramic brackets bonded with Ortho Lite Cure; Group 3 (G3) = metallic brackets bonded with Transbond Color Change (3M, Monrovia, CA, USA); Group 4 (G4) = ceramic brackets bonded using Transbond Color Change; Group 5 (G5) = metallic brackets bonded with Transbond XT (3M, Monrovia, CA, USA); and Group 6 (G6) = ceramic brackets bonded with Transbond XT. All teeth received prophylactic pumice stone and rubber cup for 10 seconds, washed and dried, etched with 37 % phosphoric acid according to the manufacturer's recommendations, then the primer was applied. The resin was applied at the base of the bracket and the same were placed in the center of the buccal surface of the teeth with slight hand pressure. The excess material was removed with an explorer probe. In G1, the adhesive was polymerized for 20 seconds on incisal and lingual aspects. In G2, the cure time was 20 seconds on the buccal aspect. In G3 and G5, the polymerization time was 10 seconds on mesial and distal on each bracket. In G4 and G6, the cure time was 10 seconds applied to the buccal surface. After the bonding procedure, the samples were stored in a closed container with 100% relative humidity at 23 °C for one hour and then immersed in distilled water for 23 hours.

The samples were tensioned with two segments of 0.010-in orthodontic wire tied on proximal wing and bent in the central region of the buccal surface to apply force perpendicular to the base of the bracket. The opposite end of the wire was connected to a universal testing machine (Applied Test Systems®, ATS-1105c, Butler, PA, USA). Displacement rate used was 0.5 mm/min. After bonding, all samples were analyzed by optical microscope (Olympus S7CTV, Center Valley, PA, USA) with a magnification of 10X to evaluate the adhesive remnant index (ARI) according to Artun and Bergland[3] (Table 1). To illustrate the debonding pattern, photographs taken with the optical microscope with a 20X magnification were made (Fig 1).

Statistical analysis was performed using SPSS® 10.0 software. To verify the normality of the data, we used the Kolmogorov-Smirnov test. In order to

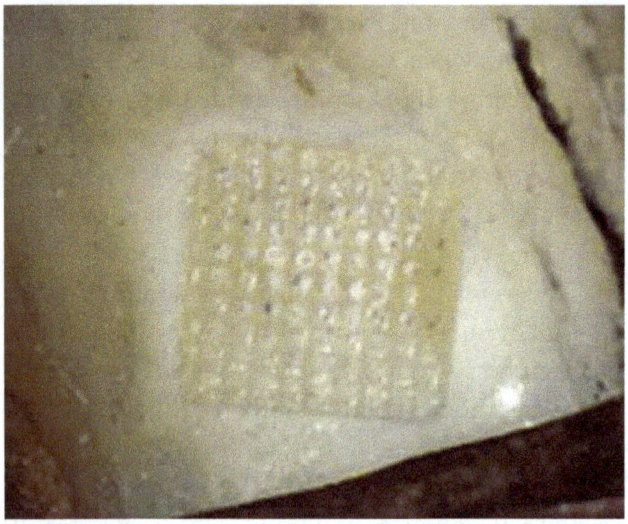

Figure 1 - Illustration of the ARI score 3 (20X magnification).

Table 1 - Adhesive remnant index (ARI).

Score	Quantity of adhesive bonded to enamel
0	No adhesive left on the tooth
1	Less than half of the adhesive left on the tooth
2	More than half of the adhesive left on the tooth
3	All adhesive left on the tooth with a distinct impression of the bracket mesh

Table 2 - Comparison of bond strength (MPa) between the groups ($p < 0.01$).

Group	n	Mean*	SD
G1	25	2.47^{a}	1.66
G2	30	2.75^{a}	1.64
G3	30	4.26^{b}	1.20
G4	25	4.22^{b}	1.12
G5	30	5.62^{c}	0.75
G6	30	5.95^{c}	0.91

* Different letters represent statistical difference ($p < 0.01$).

Table 3 - ARI comparison between groups.

Group	Index 0		Index 2		Index 3		Total	
	n	%	n	%	n	%	n	%
G1	5	20.0	2	8.0	18	72.0	25	100.0
G2	8	26.6	4	13.3	18	60	30	100.0
G3	1	3.3	6	20	23	76.6	30	100.0
G4	-	-	4	13.3	21	70	25	100.0
G5	2	6.6	5	16.6	23	76.6	30	100.0
G6	1	3.3	3	10	26	86.6	30	100.0
Total	17	10	24	14.11	129	75.88	170	100.0

compare the results of the bond strength, analysis of variance (ANOVA) and the Tukey test were used. To compare the results of the ARI between different groups it was used the Kruskal-Wallis test.

RESULTS

The results of this study are shown in Tables 2 and 3. In G1 and G4, five specimens were excluded because of discrepancies in the obtained values.

The results show no statistical difference between the groups where the same adhesive was used for bonding ceramic and metallic brackets. However, there was significant difference between the three brands of adhesive used. The groups bonded with Transbond XT (G5 and G6) showed the highest adhesion, followed by the groups bonded with Transbond Color Change (G3 and G4). The worst results were obtained with the Ortho Lite Cure resin (G1 and G2). The results for the ARI showed no significant difference between the groups and the most frequent result was the resin completely bonded to enamel surface after debonding (Fig 1).

DISCUSSION

The bond strength between brackets and enamel has been extensively researched over the past two decades. However, some issues still persist for the choice of adhesive by the orthodontist, especially due to the large amount of materials available in the market. The main issues fall back on the safety of the procedure, cost-benefit and efficacy of the product. Plaque accumulation around the brackets is an important issue, since the orthodontic appliances may be responsible for caries and gingival disease.[2,17] Thus, the colored adhesives can be an important tool in reducing the excess of material and dental plaque.

In the present study, when the results of the ARI are evaluated, we note that for all groups the most common result was the score 3, where all the adhesive remains in the enamel after debonding. Olsen et al[18] reported that the ARI index 3 is the safest, where the chance of dental damage is less likely. Therefore, we can conclude that the tensile strength obtained with both resins, traditional and colored, is safe.

When the bond strength is analyzed, it can be concluded that there was no differences between metallic and ceramic brackets when the same adhesive was used, which gives the orthodontist the possibility to safely bond ceramic brackets. This fact brings tranquility, due to the increasing demand for esthetic orthodontic brackets in clinics. The bond strength obtained in G1 and G2 was too low to orthodontic use.[9,14,19] The adhesive strength for G3 and G4 was a bit low for bonding orthodontic accessories, but it was acceptable.[22] The tensile strength shown in G5 and G6 was adequate according to Aasrum et al.[1] However, while Reynolds[21] recommends shear strength of 7 MPa, he also relates the difficulty of establishing the optimal adhesive strength between bracket and tooth enamel. Other studies have also demonstrated the difficulty of establishing a numerical value for bonding strength when it depends on many factors such as experimental procedures,[11] adhesive thickness,[8] bonding procedures,[6] type of adhesive used,[2,18] and the direction and type of applied force,[13] and other factors. Therefore, the comparison of results becomes difficult. This raises some questions as: Are we basing our clinical choices properly, or should further studies be conducted to clarify these issues? Murray and Hobson[15] as well as Eliades et al,[7] report the difficulty of comparing the results obtained in *in vitro* tests to the *in vivo* reality. According to these authors, methods for assessing the influence of the environment on intraoral adhesive strength of brackets to enamel should also be developed. The discrepancy between the results of this study and the results reported in the literature may be due to the different methodologies used, but probably the presence of colored pigments in orthodontic resins must reduce the bond strength of these materials.

A clinical observation noticed by the operator was that the Ortho Lite Cure orange pigment does not differentiate from tooth enamel color and it is not very useful in removing the excess of material. The pigments present in the Color Change Transbond are quite distinct from enamel and assist in the removal of resin excess, but their sandy consistency is not very pleasant to work with.

Further studies with these materials must be conducted to obtain more information about the shear strength. The impact of these adhesives on plaque accumulation must also be thoroughly investigated in order to determine whether or not they have a positive effect on plaque reduction during orthodontic treatment. Since these adhesives are more expensive than traditional ones, the benefits should be significant. It is recommended that more studies be conducted to investigate the ideal adhesion strength of orthodontic accessories in human enamel.

CONCLUSIONS

The results of this study demonstrated:

a) Tensile strengths of metallic and ceramic brackets were similar when the same adhesive was used.

b) Transbond XT adhesive had the highest bond strength, followed by Transbond Color Change adhesive, which presented clinically acceptable resistance values.

c) The worst results in terms of tensile strength were obtained with the Ortho Lite Cure adhesives, which were considered low for orthodontic use.

d) Further studies must be conducted on the clinical use of colored adhesives.

REFERENCES

1. Aasrum E, Ng'ang'a PM, Dahm S, Ogaard B. Tensile bond strength of orthodontic brackets bonded with a fluoride-releasing light-curing adhesive. An in vitro comparative study. Am J Orthod Dentofacial Orthop. 1993 Jul;104(1):48-50.
2. Abu Alhaija ESJ, Al-Wahadni AMS. Evaluation of shear bond strength with different enamel pre-treatments. Eur J Orthod. 2004;26(2):179-84.
3. Artun J, Bergland S. Clinical trials with crystal growth conditioning as an alternative to acid-etch enamel pretreatment. Am J Orthod. 1984;85(4):333-40.
4. Bishara SE, Fonseca JM, Fehr DE, Boyer DB. Debonding forces applied to ceramics brackets simulating clinical conditions. Angle Orthod. 1994:64(4):277-82.
5. Britton J, McInnes P, Weinberg R, Ledoux W, Retief D. Shear bond strength of ceramic orthodontic brackets to enamel. Am J Orthod Dentofacial Orthop. 1990;98(4):348-53.
6. Chung CH, Cuozzo PT, Mante FK. Shear bond strength of a resin-reinforced glass ionomer cement an in vitro comparative study. Am J Orthod Dentofacial Orthop. 1999;115(1):52-4.
7. Eliades G, Eliades T, Brantley WA, Watts DC, editors. Dental materials in vivo: aging and related phenomena. Chicago: Quintessence; 2003. p. 3-23.
8. Evans LB, Powers JM. Factors affecting in vitro bond strength of no-mix orthodontic cements. Am J Orthod. 1985;87(6):508-12.
9. Habibi M, Nik TH, Hooshmand T. Comparison of debonding characteristics of metal and ceramic orthodontics brackets to enamel: an in vitro study. Am J Orthod Dentofacial Orthop. 2007;132(5):675-9.
10. Huser MC, Baehni PC, Lang R. Effects of orthodontic bands on microbiologic and clinical parameters. Am J Orthod Dentofacial Orthop. 1990;97(3):213-8.
11. Kanemura N, Sano H, Tagami J. Tensile bond strength to and SEM evaluation of ground and intact enamel surfaces. J Dent. 1999;27(7):523-30.
12. Katona TR, Chen J. Engineering and experimental analyses of the tensile loads applied during strength testing of direct bonded orthodontic brackets. Am J Orthod Dentofacial Orthop. 1994;106(2):167-74.

13. Klocke A, Kahl-Nieke B. Influence of force location in orthodontic shear bond strength testing. Dent Mater. 2005;21(5):391-6.
14. Lopez JI. Retentive shear bond strengths of various bonding attachment bases. Am J Orthod. 1980;77(6):669-78.
15. Murray SD, Hobson RS. Comparison of in vivo and in vitro shear bond strength. Am J Orthod Dentofacial Orthop. 2003;123(1):2-9.
16. Naranjo AA, Triviño ML, Jaramillo A, Betancourth M, Botero JE. Changes in the subgingival microbiota and periodontal parameters before and 3 months after bracket placement. Am J Orthod Dentofacial Orthop. 2006;130(3):275.e17-22.
17. Oesterle LJ, Shellhart WC, Belanger GK. The use of bovine enamel in bonding studies. Am J Orthod Dentofacial Orthop. 1998;114(5):514-9.
18. Olsen ME, Bishara SE, Damon P, Jakobsen JR. Evaluation of Scotchbond multipurpose and maleic acid as alternative methods of bonding orthodontic brackets. Am J Orthod Dentofacial Orthop. 1997;111(5):498-501.
19. Pickett KL, Sadowsky PL, Jacobson A, Lacefield W. Orthodontic in vivo bond strength: comparison with in vitro results. Angle Orthod. 2001;71(2):141-8.
20. Retief DH, Harris BE, Bradley EL, Denys FR. Pyruvic acid as an etching agent in clinical dentistry. J Biomed Mater Res. 1985;19(3):335-48.
21. Reynolds IR. A review of direct orthodontic bonding. Brit J Orthod. 1975;2(3):171-8.
22. Sharma-Sayal SK, Rossouw PE, Kulkarni GV, Titley KC. The influence of orthodontic bracket base design on shear bond strength. Am J Orthod Dentofacial Orthop. 2003;124(1):74-82.
23. Van Noort R, Noroozi S, Howard IC, Cardew G. A critique of bond strength measurements. J Dent. 1989;17(2):61-7.

20

The influence of distal-end heat treatment on deflection of nickel-titanium archwire

Marcelo Faria da Silva[1], Célia Regina Maia Pinzan-Vercelino[2], Júlio de Araújo Gurgel[2]

Objective: The aim of this *in vitro* study was to evaluate the deflection-force behavior of nickel-titanium (NiTi) orthodontic wires adjacent to the portion submitted to heat treatment. **Material and Methods:** A total of 106 segments of NiTi wires (0.019 x 0.025-in) and heat-activated NiTi wires (0.016 x 0.022-in) from four commercial brands were tested. The segments were obtained from 80 archwires. For the experimental group, the distal portion of each segmented archwire was subjected to heat treatment (n = 40), while the other distal portion of the same archwire was used as a heating-free control group (n = 40). Deflection tests were performed in a temperature-controlled universal testing machine. Unpaired Student's t-tests were applied to determine if there were differences between the experimental and control groups for each commercial brand and size of wire. Statistical significance was set at $p < 0.05$. **Results:** There were no statistically significant differences between the tested groups with the same size and brand of wire. **Conclusions:** Heat treatment applied to the distal ends of rectangular NiTi archwires does not permanently change the elastic properties of the adjacent portions.

Keywords: Orthodontic wires. Heat treatment. Mechanical properties.

[1] Private practice, Palmas, Tocantins, Brazil.

[2] Assistant Professor, Universidade Ceuma, Department of Orthodontics, São Luís, Maranhão, Brazil.

» The authors report no commercial, proprietary or financial interest in the products or companies described in this article.

Júlio de Araújo Gurgel
E-mail: jagurgel@marilia.unesp.br

INTRODUCTION

Nickel-titanium (NiTi) wires are commonly used in the early stages of orthodontic treatment because they release light constant forces that are appropriate for alignment and leveling. Among the types of NiTi wires, heat-activated NiTi wires stand out because their action is influenced by temperature.[1] These types of wire exhibit crystallographic transformation under controlled temperatures. However, the austenite finish temperature (Af) of heat-activated NiTi wires has shown variability among commercial brands.[2]

NiTi archwires are used for the initial leveling phase of orthodontic treatment performed with conventional or self-ligating brackets. Self-ligating systems reduce friction, thereby allowing shifting, especially of thin or rectangular wires.[3] This may result in incisor protrusion and/or in protruding wire in the distal portion of molar tubes. This last fact may cause impingement of the oral tissue surrounding the distal portion of molar tubes. To minimize this injury, crimpable stops are recommended, as they are placed over the archwire in any interbracket spaces so as to limit the shift of archwires.[3] Another clinical procedure to limit archwire shifting is to heat the ends of archwire, allowing it to become formable. At room temperature, heat treatment causes reduction in stiffness of metal alloys. Excessive heating of the wire leads to loss of tempering of the alloy and facilitates bending as a consequence of changes caused to the mechanical properties of the wire. Clinical orthodontists usually carry out heat treatment with a blowtorch or a conventional cigarette lighter. For NiTi wires, heat treatment at ± 650 °C causes loss of mechanical properties.[4]

Following heat treatment in the distal ends, the wires are cinched back to the lingual or gingival sides. However, this effective and easy-to-perform technique requires scientific validation due to influences caused to the mechanical properties of the adjacent segment of the treated archwire.

Studies have shown that exposure of NiTi wires to temperatures of 500 °C and 600 °C alters their mechanical properties, reducing the force released in deflection tests.[4,5,6] Because metal alloys are good thermal conductors, it is understood that tempering orthodontic wires leads to heat dissipation at other portions of the archwire. Thus, heat treatment of the distal end of NiTi wires is a matter of concern because it may negatively affect deflection of the area adjacent to heat treatment, which might include molar and premolar regions.

This *in vitro* study analyzed the force present in different commercial brands of NiTi wires in a deflection test. The null hypothesis was that heat treatment of the distal ends of NiTi orthodontic archwires does not alter deflection in the adjacent area.

MATERIAL AND METHODS

Sample size was calculated using Gpower™, version 3.1 software (University of Düsseldorf, Düsseldorf, Germany). The parameters adopted were the following: significance level α of 5%; test power of 70%; and effect size equal to 1. A sample size (n) of 10 specimens in each group was determined. The following archwires were used in this study: 40 NiTi heat-activated archwires from the same lot with cross sections of 0.016 x 0.022-in and 40 NiTi arches from the same lot with cross sections of 0.019 x 0.025-in (Table 1). Thus, four brands were selected for evaluation, with one rectangular cross section evaluated for each type of NiTi archwire.

The samples were obtained by cutting 28 mm of both straight distal portions of each archwire. The segment without heat treatment comprised the control group. In the experimental group, heat treatment was carried out and resulted in distal segment annealing. Initially, a 5-mm length was selected at the end of each segment, and heat treatment was performed for three seconds, with the aid of a miniature gas orthodontic blowtorch (Ortho-Gas GB-2001, Blazer S.A., Guangzhou, China), causing the wire to become red hot. The duration of heat treatment, the flame and the temperature were all calibrated. The flame was standardized by a blue color measuring 20 mm in height. Flame temperature was controlled with the aid of a portable temperature gauge (Termopar, Novus - Smart Meter, Porto Alegre, Rio Grande do Sul, Brazil), so as to stabilize temperature at 650 °C. All specimens comprising the experimental group were positioned over the flame, as described above, until it acquired a red-hot color, indicating that annealing had been achieved. The samples were placed in plastic containers and labeled for test operator blinding. Thus, 80 specimens

Table 1 - Complete description of specifications of the nickel-titanium (NiTi) wires tested.

Groups		Commercial name	Manufacturer
0.016 x 0.022-in	E	Thermal*	Shenzhen Superline Technology, Shenzhen, China. (distributed by Eurodonto™, Paraná, Brazil)
	M	Thermo Plus*	Dental Morelli™, Sorocaba, São Paulo, Brazil
	O	Flexy Thermal Smart 37 °C	Beijing Smart Technology™, Beijing, China. (distributed by Orthometric™, Marília, São Paulo, Brazil)
	U	Nitinol heat-activated*	3M™/Unitek™, Monrovia, California, USA.
0.019 x 0.025-in	E	Super Elastic	Shenzhen Superline Technology™, Shenzhen, China. (distributed by Eurodonto™, Paraná, Brazil)
	M	Super Elastic	Dental Morelli™, Sorocaba, São Paulo, Brazil
	O	Flexy Super Elastic	Beijing Smart Technology™, Beijing, China. (distributed by Orthometric™, Marília, São Paulo, Brazil)
	U	Nitinol Superelastic	3M™/Unitek™, Monrovia, California, USA

*No information about the transformation temperature is disclosed on the package.

from the control group and 80 specimens from the experimental group were generated.

A three-point bending test was carried out for the specimen wires (n = 10). All samples were loaded under the same protocol and according to ISO/CD 15841.[7] A metallic device consisting of two 5-mm diameter pins welded vertically 14 mm apart was used. A maxillary premolar metallic bracket was attached to one of the pins, and a simple tube specifically designed for maxillary molars was attached to the other pin. Both attachments had a 0.22 slot without torque and angulation (Morelli™, Sorocaba, São Paulo, Brazil).

Each specimen was placed under the bracket and the attachment so that the distance between the distal end of each bracket and the wire was the same on both sides. The experimental wires were attached to the bracket by gray elastic ligature in modules (Morelli™, Sorocaba, São Paulo, Brazil). Then, the test device was adapted to a universal testing machine inside a thermal chamber (EMIC™, São José dos Pinhais, Paraná, Brazil) at a temperature of 36 °C.

Each wire was first loaded to a deflection of 3.1 mm (activation) and then unloaded (deactivation) at a rate of 1 mm/min with a load cell of 50 N (EMIC™, Model DL 2000, São José dos Pinhais, Brazil). Both force and deflection (activation and deactivation at 1.0 mm) were compared.

Statistical analysis was performed by Statistica version 5.1 software (StatSoft Inc., Tulsa, USA) to examine the effect of heat treatment on the specimens of the same wire type. Data were examined for normality with the Kolmogorov-Smirnov test. The mean values for activation and deactivation were analyzed by t-test to test for a significant difference after heat treatment ($p < 0.05$).

RESULTS

The values achieved by the 0.019 x 0.025-in wires during activation and deactivation were higher than those for the smaller-diameter (0.016 x 0.022-in) wires. This effect was due to differences in cross-section and stiffness.

Deflection force at activation and deactivation of 1 mm did not show significant difference among wires, with similar cross-sections for either the experimental or control groups ($p > 0.05$) (Table 2).

The four commercial wire brands showed mean deactivation forces of 1.6 N for the 0.016 x 0.022- in wires and 6.2 N for the 0.019 x 0.025-in wires.

Table 2 - Force (Newton) for activation and deactivation measured at 1 mm deflection for control and experimental samples (0.016 x 0.022-in heat-activated NiTi).

Wire	Cross section	ACTIVATION			DEACTIVATION		
		Control	Experimental	*p* value	Control	Experimental	*p* value
E	**0.016 x 0.022-in**	7.50 (0.65)	6.60 (1.99)	0.186	1.81 (0.31)	1.63 (0.68)	0.456
M	**0.016 x 0.022-in**	7.16 (0.44)	7.09 (0.54)	0.761	2.24 (0.19)	1.96 (0.46)	0.096
O	**0.016 x 0.022-in**	5.63 (0.41)	5.60 (0.44)	0.877	1.30 (0.36)	1.24 (0.36)	0.737
U	**0.016 x 0.022-in**	5.84 (0.37)	5.98 (0.76)	0.633	1.23 (0.24)	1.36 (0.29)	0.293

*Significance set at 5%.

Table 3 - Force (Newton) for activation and deactivation measured at 1 mm deflection for control and experimental samples (0.019 x 0.025-in NiTi).

Wire	Cross section	ACTIVATION			DEACTIVATION		
		Control	Experimental	*p* value	Control	Experimental	*p* value
E	**0.019 x 0.025-in**	14.31 (0.46)	14.09 (0.81)	0.457	5.62 (0.32)	5.49 (0.31)	0.361
M	**0.019 x 0.025-in**	15.18 (0.92)	15.14 (0.80)	0.920	7.44 (0.44)	7.60 (0.51)	0.470
O	**0.019 x 0.025-in**	12.83 (1.71)	13.64 (0.65)	0.175	5.44 (0.49)	5.27 (0.18)	0.306
U	**0.019 x 0.025-in**	14.32 (0.89)	13.29 (2.72)	0.269	6.24 (0.65)	6.43 (0.34)	0.422

*Significance set at 5%.

In general, for the 0.016 x 0.022-in wires, it was observed that both activation and deactivation values were lower in the experimental group than in the control group (Table 2). An exception to this rule was observed for the "U" wires which showed higher mean values in the experimental group (5.98 N) compared to the control group (5.84 N). Additionally, during deactivation, the means for the experimental group (1.36 N) tended to be higher than in the control group (1.23 N). No significant difference was observed in these values between the control and experimental groups ($p > 0.05$) (Table 2).

Regarding 0.019 x 0.025-in wires (Table 2), during activation, only the "O" brand wires had higher mean values in the experimental group (13.64 N) compared to the control group (12.83 N). However, a similar result was not found for deactivation. For the experimental group, the "U" and "M" wires achieved values of 7.60 N and 6.43 N, respectively, and the control group achieved values of 7.44 N and 6.24 N, respectively. No significant difference was observed between the control and experimental groups ($p > 0.05$) (Table 2).

DISCUSSION

The results of this study showed that heat treatment of the tested NiTi wires ends did not alter the deflection of the adjacent portions of orthodontic archwires. Therefore, there was no change in the deflection of NiTi wires in the region adjacent to where heat treatment had been used to cinch back the wire at the molar tube. These data reveal that heat treatment applied to the distal end of rectangular NiTi wires does not compromise the deflection force in the second premolar region.

According to the methods used in the present study, heat treatment should be performed at the final 5 mm of NiTi wires, whether conventional or heat-activated. In clinical practice, performing heat treatment in the distal end of a wire is usually a simple procedure for every orthodontist. To eliminate measurement bias in our study, we used a miniature orthodontic gas blow-torch that had been previously calibrated under controlled temperatures.

The NiTi orthodontic wires exposed to temperatures of 500 °C showed changes in some of their mechanical properties. However, when wires are exposed to temperatures of 600 °C, the properties are completely lost.[4] In this study, heat treatment was performed at a temperature of 650 °C until the wire became red-hot. The same procedure is used by orthodontists who wish to easily bend an orthodontic wire of a different alloy.

The objective of the present study was not to compare commercial brands, but to compare the effects of heat treatment on different cross-section and brands of wires. However, for Unitek™/3M™ 0.016 x 0.022-in wires, an insignificant increase in stiffness was observed in the experimental group. This change did not appear to be sufficient to hinder tooth movement. For the 0.016 x 0.022-in wires (Eurodonto™, Morelli™, Orthometric™), activation and deactivation values were lower in the experimental group compared to the control group, indicating that heat treatment caused no significant changes in adjacent regions (Table 2). Because these differences between groups were not statistically significant, it should be understood that the reduction in force necessary for deflection was not significant to orthodontic movement.

Only during activation Orthometric 0.019x0.025-in NiTi wires exhibited higher mean values for the experimental group compared to the control group. Similar results were not observed for deactivation. Nevertheless, for Unitek™/3M™ and Morelli™ wires, the experimental group showed higher values than those of the control group for deactivation. This difference would indicate that heat treatment causes a slight increase in stiffness for some NiTi wires (Table 2).

In this study, heat treatment in the distal portion of NiTi wires did not influence deflection for various tested brands. Thus, it seems clear that orthodontists can select the NiTi wire of their choice and anneal any desired spot (cinched back) to the archwire. Clinicians should prevent soft-tissue irritation caused by swiveling of the archwire; this should be the standard of care during severe anterior crowding correction. Crowding correction with NiTi wires is efficiently performed between appointments when wire excess is common in the distal region of molar tubes. For rectangular archwires, correct leveling and alignment allowed shifting of the archwire, leading not only to soft tissue irritation, but also to arch distortion and asymmetry. Although crimpable stops are the most commonly indicated methods to avoid archwire shifting, they partially retain the archwire due to interbracket distance, thus allow free space for shifting. Heating the distal ends of NiTi archwires is advantageous due to being an inexpensive, rapid and simple procedure. This fact is particularly important for treatment performed with self-ligating systems because low friction allows archwire shifting.[3,8,9]

Although there are many studies in the literature on the deflection of NiTi wires,[1,4,10,11] to the best of our knowledge, no previous study has determined the influence of thermal treatment in NiTi wires or in heat-activated NiTi wires. In the future, laboratory and clinical research can examine the aspects highlighted in this study in greater detail.

Although values obtained for *in vitro* experiments do not always coincide with clinical reality, they provide a means of comparison with other studies and guide the selection of the best material for a given stage of treatment.[12,13] The present study demonstrated that heat treatment of distal ends can be performed with heat-activated and conventional rectangular NiTi wires without any risk of detrimentally affecting alignment or leveling of teeth adjacent to the area chosen for heat treatment.

CONCLUSIONS

Based on the methods used in this *in vitro* study, we conclude that heat treatment does not permanently change the elastic properties of adjacent areas in conventional or heat-activated rectangular NiTi archwires.

REFERENCES

1. Gurgel JA, Kerr S, Powers JM, LeCrone V. Force-deflection properties of superelastic nickel-titanium archwires. Am J Orthod Dentofacial Orthop. 2001 Oct;120(4):378-82.
2. Lombardo L, Toni G, Stefanoni F, Mollica F, Guarneri MP, Siciliani G. The effect of temperature on the mechanical behavior of nickel-titanium orthodontic initial archwires. Angle Orthod. 2013 Mar;83(2):298-305.
3. Ludwig B, Gasl B, Lietz T. Auxiliary equipment and techniques. In: Ludwig B, Bister D, Baumgaertel S. Self-ligating brackets in orthodontics. Vicenza: Thieme; 2012. p. 173-205.
4. Khier SE, Brantley WA, Fournelle RA. Bending properties of superelastic and nonsuperelastic nickel-titanium orthodontic wires. Am J Orthod Dentofacial Orthop. 1991 Apr;99(4):310-8.

5. Yoneyama T, Doi H, Kobayashi E, Hamanaka H. Super-elastic property of Ti-Ni alloy for use in dentistry. Front Med Biol Eng. 2000;10(2):97-103.
6. Berger J, Waram T. Force levels of nickel titanium initial archwires. J Clin Orthod. 2007 May;41(5):286-92.
7. International Organization for Standardization. Wires for use in orthodontics. ISO 15841. UNE-EN ISO; 2007. p. 1-12.
8. Damon DH. The rationale, evolution and clinical application of the self-ligating bracket. Clin Orthod Res. 1998 Aug;1(1):52-61.
9. Nakano H, Satoh K, Norris R, Jin T, Kamegai T, Ishikawa F, et al. Mechanical properties of several nickel-titanium alloy wires in three-point bending tests. Am J Orthod Dentofacial Orthop. 1999 Apr;115(4):390-5.
10. Ong E, Ho C, Miles P. Alignment efficiency and discomfort of three orthodontic archwire sequences: a randomized clinical trial. J Orthod. 2011 Mar;38(1):32-9.
11. Bartzela TN, Senn C, Wichelhaus A. Load-deflection characteristics of superelastic nickel-titanium wires. Angle Orthod. 2007 Nov;77(6):991-8.
12. Burstone CJ. Variable-modulus orthodontics. Am J Orthod. 1981 Jul;80(1):1-16.
13. Hayashi K, Araki Y, Mizoguchi I. Nonlinear large-deflection analysis of orthodontic wires. Angle Orthod. 2004 Feb;74(1):112-7.

21

Effects of surface treatment of provisional crowns on the shear bond strength of brackets

Josiane Xavier de Almeida[1], Mauren Bitencourt Deprá[1], Mariana Marquezan[2], Luciana Borges Retamoso[3], Orlando Tanaka[4]

Objective: To assess the adhesive resistance of metallic brackets bonded to temporary crowns made of acrylic resin after different surface treatments. **Methods:** 180 specimens were made of Duralay and randomly divided into 6 groups (n = 30) according to surface treatment and bonding material: G1 – surface roughening with Soflex and bonding with Duralay; G2 – roughening with aluminum oxide blasting and bonding with Duralay; G3 – application of monomer and bonding with Duralay; G4 – roughening with Soflex and bonding with Transbond XT; G5 – roughening with aluminum oxide blasting and bonding with Transbond XT and G6: application of monomer and bonding with Transbond. The results were statistically assessed by ANOVA/Games-Howell. **Results:** The means (MPa) were: G1= 18.04, G2= 22.64, G3= 22.4, G4= 9.71, G5= 11.23, G6= 9.67. The Adhesive Remnant Index (ARI) ranged between 2 and 3 on G1, G2 and G3 whereas in G4, G5 and G6 it ranged from 0 to 1, showing that only the material affects the pattern of adhesive flaw. **Conclusion:** The surface treatment and the material influenced adhesive resistance of brackets bonded to temporary crowns. Roughening by aluminum blasting increased bond strength when compared to Soflex, in the group bonded with Duralay. The bond strength of Duralay acrylic resin was superior to that of Transbond XT composite resin.

Keywords: Acrylic resins. Orthodontic brackets. Shear bond strength.

[1] Graduated in Dentistry, Catholic University of Paraná (PUCPR).
[2] PhD student in Orthodontics, Federal University of Rio de Janeiro (UFRJ).
[3] PhD in Dental Materials, Catholic University of Rio Grande do Sul (PUCRS).
[4] Postdoc in Orthodontics, Saint Louis University and Federal University of Juiz de Fora. Full professor at PUCPR.

» The authors report no commercial, proprietary or financial interest in the products or companies described in this article.

Orlando Tanaka
Rua Imaculada Conceição, 1155 – Curitiba/PR — Brazil
CEP: 80215-901 – E-mail: tanakaom@gmail.com

INTRODUCTION

The technique of directly bonding orthodontic appliances by means of acid conditioning and composite resin became universal in the 90s.[8] Since then, many researches have been developed with the aim of verifying the resistance of metallic brackets on dental enamel.[2] Bonding in Orthodontics, although temporary, must be resistant enough to withstand orthodontic and occlusal forces.[18]

As a result of developments in technology regarding continuing education and communication in orthodontics, there has been an increase in the demand of adult patients seeking orthodontic treatment in the last few years, and it is not unusual to find amalgam restorations, incrustations in gold, ceramic crowns and fixed prosthesis in these patients.[20]

Orthodontics is oftentimes an intermediate stage to oral rehab. Thus, it becomes necessary to perform bracket bonding in temporary crowns which are generally made of self-etching acrylic resin. Newman[11] asserted that the materials and techniques available are capable of effectively bonding accessories to the surface of materials other than enamel.

According to Zachrisson,[21] acrylic resin is recommended for bonding on acrylic surfaces because its bonding strength is greater than that obtained with other bonding agents.

Some works in the literature focus on bracket bonding on surfaces of gold, amalgam, resin and porcelain, however, there are a few references about bonding on acrylic resin present in temporary crowns.[3,12] Therefore, this work aims at assessing bond strength between brackets and acrylic resin after different surface treatments using two distinct bonding materials.

MATERIAL AND METHODS

The specimens were made of self-etching acrylic resin (Duralay/Reliance, Worth, USA). Polymethylmethacrylate and methylmethacrylate were mixed in the proportions recommended by the manufacturer (3 powder:1 fluid) in a glass recipient with lid until the mixture reached the plastic phase. Afterwards, resin was poured into standardized aluminum rings (20 x 20 mm). With resin polymerization, the specimens were removed and regularized under refrigeration in 400, 600 and 1200 wet sandpaper. After the use of sandpapers, the specimens were polished with felt disc and calcium carbonate in a bench vise.

The 180 specimens were randomly divided into 6 groups (G1 to G6), according to the surface treatment and material used for bonding (Table 1).

G1 and G4 samples had their surface roughened with coarse sandpaper disc (Soflex) during 2 minutes, rinsed with air/water blasting for 15 seconds and dried with air blasting for another 15 seconds.

G2 and G5 samples had their surface roughened with 45-µm aluminum oxide blasting during 45 seconds, rinsed with air/water blasting for 15 seconds and dried with air blasting for another 15 seconds.

As for G3 and G6 samples, monomer was applied to the surface of specimens central region. To this end, monomer was dropped on a disposable brush which remained in contact with the acrylic surface for 5 seconds.

Thereafter, excess was removed with air blasting and orthodontic bonding was performed by a single operator, as follows.

On groups G1, G2 and G3, Duralay® acrylic resin (Reliance) was the material used for bonding. It was inserted in the base of the brackets by means of the brush technique, with accessories positioned and subjected to 400 gF of pressure measured by a dynamometer (ETM). In order to maintain the proportion recommended by the manufacturer, 1g of powder was mixed with 0.5 ml of fluid in a Dappen dish. This measure was used for the bonding of two specimens. Excess was removed with the aid of a probe. After bracket bonding, the specimens were immediately stored in distilled water at 37°C for 24 hours.[9,13]

Conditioning was performed with phosphoric acid at 37% (Dentalville, Joinville, Brazil) for 15 seconds on the specimens of G4, G5 and G6. After that, the surfaces were rinsed with air/water blasting for 15 seconds

Table 1 - Division of groups according to surface preparation and bonding resin.

Group	Surface preparation	Bonding resin
G1	Soflex sandpaper disc	Duralay
G2	Aluminum oxide	Duralay
G3	Monomer	Duralay
G4	Soflex sandpaper	Transbond XT
G5	Aluminum oxide	Transbond XT
G6	Monomer	Transbond XT

and dried with air blasting for another 15 seconds, followed by the application of Transbond adhesive (3M/ Unitek®). Transbond XT® (3M/Unitek®) light-activated resin was inserted in the base of the brackets (3M/ Unitek®) according to the manufacturer's instructions. It was positioned and subjected to 400 gF of pressure measured by a dynamometer (ETM) (Fig 1). Excess was removed with the aid of a probe and the resin was light-activated for 40 seconds, 10 seconds in each face. Once bracket bonding had been finished, the specimens were stored in distilled water at 37°C for 24 hours.[9,13]

The specimens were subjected to shear test with guillotine system at a speed of 0.5 mm/min in a Universal Testing Machine (EMIC DL500, São José dos Pinhais, Paraná, Brazil) connected to a computer (Fig 2). Strength value was obtained at the moment of bond rupture. Then, it was recorded and converted into MPa by means of specific calculations.

Bond failure was observed by a single operator through a stereomicroscope with magnification of 40X. The Adhesive Remnant Index (ARI) was analyzed as suggested by Årtun and Bergland,[1] where 0 indicates no adhesive remnant in the dental structure; 1, less than half of remnant in the dental structure; 2, more than a half of remnant in the dental structure and 3, all the adhesive remnant adhered to the bracket base.

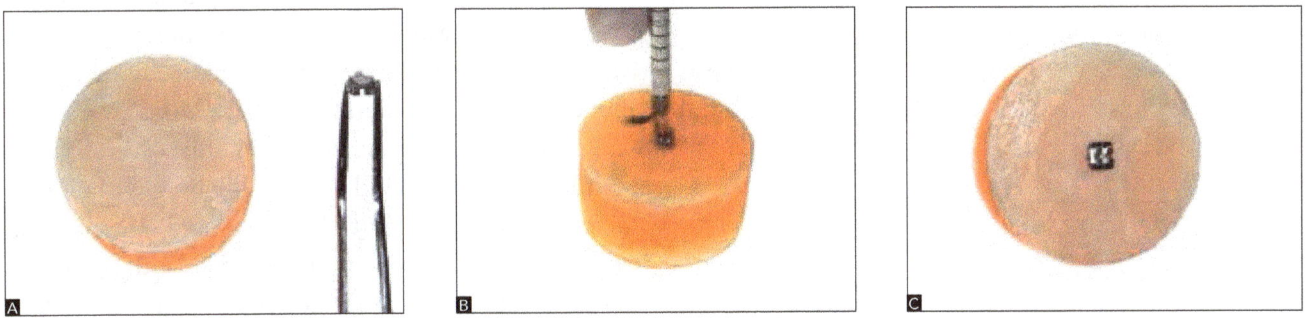

Figure 1 - Sequence of bonding. **A)** bonding material applied to the base of the bracket, **B)** pressure of 400 gF applied at the moment of bonding to standardize the material thickness, **C)** specimen.

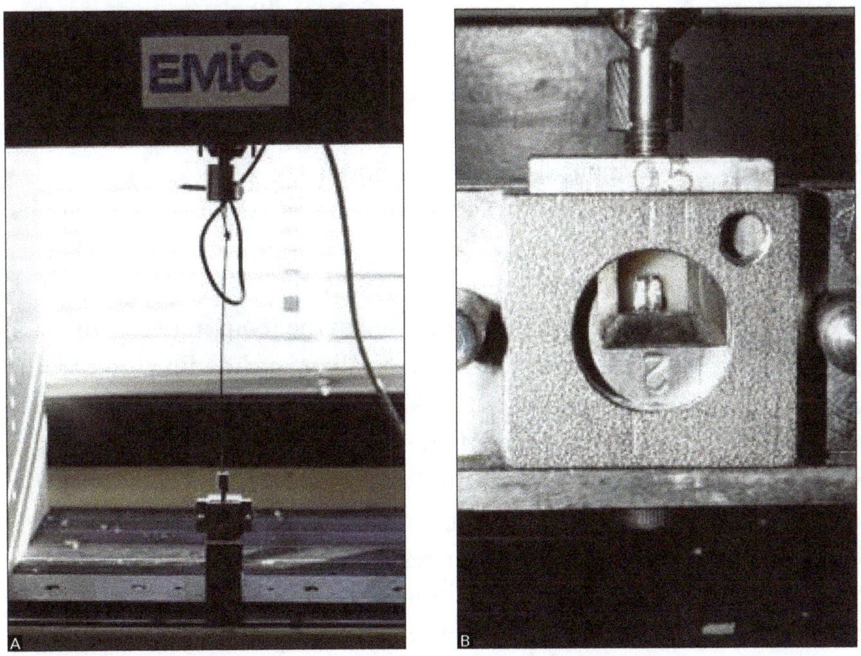

Figure 2 - **A)** shear bond strength test, **B)** specimen positioned in the testing machine

RESULTS

Kolmogorov-Smirnov static test revealed that variables related to bond strength presented normal distribution, except for G1. Comparison of mean values was performed through two-way ANOVA.

The yielded results showed that the value of F was statistically significant ($p < 0.05$) for the variables "material" and "treatment". Thus, Games-Howell test of multiple comparison was used to identify the differences, since the measures did not present homogeneous distribution (Levene test) (Table 2).

The Adhesive Remnant Index (ARI) in G1, G2 and G3 ranged between 2 and 3, whereas in G4, G5 and G6 it ranged between 0 and 1. As distribution was not normal, Kruskal Wallis test was used. No significant difference ($p > 0.05$) was found for surface treatment. Mann-Whitney U test showed significant difference ($p < 0.05$) with regard to the material used for bonding. Duralay had bond strength increased (Table 3).

The Spearman coefficient of linear correlation was 0.5, which shows a regular correlation between bond strength and ARI.

Table 2 - Mean, standard deviation and p value for adhesive resistance of groups..

Group	Mean ± standard deviation	Statistics
G1	18.04 ± 3.46	A
G2	22.64 ± 4.04	B
G3	22.41 ± 3.95	A, B
G4	9.71 ± 2.11	C
G5	11.23 ± 2.75	C
G6	9.67 ± 1.95	C

Different letters indicate statistically significant difference for the Games-Howell test ($p < 0.05$).

Table 3 - Mean, standard deviation and p value for the Adhesive Remnant Index (ARI) of groups.

Group	Mean ± standard deviation	Statistics
G1	2.84 ± 0.46	A
G2	2.94 ± 0.09	A
G3	2.70 ± 0.95	A
G4	0.71 ± 0.09	B
G5	0.03 ± 0.05	B
G6	0.77 ± 0.15	B

Different letters indicate statistically significant difference for Mann-Whitney U test ($p < 0.05$).

DISCUSSION

After acid conditioning was discovered,[3] the processes of adhesion to dental surfaces have improved. Adhering brackets to enamel or other structures depends on some factors such as preparation of the surface, adhesive and material used for bonding, among others.[19]

In this study, it was observed that pre-treating the acrylic resin surface affects bond strength. In the group in which the surface was roughened by aluminum oxide blasting, the adhesive resistance was statistically superior ($p < 0.05$) to the surface treated with Soflex, when bonding was performed with Duralay. It is probable that aluminum oxide was capable of creating deeper slots that caused the bonding material to adhere to the acrylic resin, making the bond between bracket and bonding material the weak link of the adhesive process.[5]

Surface preparation by chemical variation was performed in accordance with Cunningham and Benington[8] and Takahashi et al,[17] who recommended the use of dichloromethane solvent to increase acrylic resin bond strength. Thus, in this research, the prior application of monomer generated an adhesive resistance similar to that obtained after roughening with Soflex, a fact that disagrees with Spratley[16] and Chung et al,[7] who asserted that wetting the surface with monomer alone would not increase adhesive resistance in denture base. Additionally, they indicated the necessity of rugosities on the surface of prosthesis in order to obtain an acceptable adhesive resistance. This difference is probably due to the level of strength to which it will be subjected because, in previous works, the prosthesis were subjected to masticatory loads, different from the present research in which the level of applied strength was lower.

The surface treatment did not change the adhesive resistance when the composite resin was used as bracket bonding material. This can be explained by the short-term storage of the temporary crown made of acrylic resin before bracket bonding. According to Gegauff and Wilkerson,[10] 24 hours of storage is not capable of altering the mechanical properties of the acrylic, thus, resistance remains even with the use of different surface preparations.

The adhesive resistance of brackets bonded to temporary materials must be strong enough to resist dental movement without debonding the orthodontic accessory, and weak enough to be removed without damaging the surface after orthodontic treatment is finished.[4] According to Reynolds[15] and Whitlock et al[18] clinically acceptable adhesive resistance ranges between 5 and 8 MPa, which indicates that any surface treatment used in this research can be clinically used. Moreover, acrylic or composite resin maintains bond strength above the level accepted for clinical use.[15,18]

The present research obtained increase in the shear bond strength when bracket bonding was performed with acrylic resin. This can be explained by the fact that no other material was used, since adhesive resistance increases when materials of similar chemical components are used,[6] because material's cohesive power is substantially higher than adhesion strength obtained by adding another bonding agent. Thus, the results of the present study agree with Zachrisson[21,22] who asserted that acrylic is the recommended bonding material for bonding performed in acrylic surfaces, regardless of the type of bracket. However, this increase in bond strength (18.04 to 22.64 MPa) favors the integrity of the temporary crown surface, since the adhesive remnant remains in the restoration. In this situation, the ARI ranged between 2 and 3.

On the groups bonded with Transbond XT composite resin, the adhesive resistance was statistically lower. This procedure is similar to repairs carried out on acrylic prosthesis. When a relatively new material has been just polymerized and polished, it presents slightly over 50% of non-reactive methacrylate groups. However, as time goes by, there will be less non-reactive methacrylate groups, which will generate few crosslinks with the new material inserted and reduction in the capacity of the monomer in penetrating the matrix. Thus, resistance between the temporary crown material and the resin inserted in the base of the bracket is reduced in about 50%.[10]

Reduction in adhesive resistance makes it difficult to remove the accessory without damaging the temporary restoration because failure occurs in the interface temporary crown/resin, a fact that is confirmed by the Adhesive Remant Index, which ranged between 0 and 1.

The outstanding differences obtained on ARI showed an opposite pattern of debonding, which resulted in regular correlation between this index and the adhesive resistance. Thus, it can be asserted that adhesive resistance increases with acrylic resin being used as bonding material. As a consequence, the amount of material on the temporary crown also increases, facilitating the preservation of the buccal surface. However, the material will need to be mechanically removed by the professional. Despite the differences found in shear bond strength of brackets bonded to temporary crowns made with acrylic resin, additional studies are warranted to further investigate this topic.

CONCLUSION

Both the surface treatment and material influenced bond strength of metallic brackets bonded to temporary crowns made with self-etching acrylic resin. Roughening performed with aluminum oxide blasting increased bond strength when compared to Soflex, in the group bonded with Duralay. Bond strength of Duralay acrylic resin was superior to that of Transbond XT composite resin.

REFERENCES

1. Artun J, Bergland S. Clinical trials with crystal growth conditioning as an alternative to acid-etch enamel pretreatment. Am J Orthod. 1984;85(4):333-40.
2. Bengtson NG, Bengtson AL, Carvalho DS, Rossetto SM. Estudo comparativo da força adesiva de quatro materiais para colagem de braquetes. Rev Dental Press Ortod Ortop Facial. 2003;8(3):43-7.
3. Bisaggio GKGC, Marassi C. Colagem direta de braquetes ortodônticos - uma revisão [monografia]. Rio de Janeiro (RJ): UNIGRANRIO; 2003.
4. Buonocore MG. A simple method of increasing the adhesion of acrylic filling materials to enamel surface. J Dent Res. 1955;34(6):849-53.
5. Chay SH, Wong SL, Mohamed N, Chia A, Yap AU. Effects of surface treatment and aging on the bond strength of orthodontic brackets to provisional materials. Am J Orthod Dentofacial Orthop. 2007;132(5):577.e7-11.
6. Chen HL, Lai YL, Chou IC, Hu CJ, Lee SY. Shear bond strength of provisional restoration materials repaired with light-cured resins. Oper Dent. 2008;33(5):508-15.
7. Chung RW, Clark RK, Darvell BW. The bonding of cold-cured acrylic resin to acrylic denture teeth. Aust Dent J. 1995;40(4):241-5.
8. Cunningham JL, Benington IC. An investigation of the variables which may affect the bond between plastic teeth and denture base resin. J Dent. 1999;27(2):129-35.
9. Fox NA, McCabe JF, Buckley JG. A critique of bond strength testing in orthodontics. Br J Orthod. 1994;21(1):33-43.
10. Gegauff AG, Wilkerson JJ. Fracture toughness testing of visible light- and chemical-initiated provisional restoration resins. Int J Prosthodont. 1995;8(1):62-8.
11. Newmam GV. Bonding to porcelain. J Clin Orthod. 1983;17(1):53-5.
12. Noronha MP, Masioli DLC, Almeida MAO. A influência do silano na colagem de braquetes metálicos em superfície de resina acrílica. Braz Oral Res. Supplement. Proceedings of the 22nd Annual SBPqO Meeting. São Paulo, 2005. v. 19, p. 114.
13. Pashley DH, Tay FR. Aggressiveness contemporary self-etching adhesives: Part II. Dent Mater. 2001;17(5):430-44.

14. Phillips RW. Restorative resins: repair of composites. In: Dyson J, editor. Skinner's science of dental materials. Philadelphia: W. B. Saunders; 1991. p. 235.
15. Reynolds IR. A review of direct orthodontic bonding. Br J Orthod. 1975;2(3):171-8.
16. Spratley MH. An investigation of the adhesion of acrylic resin to dentures. J Prosthet Dent. 1987;58(3):389-92.
17. Takahashi Y, Chai J, Takahashi T, Habu T. Bond strength of denture teeth to denture base resins. Int J Prosthodont. 2000;13(1):59-65.
18. Whitlock BO, Eick JD, Ackerman RJ Jr, Glaros AG, Chappell RP. Shear strength of ceramic brackets bonded to porcelain. Am J Orthod Dentofacial Orthop. 1994;106(4):358-64.
19. Wickwire NA, Rentz D. Enamel pretreatment: a critical variable in direct bonding systems. Am J Orthod. 1973;64(5):499-512.
20. Zachrisson BU, Buyukyilmaz T. Recent advances in bonding to gold, amalgam and porcelains. Am J Orthod. 1993;27(3):661-75.
21. Zachrisson BU. Bonding in orthodontics. In: Graber TM, Swain BF. Orthodontic current and principles and techniques. St. Louis: C.V. Mosby; 1985. p. 485-563.
22. Zachrisson BU. Orthodontic bonding to artificial tooth surfaces: clinical versus laboratory findings. Am J Orthod Dentofacial Orthop. 2000;117(5):592-4.

22

Evaluation of the prototype of a new bracket-positioning gauge

Sergio Luiz Mota Júnior[1], Marcio José da Silva Campos[1], Carina Abrantes Schmitberger[2], Juliana de Andrade Vitral[3], Marcelo Reis Fraga[1], Robert Willer Farinazzo Vitral[1]

Objective: The purposes of this study were to present a prototype of a bracket-positioning gauge, which makes vertical inclination of the instrument difficult, allowing a reduction of vertical bracket positioning error, and to test its accuracy in bracket positioning by groups of individuals with different clinical experience and in specific groups of teeth. **Methods:** For the testing of the prototype, four groups of six participants each were used: Group 1 was composed of undergraduate students in the dental school, who had no previous experience in bonding orthodontic attachments; Group 2 was composed of orthodontic graduate students in the dental school; Group 3 consisted of orthodontists with a maximum of 5 years of clinical experience; Group 4 comprised orthodontists with more than 5 years of clinical experience. A typodont was simulated with a Class I crowded malocclusion, which reproduced the same occlusal characteristics for all groups to be bonded. All participants were instructed to bond 0.022×0.028-in Edgewise brackets on the labial surfaces of the upper and lower incisors, canines, and premolars at a height of 4 mm from the incisal edge or the labial cusp tip. **Results:** Only the mean value of Group 1 showed statistically significant difference in the comparison with the standard measurement. In the groups of teeth, the difference was significant for the premolar and incisor groups. **Conclusion:** Clinical experience interfered with the accuracy of vertical positioning of orthodontic attachments. As for the groups of teeth, premolars, followed by canines and incisors had the closest mean values to the standard measurement.

Keywords: Orthodontics. Orthodontic brackets. Orthodontics, corrective. Patents.

[1] Universidade Federal de Juiz de Fora, Departamento de Odontologia Social e Infantil (Juiz de Fora/MG, Brazil).
[2] Universidade Federal de Juiz de Fora, Programa de Pós-graduação em Saúde (Juiz de Fora/MG, Brazil).
[3] Universidade Federal de Juiz de Fora, Curso de Graduação em Arquitetura e Urbanismo, (Juiz de Fora/MG, Brazil).

» The authors report no commercial, proprietary or financial interest in the products or companies described in this article.

Sergio Luiz Mota Júnior
Rua Humaitá 10/303, Juiz de Fora/MG - CEP: 36.016-150 - Brasil
E-mail: sergiomotajr_orto@yahoo.com.br

INTRODUCTION

Orthodontic treatment should provide the patient with functional and aesthetic balance between dental, skeletal and facial structures.[1,2] In this process, the correct positioning of orthodontic brackets is of paramount importance for the orthodontic mechanics and treatment results.[3-9] Poorly positioned brackets may result in poor teeth alignment, torque alterations,[10-17] changes in arch length,[18] distortions in bracket prescription,[19] as well as occlusal interferences that can compromise masticatory function.[7,10,18]

For some authors, brackets should be centered on the crown of the tooth,[3,20] whereas others recommend placing the brackets at specific heights for each tooth or group of teeth.[7,10,13,16,21-25] Bracket positioning, however, is influenced by the operator and tooth morphology.[2,26-29]

Studies show that gauges used for bracket placement, when used with the wrong inclination, may interfere with the correct bracket height.[9,19,28,29] The Boone gauge, one of the most used bracket positioning devices, allows inadequate inclination of the instrument when positioning orthodontic attachments, regardless of the operator's clinical experience.[30]

The purposes of this study were to present a prototype of a bracket-positioning gauge, which makes undesirable vertical inclination of the instrument more difficult than with other gauges, allowing a reduction of vertical bracket positioning error; and to test its accuracy in bracket positioning by groups of individuals with different clinical experience and in specific groups of teeth.

MATERIAL AND METHODS

This star-like bracket-positioning gauge was conceived at the Universidade Federal de Juiz de Fora, with funding from FAPEMIG. The gauge was machined and assembled at Robtec industry in the city of Diadema, São Paulo, Brazil. It consists of a star-like metal base with four points, which allow the placement of orthodontic attachments at the heights of 3.5mm, 4.0mm, 4.5mm, and 5.0mm (Fig 1). In order to minimize bracket-positioning error caused by incorrect vertical inclination of the instrument, on each point end of the gauge there are two pins stuck on a sliding base that should contact the labial surface of the tooth above and below the bracket. It has a nickel-titanium coil spring adapted posteriorly to the sliding base, which allows the operator to push the instrument towards the tooth, approaching the central pin toward the bracket (Fig 2). The measuring point end of the gauge should be positioned in a way that the metal base touches the incisal edge or the labial cusp tip of the tooth until the central pin reaches the bracket slot (Fig 3). After the force ceases, the pins and the sliding base return to their original position (Fig 2).

The methodology used in the present study to assess vertical bracket positioning was the same as that described in a previous report by Mota Júnior et al.[30]

In order to test the new gauge, four groups of volunteers were formed according to their clinical experience in orthodontics (Tab 1).

Comparisons between the groups of teeth were made between incisors, canines, and premolars.

For standardization in assembling a Class I malocclusion for bracket placement (Fig 4A), an acetate impression tray was fabricated to mount the teeth in a typodont (Fig 4B). Teeth were mounted in such a way that the gauge could be used without interference.

Before bracket placement procedure, a video with the instructions on how to use the bracket-positioning gauge was presented. Each participant was instructed to place the 0.022x0.028-in Edgewise brackets (380-0021; American Orthodontics, Sheboygan, Wis, USA) on the labial surface of the maxillary and mandibular incisors, canines, and premolars (20 bonded teeth per subject), at a height of 4mm from the incisal edge or labial

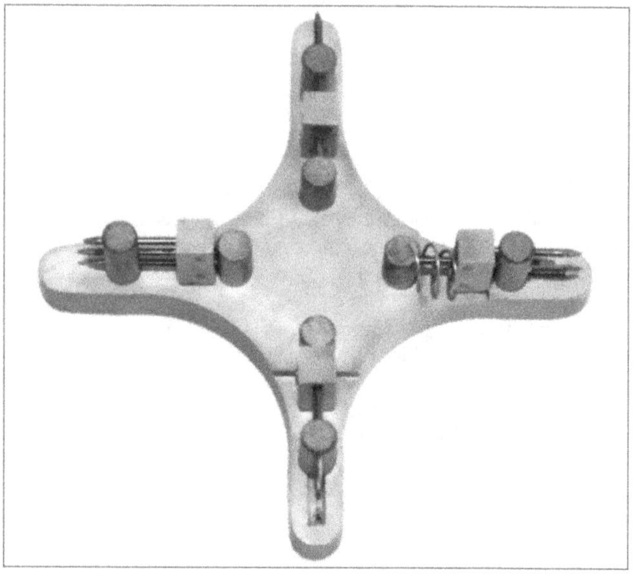

Figure 1 - Prototype of bracket-positioning gauge.

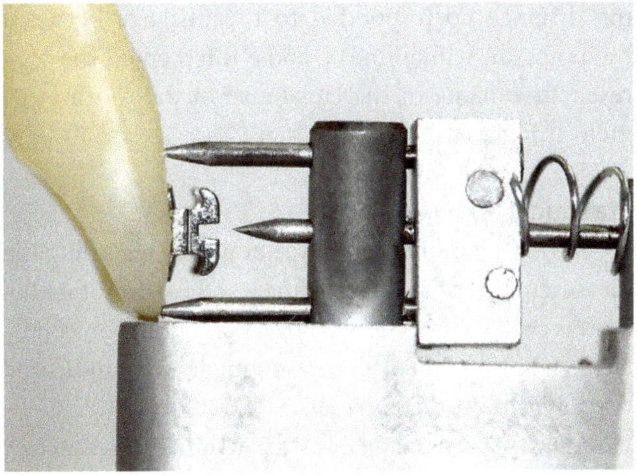

Figure 2 - Lateral view of the active point end of the prototype.

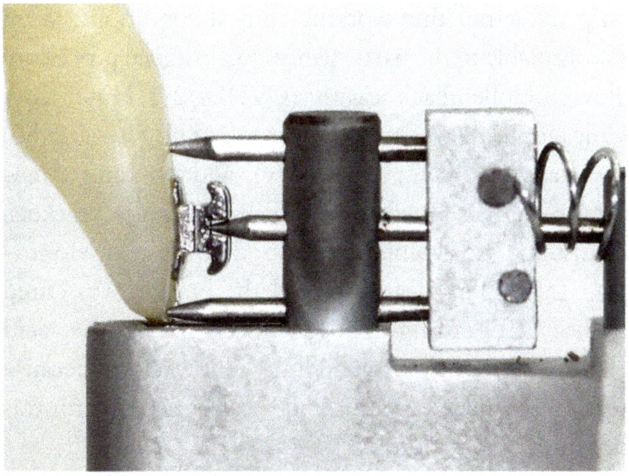

Figure 3 - Lateral view of the active point end of the prototype with central pin inserted into bracket slot.

Table 1 - Distribution of groups of participants, number of participants, and number of teeth in each group.

Group	Participants	Number of participants	Number of teeth
1	Undergraduate students with no clinical experience in orthodontics	6	120
2	Orthodontics graduate students	6	120
3	Orthodontists with a maximum of 5 years of clinical experience	6	120
4	Orthodontists with more tan 5 years of clinical experience	6	120

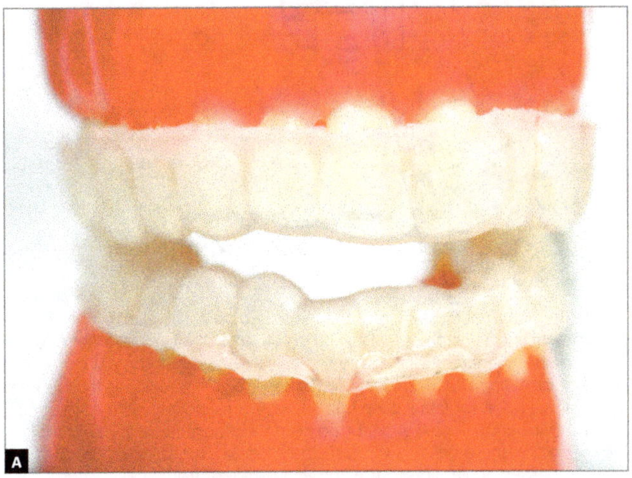

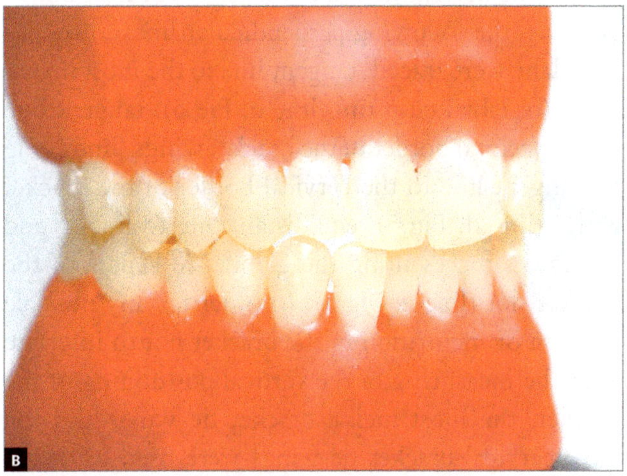

Figure 4 - View of typodont with acetate impression tray (**A**) and with simulated malocclusion (**B**).

cusp tip, simulating working clinical conditions. Were also available to the participants: non-surgical procedure gloves, Hollemback carver (CVHL1/29; Hu-Friedy, Chicago, Ill, USA), mouth mirror (M8H; Hu- Friedy), tweezers (DPU17; Hu-Friedy), and bonding tweezers (678-212; Hu-Friedy). For bonding the brackets, Transbond XT composite resin (3M Unitek, Monrovia, Calif, USA) was used and the bracket was cured with a LED curing light for 5 seconds. Neither acid etching of enamel nor a bonding agent was used because teeth were made of plastic and shear bond strength was not under evaluation.

In order to standardize the photographs, teeth were removed from the typodont and inserted into a device with holes filled with self-polymerized acrylic resin (Coldpac Ortho Resin; Yates Motloid, Chicago, Ill, USA) (one hole for each tooth), keeping the mesial surface of the tooth parallel to and facing towards the camera lens. A Canon EOS XSi digital camera of 13 megapixel, with a macro lens of 100mm (2756B001; Canon, Oita, Kyushu, Japan), shutter speed of 1/100 and aperture of f/2.8 was positioned with the camera lens 20cm from the object to be photographed.[30] A millimeter ruler (CLR6; Hu-Friedy) was inserted in the photographed field to determine the real dimensions of the images in the Keynote software for Mac Os (Version 6.1, Keynote for Mac; Apple, Cupertino, Calif, USA).[30]

The determination of the representative plane of the labial surface of the teeth (line a, Fig 5) was done with the mesial view using the union of the most anterior point of the cementoenamel junction and the most incisal point (or labial cusp tip) of the tooth (Fig 5). For the determination of the height of the bonded brackets, the following perpendicular lines to the labial plane were traced: tangent line to the most incisal point (or labial cusp tip) (line b, Fig 5), tangent line to the occlusal border of the bracket wings (line c, Fig 5), tangent line to the cervical border of the bracket wings (line d, Fig 5), equidistant line to lines c and d (Fig 5), representing the geometric center of the bracket slot (line e, Fig 5). In order for any possible rotation or inclination of the bracket not to interfere with the measuring of the vertical positioning of the bracket, the most incisal bracket tie wings and the most cervical bracket tie wings were used to determine the geometric center of the bracket. The bonding distance corresponded to the distance between the points in which lines b and e intercepted the representative plane of the labial face of the tooth (segment f, Fig 5).[30]

Statistical analysis

To test the calibration of the evaluator regarding the measurements of the digital images, the error of method was calculated using the intraclass correlation coefficient (ICC), in which all measurements were measured twice with a 30-day interval.

For the statistical analysis the Minitab software for Windows (version 17; Minitab, State College, Pa, USA) was used. The Anderson-Darling test was applied to evaluate the normality of data. For the comparison of the values obtained in each group of participants and for the groups of teeth with the established standard pattern (4mm), the Student's t-test was performed. Homogeneity of variances was evaluated using Bartlett's test with a level of significance of 95%.

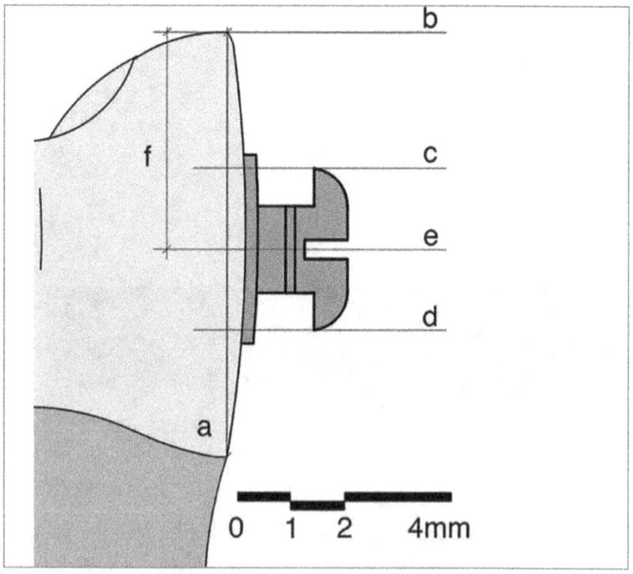

Figure 5 - Schematic drawing of the lines used for the evaluation of bracket positioning: line a = representative line of the labial plane (most anterior point of the cementoenamel junction to the most incisal point (or labial cusp tip) of the tooth); line b = perpendicular line to the line a, passing through the most incisal point (or labial cusp tip); line c = perpendicular line to the line a passing through the most superior point of the bracket; line d = perpendicular line to the line a passing through the most inferior point of the bracket; line e = perpendicular line to the line a, equidistant from lines c and d; segment f = bracket placement height.

RESULTS

The analysis of the calibration procedure showed excellent agreement between evaluations (ICC=0.995). The sample showed normal distribution ($p>0.05$) for the Anderson- Darling normality test.

Table 2 presents the values concerning bonding heights in each group of participants (groups 1-4) and the respective p values (Student's t test) in comparison with the standard measurement (4mm).

Figure 6 shows the results of Bartlett's test, indicating that at least one group of participants showed statistically significant difference when compared to the homogeneity of variance ($p=0.014$) of the four groups under study.

Table 3 shows the values of the bonding heights of each group of teeth (incisors, canines, and premolars) and the respective p values (Student's t test) in comparison with the standard measurement (4mm).

Figure 7 demonstrates the results of Bartlett's test, indicating that there was no statistically significant difference in the comparison of homogeneity of variances in the groups of teeth ($p=0.130$).

Table 2 - Means, standard deviations, variances, minimum, maximum and p value for each group of participants.

Group	n	Mean	Standard deviation	Variance	Minimum	Maximum	p value
1	120	3.737	0.359	0.129	3.037	4.683	<0.05*
2	120	3.996	0.312	0.097	3.376	4.936	0.900
3	120	3.995	0.303	0.092	2.987	4.743	0.882
4	120	4.039	0.267	0.071	3.026	4.868	0.106

* Statistically significant difference.

Table 3 - Means, standard deviations, variances, minimum, maximum and p value for each group of teeth.

Group of teeth	n	Mean	Standard deviation	Variance	Minimum	Maximum	p value
Incisors	192	3.877	0.308	0.095	3.026	4.743	<0.05*
Canines	96	4.060	0.312	0.098	3.205	4.743	0.061
Premolars	192	3.948	0.352	0.125	2.987	4.936	<0.05*

* Statistically significant difference.

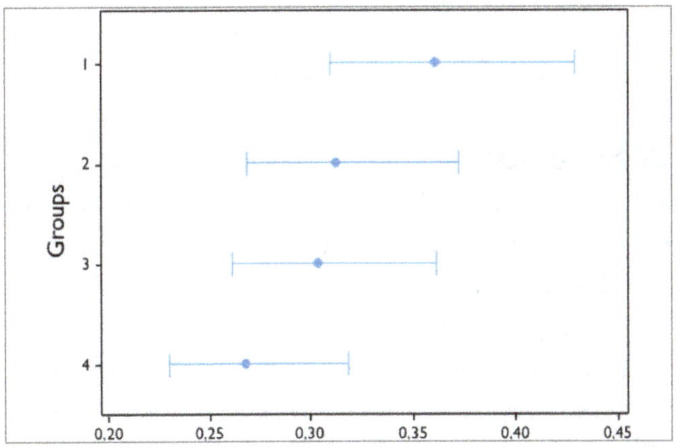

Figure 6 - Bartlett's test to evaluate the homogeneity between the variances in groups 1, 2, 3 and 4.

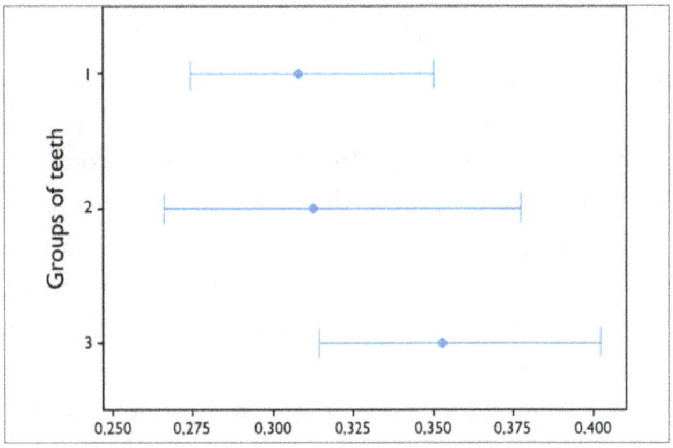

Figure 7 - Bartlett's test to evaluate the homogeneity between the variances in the groups of incisors (1), canines (2), and premolars (3).

DISCUSSION

During installation of orthodontic appliance, it is desirable that the brackets be placed in specific positions on the surface of the tooth. Visual acuity[26,28] as well as bracket-positioning gauges[4-8,27,30] may fail to position orthodontic attachments vertically. The most often used bracket-positionig gauges are the star-like gauge (also known as Boone gauge) and the pole-like gauge (also known as height bracket-positioning gauge).[19] In case orthodontic attachments are not properly positioned on the surface of the tooth, compensations in the archwire or replacement of orthodontic attachments will be required,[16] increasing chair and treatment time.[10,12-14,16-18]

In order to minimize the errors on the vertical positioning of the brackets caused by the malposition of the gauge, a prototype bracket-positioning gauge, whose main characteristic is to make it difficult for the operator to incline the instrument during its use, was developed. By positioning the upper and lower end points of the star-like stainless steel bracket-positioning gauge on the surface of the tooth, it allows its central end point to be inserted into the bracket's slot in a perpendicular way to the labial surface of the tooth. The prototype was manufactured with a thicker base than that of the initial project because of the machining process used.

According to Armstrong et al,[28] one should use the distance from the incisal edge (or labial cusp tip) of the tooth to the center of the bracket as reference for bonding height. By using this reference measurement during the prototype test, only group 1 showed statistically significant difference ($p<0.05$) in the comparison of the mean (3.737 mm) with the standard measurement (4 mm). Groups 2, 3, and 4 showed means with no significant differences ($p>0.05$) when compared to the standard measurement: 3.996 mm, 3.995 mm, and 4.039 mm, respectively. When comparing these results with those from tests using similar methodology with the Boone gauge,[30] it can be noted that, in all groups of participants, bracket placement with the prototype presented results closer to the standard measurement of 4 mm, except the group consisted of undergraduate students with no previous experience in bonding brackets. Besides, this group showed significant greater variance than the other groups ($p<0.05$) in both studies.

For those subjects with experience in bonding orthodontic attachments (groups 2, 3 and 4), the values of the means did not reveal any relationship with bonding accuracy and clinical experience. Regardless of the clinical experience in Orthodontics, the mean of bonding height was very close to the standard measurement, with no significant differences. Armstrong et al[29] compared the accuracy of bracket placement by orthodontists and inexperienced dental students and concluded that the vertical accuracy of bracket placement was not related to clinical experience. Mota Júnior et al,[30] in turn, evaluating four groups of subjects with different clinical experience in bonding brackets, drew the same conclusion.

However, in this type of evaluation the variance in each group seems to be more important than the mean.[30] The use of this prototype yielded smaller variances in Groups 1, 3, and 4 in comparison with the results from the study with the Boone gauge using similar methodology.[30] As for clinical experience, the prototype study showed that the longer the clinical experience, the lower the variance in the groups. In the assessment of homogeneity of variances between the groups of subjects, the Bartlett's test demonstrated that there was statistically significant difference ($p<0.05$) for Group 1 in relation to the other groups. Despite the fact that no participant in the sample had previous experience with the instrument, clinical experience, associated with the characteristics of the instrument itself, seems to have influenced the better vertical accuracy of bracket placement.

The evaluation of the groups of teeth showed that premolars had the closest means to 4mm, followed by canines and incisors. Despite that, the difference was significant for the groups of premolars and incisors. Although the incisors showed the most distant means to the standard measurement, they showed smaller variance (0.095). For all groups of teeth, the variances found in the present study were smaller than those found by Mota Júnior et al:[30] 0.115, 0.109, and 0.135, for the incisors, canines, and premolars, respectively.

CONCLUSION

The prototype demonstrated vertical accuracy for bonding orthodontic brackets.

Clinical experience interfered with vertical accuracy of bracket placement.

As for the groups of teeth, the closest means to the standard measurement were those from the premolars, followed by canines and incisors. There was no difference in the homogeneity of variances.

Authors contribution

Conception or design of the study: SLMJ, JAV, MJSC, RWFV. Data acquisition, analysis or interpretation: SLMJ, CAS, RWFV. Writing the article: SLMJ, MRF. Critical revision of the article: SLMJ, MJSC, RWFV. Final approval of the article: SLMJ. Obtained funding: RWFV. Overall responsibility: RWFV.

REFERENCES

1. Jarabak JR. Development of a treatment plan in the light of one´s concept of treatment objectives. Am J Orthod. 1960 July;46(7):481-514.
2. Mestriner MA, Enoki C, Mucha JN. Normal torque of the buccal surface of mandibular teeth and its relationship with bracket positioning: a study in normal occlusion. Braz Dent J. 2006;17(2):155-60.
3. Andrews LF. The straight-wire appliance, origin, controversy, commentary. J Clin Orthod. 1976 Feb;10(2):99-114.
4. Droschl H, Bantleon HP. Bracket positioning gauge. J Clin Orthod. 1986 Apr;20(4):266-8.
5. Diamond M. Precision bracket placement instrument. J Clin Orthod. 1989 Aug;23(8):556-9.
6. Samuels RH. A new bracket-positioning instrument. J Clin Orthod. 2000 Aug;34(8):482-3.
7. Carlson SK, Johnson E. Bracket positioning and resets: five steps to align crowns and roots consistently. Am J Orthod Dentofacial Orthop. 2001 Jan;119(1)76-80.
8. Geron S. A new instrument for controlled bracket positioning. J Clin Orthod. 2002 Apr;36(4)206-7.
9. Ousehal L, Lazrak L. The accuracy of brackets placement in direct bonding technique: a comparison between the pole-like bracket positioning gauge and the star-like positioning bracket gauge. OJST. 2011 Dec;1(4):121-5.
10. McLaughlin RP, Bennett JC. Bracket placement with the preadjusted appliance. J Clin Orthod. 1995 May;29(5)302-11.
11. Meyer M, Nelson G. Preadjusted edgewise appliances: theory and practice. Am J Orthod. 1978 May;73(5)485-98.
12. Thurow RC. Edgewise orthodontics. St Louis: Mosby; 1962.
13. Alexander RG. The vari-simplex discipline. Part 1. Concept and appliance design. J Clin Orthod. 1983 June;17(6):380-92.
14. Germane N, Bentley BE, Isaacson RJ. Three biologic variables modifying faciolingual tooth angulation by straight-wire appliances. Am J Orthod Dentofacial Orthop. 1989 Oct;96(4):312-9.
15. Germane N, Bentley BE, Isaacson RJ, Revere, JH. The morphology of canines in relation to preadjusted appliances. Angle Orthod. 1990 Spring;60(1):49-54.
16. Balut N, Klapper L, Sandrik J, Bowman D. Variations in bracket placement in the preadjusted orthodontic appliance. Am J Orthod Dentofacial Orthop. 1992 July;102(1):62-7.
17. Creekmore TD, Kunik RL. Straight wire: the next generation. Am J Orthod Dentofacial Orthop. 1993 July;104(1):8-20.
18. Hussels W, Nanda RS. Effect of maxillary incisor angulation and inclination on arch length. Am J Orthod Dentofacial Orthop. 1987 Mar;91(3):233-9.
19. Mohammadi A, Moslemzadeh SH. Comparison of the accuracy of bracket placement with height bracket positioning gauge and Boone gauge. J Dent Res Dent Clin Dent Prospects. 2011 Dec;5(4):111-8.
20. Angle EH. The latest and best in orthodontic mechanism. Dent Cosmos. 1928 Dec;70(12):1143-58.
21. Boone GN. Archwires designed for individual patients. Angle Orthod. 1963 July;33(3):178-85.
22. Tweed CH. Clinical orthodontics. St Louis: Mosby; 1966.
23. Ricketts MR. Bioprogressive therapy as an answer to orthodontic needs. Part I. Am J Orthod. 1976 Sept;70(3):241-68.
24. Dellinger EL. A scientific assessment of the straight-wire appliance. Am J Orthod. 1978 Mar;73(3):290-9.
25. Roth RH. The Straight-wire appliance 17 years later. J Clin Orthod. 1987 Sept;21(9):632-42.
26. Fowler PV. Variations in the perception of ideal bracket location and its implications for the pre-adjusted edgewise appliance. Br J Orthod. 1990 Nov;17(4):305-10.
27. Eliades T, Gioka C, Papaconstantinou S, Bradley TG. Premolar bracket position revised: proximal and occlusal contacts assessment. World J Orthod. 2005 Summer;6(2):149-55.
28. Armstrong D, Shen G, Petocz PA, Darendeliler MA. A comparison of accuracy in bracket positioning between two techniques - localizing the centre of the clinical crown and measuring the distance from the incisal edge. Eur J Orthod. 2007 Oct;29(5):430-6.
29. Armstrong D, Shen G, Petocz P, Daredeliler MA. Accuracy of bracket placement by orthodontists and inexperienced dental students. Aust Orthod J. 2007 Nov;23(2):96-103.
30. Mota Júnior SL, Vitral JA, Schimitberger CA, Machado DB, Avelar JC, Fraga MR, et al. Evaluation of the vertical accuracy of bracket placement with the Boone gauge. Am J Orthod Dentofacial Orthoped. 2015 Nov;148(5):821-6.

23

Bonding brackets on white spot lesions pretreated by means of two methods

Julia Sotero Vianna[1], Mariana Marquezan[2], Thiago Chon Leon Lau[3], Eduardo Franzotti Sant'Anna[4]

Objective: The aim of this study was to evaluate the shear bond strength (SBS) of brackets bonded to demineralized enamel pretreated with low viscosity Icon Infiltrant resin (DMG) and glass ionomer cement (Clinpro XT Varnish, 3M Unitek) with and without aging. **Methods:** A total of 75 bovine enamel specimens were allocated into five groups (n = 15). Group 1 was the control group in which the enamel surface was not demineralized. In the other four groups, the surfaces were submitted to cariogenic challenge and white spot lesions were treated. Groups 2 and 3 were treated with Icon Infiltrant resin; Groups 4 and 5, with Clinpro XT Varnish. After treatment, Groups 3 and 5 were artificially aged. Brackets were bonded with Transbond XT adhesive system and SBS was evaluated by means of a universal testing machine. Statistical analysis was performed by one-way analysis of variance followed by Tukey post-hoc test. **Results:** All groups tested presented shear bond strengths similar to or higher than the control group. Specimens of Group 4 had significantly higher shear bond strength values ($p < 0.05$) than the others. **Conclusion:** Pretreatment of white spot lesions, with or without aging, did not decrease the SBS of brackets.

Keywords: Dental caries. Orthodontic brackets. Shear bond strength.

[1] Private practice, Rio de Janeiro, Rio de Janeiro, Brazil.

[2] Postdoc resident, Universidade Federal do Rio de Janeiro (UFRJ), Department of Pediatric Dentistry and Orthodontics, Rio de Janeiro, Rio de Janeiro, Brazil. Dentist, Universidade Federal de Santa Maria (UFSM), Department of Restorative Dentistry, Santa Maria, Rio Grande do Sul, Brazil.

[3] PhD resident, Universidade Federal do Rio de Janeiro (UFRJ), Rio de Janeiro, Rio de Janeiro, Brazil.

[4] Professor, Universidade Federal do Rio de Janeiro (UFRJ), Rio de Janeiro, Rio de Janeiro, Brazil.

» The authors report no commercial, proprietary or financial interest in the products or companies described in this article.

Eduardo Franzotti Sant'Anna
E-mail: eduardofranzotti@ortodontia.ufrj.br

INTRODUCTION

White spot lesions around orthodontic brackets are a clinical problem arising during and after orthodontic treatment.[1] They are associated with plaque accumulation due to increased difficulty maintaining oral hygiene in the presence of orthodontic appliances, and modification of the quantity and quality of oral microbiota after appliance placement.[2] It is believed that approximately 50% of orthodontic patients develop these lesions,[3] and several studies have reported a significant increase in the prevalence and severity of tooth demineralization in patients during orthodontic treatment.[4-11]

The traditional method for treating white spots is to remineralize incipient lesions with the use of fluorides.[12] The remineralization process involves diffusion of calcium and phosphate ions into the subsurface lesion to restore the lost tooth structure.[13] Fluoride helps to reharden the softened tooth structure by increasing the percentage of mineral deposition, but there is controversy about whether this treatment improves the milky color of the porous enamel, or whether it only rehardens the surface layer with less effect on its appearance.[14] Treatment modalities aimed to mask white spots and render them less visible have been developed over the years.[15-18] The most recent treatment modality is based on the application of low viscosity infiltrant resins to the affected area.

Rebonding brackets is a common procedure during orthodontic treatment[19] because of the high debonding rates of orthodontic brackets resulting from mechanical and thermal stresses, or because orthodontists need to change the position of brackets.[20] White spot lesions may be found on the buccal surface of teeth during rebonding. This would lead the orthodontist to being concerned about the adequacy of the bonding procedure to these surfaces, and only a few studies have demonstrated the influence of white spot lesion treatment on the shear bond strength of brackets.[20-23]

The need for bonding brackets to surfaces treated with fluoride material or infiltrant resins may also arise in cases of orthodontic retreatment. The influence of the time elapsed between white spot lesion treatment and the bonding procedure has not been previously investigated.

The purpose of this *in vitro* study was to evaluate the shear bond strength of brackets bonded to demineralized and pretreated enamel surfaces immediately after white spot lesion treatment and after aging procedure.

MATERIAL AND METHODS

A total of 75 bovine incisor crowns were debrided, rinsed and stored in distilled water with 0.1% thymol to prevent dehydration and bacterial growth. Crowns were refrigerated at 5 °C before the experiment. The teeth were embedded in cylindrical molds (25 mm in diameter, Tigre, Joinville, Brazil). The labial surfaces of the crowns were pressed against a glass plate, and the molds were filled with self-curing acrylic resin (JET-Classic, Campo Limpo, Brazil). The enamel surfaces were ground flat and progressively polished with 400, 600 and 1200 grit abrasive papers (Polishing Machine model PLF-Fortel industry and trade LTDA, São Paulo/SP, Brazil) to obtain a flat surface. Afterwards the specimens were stored in distilled water.

The samples were randomly assigned into five groups ($n = 15$, calculated by one-tailed Student's-t test with 90% power and 5% significance level). In Group 1 (control), the enamel surface was not demineralized. In the other four groups, the surfaces were submitted to cariogenic challenge, and white spot lesions were treated. The specimens received a mask to standardize the demineralization area. The remaining tooth surfaces were covered with acid-resistant varnish (nail varnish).[24] A demineralizing solution (0.05 mol/L acetate buffer, pH 5.0, containing 1.28 mmol/L Ca, 0.74 mmol/L Pi and 0.03 µg F/mL)[25,26] was used to induce caries-like lesions on enamel. The teeth were subjected to the pH-cycling caries reversal model.[25,26] The aspect of the white spot lesions may be observed in Figure 1.

After demineralization, the specimens were stored in artificial saliva at 37 °C for 56 hours.[20] The composition of artificial saliva was hydrogen carbonate (22.1 mmol/L), potassium (16.1 mmol/L), sodium (14.1 mmol/L), hydrogen phosphate (2.6 mmol/L), boric acid (0.8 mmol/L), calcium (0.7 mmol/L), thiocyanate (0.4 mmol/L) and magnesium (0.2 mmol/L), with pH ranging between 7.4 and 7.8.[29] Artificial saliva may have induced some degree of remineralization of the lesions by incorporation and precipitation of minerals[12] during this time interval, which may also happen to white spots in a natural oral environment.

White spot lesions were treated in Groups 2 and 3, using Icon (DMG, Hamburg, Germany), a low viscosity infiltrant resin (Fig 2A). Groups 4 and 5 were treated with Clinpro XT Varnish (3M

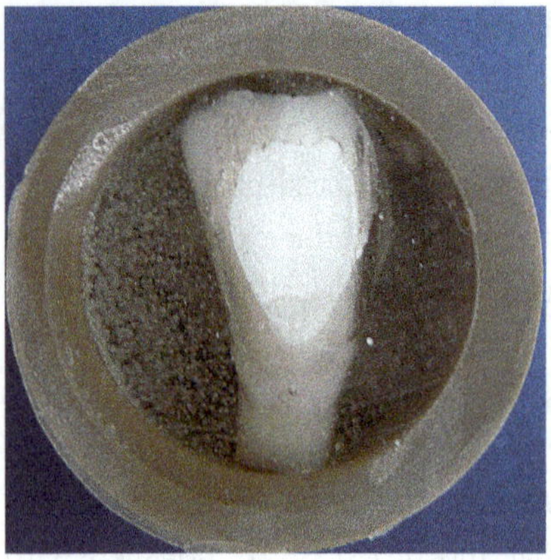

Figure 1 - Aspect of the enamel after cariogenic challenge. Compare white spot lesion with healthy enamel (lower portion) previously protected with nail polish.

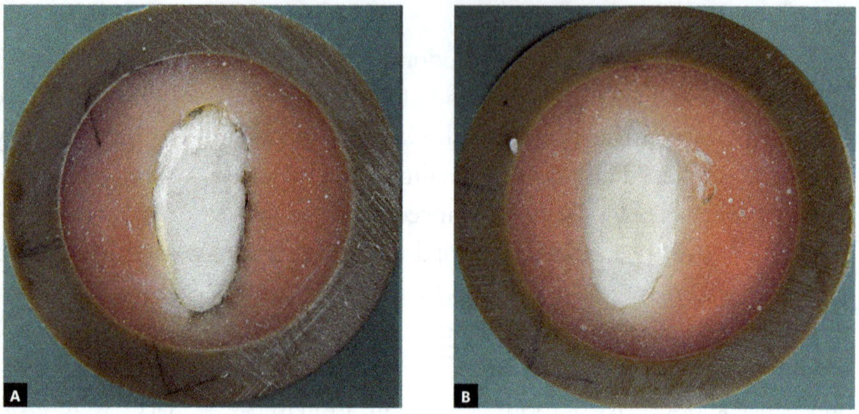

Figure 2 - Enamel treated with Icon infiltration treatment (A) and ClinproXT Varnish (B).

Table 1 - Groups, material and application protocols used in the present experiment.

<table>
<tr><th>Group</th><th>n</th><th>Material</th><th>Manufacturer</th><th>Composition</th><th>Lot #</th><th>Application</th><th>Aging</th></tr>
<tr><td>1</td><td>15</td><td>-</td><td>-</td><td>-</td><td>-</td><td>-</td><td>No</td></tr>
<tr><td rowspan="2">2</td><td rowspan="2">15</td><td rowspan="3">Icon</td><td rowspan="3">DMG (Hamburg, Germany)</td><td>Icon-Etch: hydrochloric acid salicylic pyrogenic acid.</td><td rowspan="3">632178</td><td>Applied for 120 s.</td><td rowspan="2">No</td></tr>
<tr><td>Icon-Dry: 99% ethanol.</td><td>Applied for 30 s with air drying.</td></tr>
<tr><td>3</td><td>15</td><td>Icon-Infiltrant: resin matrix based on methacrylates, primers and additives.</td><td>Applied for 180 s, reapplied for 60 s, cured for 40 s.</td><td>Yes</td></tr>
<tr><td>4</td><td>15</td><td rowspan="2">Clinpro XT Varnish</td><td rowspan="2">3 M Unitek (Landsberg, Germany)</td><td rowspan="2">Silanized glass powder, silica treated with silicon, methacrylate, 2-hydroxyethyl, water, BIS-GMA, copolymer of acrylic acid and itaconic.</td><td rowspan="2">12248</td><td rowspan="2">35% phosphoric acid for 20 s, washing and air drying, mixing the components, application and curing for 20 s.</td><td>No</td></tr>
<tr><td>5</td><td>15</td><td>Yes</td></tr>
</table>

Unitek, Landsberg, Germany), a glass ionomer cement (Fig 2B). Pretreatment and application of products were performed according to the respective manufacturers' instructions (Table 1).

After white spot lesion treatment, Groups 3 and 5 were submitted to artificial aging. The aging process was achieved by exposure to an ultraviolet irradiation lamp and a tungsten filament mercury vapor atmosphere[27] with a wavelength of 365 nm, at 45 °C and relative humidity of 65% in a particular machine (Darkroom, Model SL-204, Solab, Piracicaba, Brazil)[28] for 24 hours, which is equivalent to five years of natural aging.

In sequence, brackets were bonded. Before the bonding procedures, the enamel was polished with a rubber cup and fluoride-free pumice, sprayed with water and then dried with oil-free compressed air stream. Stainless steel brackets for maxillary central incisors (Edgewise standard, slot 0.022 x 0.028-in, 12.25 mm^2 of area, Morelli, Sorocaba, Brazil) were used. The teeth were etched (35% phosphoric acid gel, 30 seconds), washed with water, and dried by air blowing. Transbond XT system (3M Unitek, Landsberg, Germany) was applied following the manufacturer's instructions. A paper mask was manufactured to standardize the bracket bonding area: a square with 16 mm^2. The brackets were placed in position with their bases parallel to the floor, pressed firmly against the enamel surface, and excess adhesive was removed with a probe. The samples were light-cured for 60 seconds (15 seconds each from cervical, incisal, mesial and distal directions) by means of Optilux appliance (Demetron Research, Danbury, USA), with a power output of 850 mW/cm^2, determined by means of a Demetron radiometer (Model 100, Demetron, Danbury, USA). Finally, the specimens were stored in distilled water (37 °C) for 24 hours.

The specimens were placed in a custom-made stabilizing stand to ensure consistency of the point of force application and direction of the debonding force. Subsequently, they were subjected to a shear load test in a universal testing machine (DL10.000, EMIC, São José dos Pinhais, Brazil). A knife-edged shearing rod was used for the test at a crosshead speed of 0.5 mm/min, and a 50 kgf load cell was used for the shear bond strength test.[30] Force was applied parallel to the buccal surface at the bracket base-enamel interface, and the shear load at the point of failure was recorded in MPa.

Statistical analysis was performed with SPSS 20.0 software (SPSS Inc, Chicago, Ill). Intergroup comparisons were made by one-way analysis of variance (ANOVA) and post hoc Tukey. The level of statistical significance was set at 0.05.

Table 2 - Mean (standard deviation) of shear bond strength (MPa) and ANOVA/Tukey results.

Group	Mean (SD)
1	11.54 (2.31) [a]
2	10.61(1.82) [a]
3	12.65 (3.20) [a]
4	18.60 (4.37) [b]
5	12.46 (2.79) [a]

Different letters indicate statistical significance ($p < 0.05$).

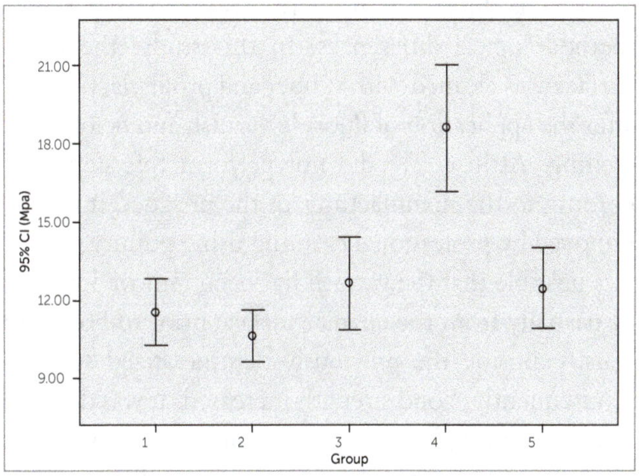

Figure 3 - Box plot for results of shear bond strength.

RESULTS

The results of the shear bond strength tests of brackets bonded to the treated surfaces showed that for specimens in Group 2, treated with Icon, the values were similar to those of the control group. In contrast, specimens in Group 4, treated with Clinpro XT Varnish, showed higher SBS values than those of the control group ($p < 0.05$). The aging process performed in Groups 3 and 5 did not adversely affect the SBS of brackets. Descriptive statistics are presented in Table 2.

DISCUSSION

In this study, an endeavor was made to simulate the clinical conditions of bonding or rebonding brackets to areas with white spot lesions treated with Clinpro XT Varnish and Icon Infiltrant. An aging process was also performed, so as to simulate material remaining in the mouth for five years and evaluate the bonding procedure to enamel treated for white spots in the past.

Clinpro XT Varnish is a glass ionomer cement that releases fluorine calcium and phosphate, and is widely indicated for treating dentinal hypersensitivity. It is an ionomer sealant that can also be used for preventing[31,32,33] and treating[33] white spot lesions, and is useful for application around orthodontic appliances,[31,32] as suggested by the manufacturer. However, this product may not solve the esthetic problem of white spot lesions on the labial surface of teeth. Icon is a very low viscosity resin, with refractive optical properties similar to those of healthy enamel, specifically indicated for cosmetic improvement and interruption of incipient caries. It is known that color stability of the Icon resin lasts for up to 12 months,[34] and its effectiveness in arresting the progression of noncavitated caries may continue for over three years after application.[35] Belli et al[24] applied abrasion tests on Icon infiltrated areas and did not note any differences in vertical wear loss when compared with original enamel.

The results of the shear bond strength tests of brackets bonded to the treated surfaces showed that for specimens in Group 2, treated with Icon, the values were similar to those of the control group. These results are compatible with those obtained by Wiegand et al[21] and Attin et al.[20] In contrast, specimens in Group 4, treated with Clinpro XT Varnish, showed higher SBS values than those of the control group ($p < 0.05$). Attin et al[20] tested another fluoride product (Clinpro White Varnish, 3M Espe, Landsberg, Germany) and found lower values than those found in this study. The difference in the results is probably due to methodological differences. In this study, the tooth surface was cleaned with rubber and prophylactic paste after the application of fluoride varnish and before acid etching. Attin et al[20] did not perform this step. According to the manufacturer of the product, it can be removed by professional cleaning using pumice. Thus, it is possible that the varnish has been removed wholly or partially from the enamel surface prior to bonding; thus, exposing the previously demineralized surface. Consequently, bond strength increased. It was decided to carry out prophylaxis prior to bonding following the methodology described by a previous study,[36] and because dentists perform this procedure routinely at the clinical practice before bracket bonding. Kimura et al[36] studied the effect of fluoride varnish treatment in the bond strength of brackets bonded to enamel using conventional and self-etching adhesives. They found no difference among groups. However, the enamel was not demineralized before fluoride varnish treatment, differing from the present study.

The accelerated artificial aging procedure was applied to Groups 3 and 5 to simulate the clinical condition in which patients had undergone white spot lesion treatment in the past; and later the orthodontist decided to bond a bracket to the infiltrated area. Accelerated aging can change the mechanical properties of resin material and reduce hardness by hydrolysis of the resin matrix. The storage solution usually used is distilled water or artificial saliva, which can infiltrate and reduce frictional forces between the polymer chains, a process known as plasticizing.[37] However, Groups 3 and 5 presented SBS values close to those of the control group. This indicated that the process of aging infiltrated areas did not adversely affect the SBS of brackets.

The infiltrated surfaces were etched with 35% phosphoric acid before the application of primer and Transbond XT, according to the recommended bonding protocol. One should take into consideration that phosphoric acid has an erosive potential on infiltrants. Thus, etching is able to partially remove the layer of the infiltrated area. However, Hammad et al[38] showed that the erosion of the infiltrated area exposed to Coke, which contains phosphoric acid, was lower than the erosion caused by natural enamel exposed to the same substance. Nevertheless, the erosion of the infiltrated surface did not appear to be capable of changing the SBS of brackets, because conventional adhesives, such as Transbond XT, are able to penetrate into carious lesions to some extent. Primer monomer formulations with increased TEGDMA (triethylene glycol dimethacrylate) and HEMA (2-hydroxyethyl methacrylate) content have a high penetration capability,[39] which most likely allows a chemical connection of the resin infiltrant to the primer.[38] Thus, it is assumed that the primer may also partially penetrate into the demineralized enamel and strengthen the outermost part of the Icon-infiltrated enamel when it is applied after preconditioning.[23]

The results of this study indicate that white spot lesion treatment with the tested dental material did not affect bracket bonding. The results should be extrapolated to clinical practice with caution, as this is a laboratory study. Further clinical researches are suggested to confirm the findings.

CONCLUSIONS

Treatment for white spots using Icon and Clinpro XT Varnish did not negatively affect the shear strength of orthodontic bonding. Simulated aging of the pretreated area also did not affect the bond strength of brackets.

REFERENCES

1. Moreira TC, Sampaio RKL. Efeitos do tratamento ortodôntico sobre o esmalte: desmineralização e pigmentação. Rev Dental Press Ortod Ortop Facial. 2001 Mar-Abr;6(2):41-8.
2. Freitas AO, Marquezan M, Nojima MC, Alviano DS, Maia LC. The influence of orthodontic fixed appliances on the oral microbiota: a systematic review. Dental Press J Orthod. 2014 Mar-Apr;19(2):46-55.
3. Souza-e-Silva CM, Parisotto TM, Steiner-Oliveira C, Kamiya RU, Rodrigues LK, Nobre-dos-Santos M. Carbon dioxide laser and bonding materials reduce enamel demineralization around orthodontic brackets. Lasers Med Sci. 2013 Jan;28(1):111-8.
4. Benson PE, Shah AA, Millett DT, Dyer F, Parkin N, Vine RS Fluorides, orthodontics and demineralization: a systematic review. J Orthod. 2005 Jun;32(2):102-14.
5. Boersma JG, van der Veen MH, Lagerweij MD, Bokhout B, Prahl-Andersen B. Caries prevalence measured with QLF after treatment with fixed orthodontic appliances: influencing factors. Caries Res. 2005 Jan-Feb;39(1):41-7.
6. Ahn SJ, Lim BS, Lee YK, Nahm DS. Quantitative determination of adhesion patterns of cariogenic streptococci to various orthodontic adhesives. Angle Orthod. 2006 Sept;76(5):869-75.
7. Kerbusch AE, Kuijpers-Jagtman AM, Mulder J, van der Sanden WJ. Prevention of white spots during orthodontic treatment with fixed appliances. Ned Tijdschr Tandheelkd. 2010 May;117(5):283-7.
8. Shungin D, Olsson AI, Persson M. Orthodontic treatment-related white spot lesions: a 14-year prospective quantitative follow-up, including bonding material assessment. Am J Orthod Dentofacial Orthop. 2010 Aug;138(2):136.e1-8; discussion 136-7.
9. Tufekci E, Dixon JS, Gunsolley JC, Lindauer SJ. Prevalence of white spot lesions during orthodontic treatment with fixed appliances. Angle Orthod. 2011;81(2):206-10.
10. Lucchese A, Gherlone E. Prevalence of white-spot lesions before and during orthodontic treatment with fixed appliances. Eur J Orthod. 2013;35(5):664-8.
11. Julien KC, Buschang PH, Campbell PM. Prevalence of white spot lesion formation during orthodontic treatment. Angle Orthod. 2013;83(4):641-7.
12. Ten Cate JM, Buijs MJ, Miller CC, Exterkate RAM. Elevated fluoride products enhance remineralization of advanced enamel lesions. J Dent Res. 2008;87(10):943-47.
13. Cochrane NJ, Cai F, Huq NL, Burrow MF, Reynolds EC. New approaches to enhanced remineralization of tooth enamel. J Dent Res. 2010;89(11):1187-97.
14. Poosti M, Ahrari F, Moosavi H, Najjaran H. The effect of fractional CO2 laser irradiation on remineralization of enamel white spot lesions. Lasers Med Sci. 2014;29(4):1349-55.
15. Paris S, Meyer-Lueckel H, Cölfen H, Kielbassa AM. Resin infiltration of artificial enamel caries lesions with experimental light curing resins. Dent Mater J. 2007 July;26(4):582-8.
16. Meyer-Lueckel H, Paris S. Improved resin infiltration of natural caries lesions. J Dent Res. 2008 Dec;87(12):1112-6.
17. Mueller J, Meyer-Lueckel H, Paris S, Hopfenmuller W, Kielbassa AM. Inhibition of lesion progression by the penetration of resins in vitro: influence of the application procedure. Oper Dent. 2006 May-Jun;31(3):338-45.
18. Ogodescu A, Ogodescu E, Talpoş S, Zetu I. Resin infiltration of white spot lesions during the fixed orthodontic appliance therapy. Rev Med Chir Soc Med Nat Iasi. 2011 Oct-Dec;115(4):1251-7.
19. Jimenez EEO, Hilgenberg SP, Rastelli MC, Rsatelli MC, Pilatti GL, Orellana B, et al. Rebonding of unused brackets with different orthodontic adhesives. Dental Press J Orthod. 2012 Mar-Apr;17(2):69-76.
20. Attin R, Stawarczyk B, Keçik D, Knösel M, Wiechmann D, Attin T. Shear bond strength of brackets to demineralize enamel after different pretreatment methods. Angle Orthod. 2012 Jan;82(1):56-61.
21. Wiegand A, Stawarczyk B, Kolakovic M, Hämmerle CH, Attin T, Schmidlin PR. Adhesive performance of a caries infiltrant on sound and demineralised enamel. J Dent. 2011 Feb;39(2):117-21.
22. Ekizer A, Zorba YO, Uysal T, Ayrikcila S. Effects of demineralizaton-inhibition procedures on the bond strength of brackets bonded to demineralized enamel surface. Korean J Orthod. 2012 Feb;42(1):17-22.
23. Naidu E, Stawarczyk B, Tawakoli PN, Attin R, Attin T, Wiegand A. Shear bond strength of orthodontic resins after caries infiltrant preconditioning. Angle Orthod. 2013 Mar;83(2):306-12.
24. Belli R, Rahiotis C, Schubert EW, Baratieri LN, Petschelt A, Lohbauer U. Wear and morphology of infiltrated white spot lesions. J Dent. 2011 May;39(5):376-85.
25. Queiroz CS, Hara AT, Paes Leme AF, Cury JA. pH-cycling models to evaluate the effect of low fluoride dentifrice on enamel de- and remineralization. Braz Dent J. 2008;19(1):21-7.
26. Maia LH, Filho HL, Araújo MV, Ruellas AC, Araújo MT. Incorporation of metal and color alteration of enamel in the presence of orthodontic appliances. Angle Orthod. 2012 Sept;82(5):889-93.
27. Doray PG, Wang X, Powers JM, Burgess JO. Accelerated aging affects color stability of provisional restorative materials. J Prosthodont. 1997 Sept;6(3):183-8.
28. Moreira AD, Mattos CT, de Araújo MV, Ruellas AC, Sant'anna EF. Chromatic analysis of teeth exposed to different mouthrinses. J Dent. 2013 Nov;41 Suppl 5:e24-7.
29. Göhring TN, Zehnder M, Sener B, Schmidlin PR. In vitro microleakage of adhesive-sealed dentin with lactic acid and saliva exposure: a radio-isotope analysis. J Dent. 2004 Mar;32(3):235-40.
30. Pithon MM, Oliveira MV, Ruellas AC, Bolognese AM, Romano FL. Shear bond strength of orthodontic brackets to enamel under different surface treatment conditions. J Appl Oral Sci. 2007 Apr;15(2):127-30.
31. Yap J, Walsh LJ, Naser-Ud Din S, Ngo H, Manton DJ. Evaluation of a novel approach in the prevention of white spot lesions around orthodontic brackets. Aust Dent J. 2014 Mar;59(1):70-80.
32. O'Reilly MT, De Jesús Viñas J, Hatch JP. Effectiveness of a sealant compared with no sealant in preventing enamel demineralization in patients with fixed orthodontic appliances: a prospective clinical trial. Am J Orthod Dentofacial Orthop. 2013 Jun;143(6):837-44.
33. Kantovitz KR, Pascon FM, Nociti FH Jr, Tabchoury CP, Puppin-Rontani RM. Inhibition of enamel mineral loss by fissure sealant: an in situ study. J Dent. 2013 Jan;41(1):42-50.
34. Feng CH, Chu XY. Efficacy of one year treatment of icon infiltration resin on post-orthodontic white spots. Beijing Da Xue Xue Bao. 2013 Feb 18;45(1):40-3.
35. Meyer-Lueckel H, Bitter K, Paris S. Randomized controlled clinical trial on proximal caries infiltration: three-year follow-up. Caries Res. 2012;46(6):544-8.
36. Kimura T, Dunn WJ, Taloumis LJ. Effect of fluoride varnish on the in vitro bond strength of orthodontic brackets using a self-etching primer system. Am J Orthod Dentofacial Orthop. 2004 Mar;125(3):351-6.
37. Ferracane JL, Berge HX, Condon JR. In vitro aging of dental composites in water--effect of degree of conversion, filler volume, and filler/matrix coupling. J Biomed Mater Res. 1998 Dec 5;42(3):465-72.
38. Hammad SM, Enan ET. In vivo effects of two acidic soft drinks on shear bond strength of metal orthodontic brackets with and without resin infiltration treatment. Angle Orthod. 2013 July;83(4):648-52.
39. Paris S, Meyer-Lueckel H, Cölfen H, Kielbassa AM. Penetration coefficients of commercially available and experimental composites intended to infiltrate enamel carious lesions. Dent Mater. 2007 Jun;23(6):742-8.

Prototype of a new tip developed to be coupled to dental light-curing units for optimizing bonding of orthodontic brackets and accessories

Sergio Luiz Mota Júnior[1], Márcio José da Silva Campos[2], Marco Abdo Gravina[3], Marcelo Reis Fraga[4], Robert Willer Farinazzo Vitral[5]

Objective: development of a new device to be coupled to light-curing units for bonding orthodontic brackets and accessories, and test its efficacy in an in vitro mechanical trial. The inner surface of the device is mirrored and is based on physical concepts of light refraction and reflection. The main advantage of such device is the reduced clinical time needed for bonding and the low possibility of contamination during the process. **Methods:** One hundred and twenty specimens were used for testing the shear bond strength of brackets bonded with the device. The Adhesive Remnant Index (ARI) was also determined. The sample was divided into 2 groups. In group 1 a halogen light-curing unit was used while in group 2 a led light-curing unit was used. Each group was then subdivided. In subgroups H1 and L1, a conventional light guide rod was used while in subgroups H2 and L2 bonding was performed with the mirrored device coupled to the tip of the guide light rod. **Results**: The values obtained for the shear bond strength and the ARI in the subgroups were compared. Results showed that there was no statistically significant difference for the shear strength ($p > 0.05$) and the ARI ($p > 0.05$) between the subgroups. **Conclusion:** The tests of mechanical trials and the ARI analysis showed that the new device fulfilled the requirements for bonding orthodontic accessories, and that the time for bonding was reduced to half, being necessary only one light exposure.

Keywords: Light-curing of dental adhesives. Orthodontic brackets. Patents. Shear strength.

[1] PhD Student in Health, Federal University of Juiz de Fora (UFJF).

[2] Post-Doctorate Student in Health,UFJF. Professor of the graduate program in Orthodontics, UFJF.

[3] MSc in PhD in Orthodontics, State University of Rio de Janeiro (UERJ). Associate professor of Orthodontics, School of Dentistry, and professor of the graduate program in Orthodontics, UFJF.

[4] MSc in Orthodontics, Pontifical Catholic University of Minas Gerais (PUC-MG). Doctorate student in Health, UFJF. Professor of the graduate program in Orthodontics, UFJF.

[5] Associate professor and program director of the graduate program in Orthodontics, UFJF.

» The author reports no commercial, proprietary or financial interest in the products or companies described in this article.

Sergio Luiz Mota Júnior
Rua Humaitá, 10 – Apto 303 – Juiz de Fora /MG – CEP: 36.016-150 – Brazil
E-mail: sergiomotajr_orto@yahoo.com.br

INTRODUCTION

The light-emitting sources for light curing of composite resins that are available in the market are halogen lamps, blue light-emitting diodes (LEDs), argon laser and xenon plasma arc.[3,20] Although the latter reduce curing time to one quarter[23] and one third,[24] respectively, in comparison to that afforded by conventional curing units, the machines are costly, which hampers their use in private dental offices.[23,24]

LED is the acronym for Light-Emitting Diode, a semiconductor diode which, when energized, emits visible light through luminescence and not through a heated filament, consuming less power and producing less heat.[18,19,20] Halogen light curing units have been replaced by LED units[2,18] due to its small number of components and lower power consumption.[6,18]

In Orthodontics, bonding brackets and accessories is time-consuming[3] and humidity control is difficult, which may lead to contamination of the enamel surface and consequent bonding failure.[21]

Based on the present conditions for bonding brackets and orthodontic accessories, combined with concepts of Optical Physics, this study aimed at developing and testing a new model of curing unit-adjusted tip, with the purpose of reducing time, achieving better quality and reducing power consumption during the bonding procedure in Orthodontics.

MATERIAL AND METHODS

Based on the existing models of curing units, of which tip contains an optical fiber filament, we developed a mirrored concave tip, based on the fact that spherical concave mirrors are polished caps which are reflective in their inner surfaces. The tip we developed (Fig 1A – upper view, 1B – lateral view) is adjusted to the tips of conventional curing units (Fig 2).

The filing of the patent application was registered with the National Institute of Industrial Property (*Instituto Nacional da Propriedade Industrial* – INPI) under the number 020110074054.

The Committee of Ethics in Animal Experimentation of the Federal University of Juiz de Fora (UFJF) approved this research project (protocol nº 025/2010).

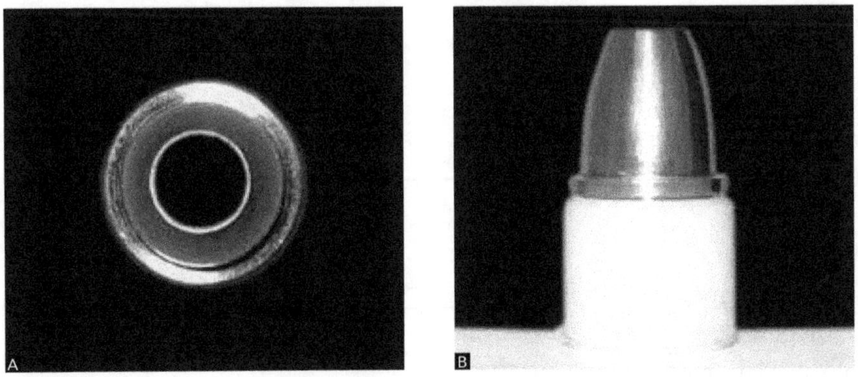

Figure 1 - **A)** Upper view, **B)** Lateral view of the new developed tip.

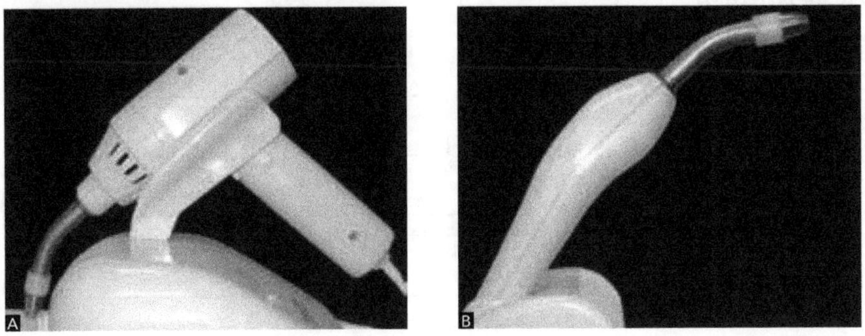

Figure 2 - **A)** Halogen light curing unit with coupled tip; **B)** LED curing unit with coupled tip.

In order to assess the performance of the tip in orthodontic bonding, we carried out the mechanical trial of shear bond strength and the analysis of the adhesive remaining index (ARI) due to their morphological and histological similarity to human teeth, 120 bovine mandibular incisors were used in this in vitro study.[11,17,22] The teeth were selected with a stereomicroscope (Stemi 2000 – C, Zeiss), at the Modern Physics Department of the Sciences Institute of the Federal University of Juiz de Fora (UFJF).

Two groups of 60 teeth each were formed. Group 1 comprised teeth of which bracket bonding was performed with a halogen-light curing unit (Dabi Atlante Ultralux), while for group 2, a LED-source curing unit (Dabi Atlante Ultraled) was used. Each group was subdivided in 2 subgroups, with 30 teeth each. In subgroups H1 and L1, the conventional tip was used, while in subgroups H2 and L2 the experimental tip we developed was used.

Bracket bonding was performed according to the instructions of the manufacturer of the composite resin (3M Transbond XT®). 120 brackets were used (Dental Morelli, reference 10.30.201).

In subgroup H1, the mesial and the distal surfaces were exposed to light for 10 seconds each. In subgroup L1, the mesial and distal surfaces were exposed to light for 5 seconds each. Light exposure was 10 seconds in subgroup H2 and 5 seconds in subgroup L2. Bonding in group 1 happened with the light held 5 mm away from the bracket-tooth interface, with an incidence parallel to the bonding surface. In group 2, the tip was positioned so as to embrace the bracket in a single incidence.

The bodies of proof for testing shear resistance were assembled[15] in a Universal Testing Machine, EMIC – DL 10000, equipped with a 50Kgf Trd 21 load cell, software Tesc version 3.04 of the Military Institute of Engineering– Rio de Janeiro – LEM DE/4. After the mechanical trial was performed, the ARI for each body of proof was determined with the Stemi 2000 – C stereomicroscope (Zeiss). The ARI indices were classified into 4 scores,[1] as shown in Table 1.

RESULTS

Table 2 shows mean values and standard deviation of each subgroup (H1, H2, L1 and L2).

Student's t test was used for comparison between subgroups. The p value for comparison between H1-H2 and L1-L2 was 0.365 and 0.176, respectively, thus, showing no statistically significant difference between the subgroups.

Figure 3 shows the distribution of values regarding the shear resistance test between groups.

The ARI distribution for each group is shown in Figure 4. The Kruskal-Wallis test was used for ARI statistical analysis. With $p > 0.05$, no statistically significant difference between groups was found.

Table 1 - Criteria for using ARI, according. (Source: Årtun et al,[1] 1984).

ARI – Adhesive Remaining Index	
Score	Frequency of remaining adhesive
0	No adhesive remaining on the dental enamel
1	Less than half of the adhesive remaining on the dental enamel
2	More than half of the adhesive remaining on the dental enamel
3	The entire adhesive remaining on the enamel, with distinct impression of the bracket mesh

Table 2 - values of shear resistance tests in MPa.

Subgroup	n	Mean ± SD
H1	30	9.89 ± 5.36
H2	30	9.01 ± 5.61
L1	30	7.01 ± 4.26
L2	30	7.63 ± 5.48
Total	120	

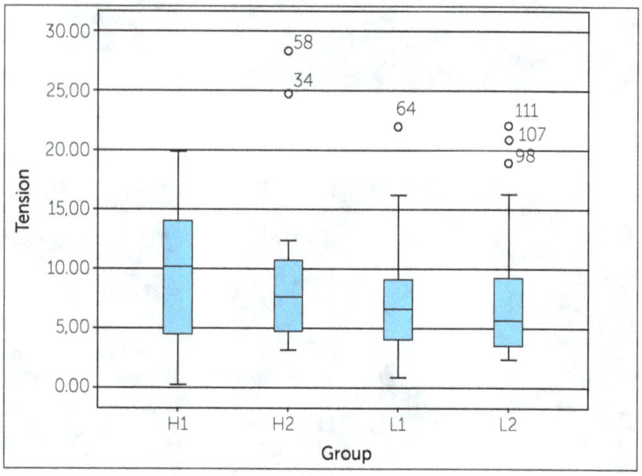

Figure 3 - Box plot diagram of shear resistance in MPa for each subgroup.

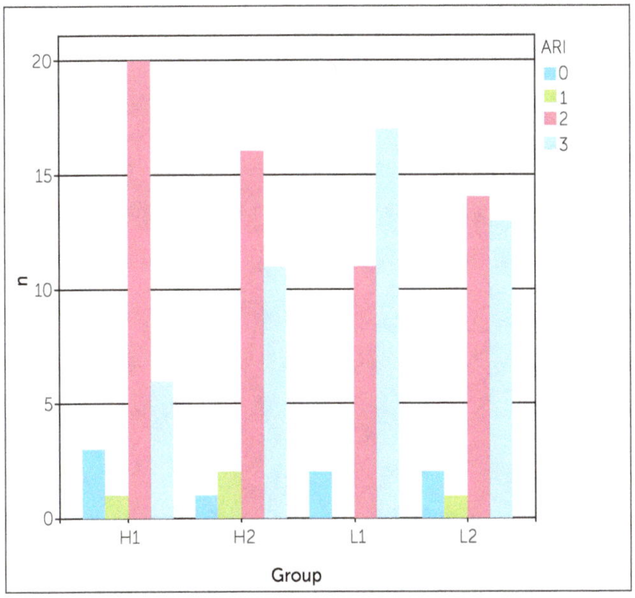

Figure 4 - Bar chart for each group, with regard to ARI incidence.

DISCUSSION

Aiming at reducing orthodontic bonding time, we developed a tip that can be coupled to curing units. This device is based on the concepts of curing unit light refraction and reflection. When visible light reaches the end of the optical fiber of the curing unit, it changes from one medium (optical fiber) to another (air), and the light ray is refracted into a medium with a lower refractive index. This refracted ray is no longer dissipated across the medium, but reflected by the inner mirrored wall of the new device. Because the new tip converges towards the bracket-tooth end, the light rays reach the composite resin in the mesial, distal, incisal/occlusal and gingival directions simultaneously, which reduces curing time up to ¼ of the time recommended by the manufacturer of traditional tips.

One of the disadvantages of using light-curing composite resins is the high number of steps that are necessary during bonding, which increases working time and the likelihood of errors and contamination during the procedure.[5,7,10,12,13,14,16] With the new tip, bonding time was reduced, consequently reducing errors caused by saliva contamination.

For subgroups H1 and L1, variation of light exposure time was in accordance with the recommendations given by the manufacturer of the 3M Transbond XT® composite resin, while for subgroups H2 and L2 it was half the time proposed by the manufacturer. The recommended times are: 20 seconds for an halogen source (10 seconds for the mesial surface and 10 seconds for the distal surface) and 10 seconds for a LED source (5 seconds for the mesial surface and 5 seconds for the distal surface).

Bond resistance corresponds to bond strength divided by the bonding interface area (mm^2). The bracket/adhesive system must resist to a minimum force of 6 MPa (megapascal) to be considered clinically successful.[4,8,9,14] All groups in this study had a mean value greater than what is required for orthodontic success.

As for the ARI assessment, the Kruskal-Wallis test showed no statistically significant difference between groups ($p > 0.05$). The majority of bodies of proof from each subgroup scored 2 or 3, with most of the adhesive remaining on the enamel surface, thus indicating that rupture occurred in the adhesive/bracket interface and not in the enamel/adhesive interface, as expected after adequate light curing.

Therefore, the shear test results and the ARI results proved both bonding techniques, either carried out with the conventional tip or with the tip developed in this study to be efficient.

CONCLUSIONS

1 – Both the mechanical trials and the ARI analysis showed that the new tip met the necessary requirements for bonding orthodontic accessories;

2 – Bonding time was reduced by half, and only a single incidence was necessary.

REFERENCES

1. Årtun J, Bergland S. Clinical trials with crystal growth conditioning as an alternative to acid-etch enamel pretreatment. Am J Orthod. 1984;85(4):333-40.
2. Barghi N, Fischer DE, Pham T. Revisiting the intensity output of curing lights in private dental offices. Compend Contin Educ Dent. 2007;28(7):380-4.
3. Bishara SE, Gordan VV, VonWald L, Olson ME. Effect of an acidic primer on shear bond strength of orthodontic brackets. Am J Orthod Dentofacial Orthop. 1998;114(3):243-7.
4. Bishara SE, VonWald L, Laffoon JF, Jakobsen JR. Effective of altering the type of enamel conditioner on the shear bond strength of a resin-reinforced glass ionomer adhesive. Am J Orthod Dentofacial Orthop. 2000;118(3):288-94.
5. Bishara SE, Laffoon JF, Vonwald L, Warren JJ. The effect of repeated bonding on the shear bond strength of different orthodontic adhesives. Am J Orthod Dentofacial Orthod. 2002;121(5):521-5.
6. Bullough JD. LED lighting systems. Lighting Answers. NLPIP. 2003 [Acesso 15 set 2011];7(3):1-23. Disponível em: http://www.lrc.rpi.edu/

programs/nlpip/lightingAnswers/led/abstract.asp.

7. Cacciafesta V, Sfondrini MF, Baluga L, Scribante A, Klersy C. Use of a self-etching primer in combination with a resin-modified glass ionomer: effect of water and saliva contamination on shear bond strength. Am J Orthod Dentofacial Orthop. 2003;124(4):420-6.
8. Cacciafesta V, Sfondrini MF, Barina E, Scribante A, Garino F, Klersy C. Effect of different light sources and guide on shear bond strength of brackets bonded with 2 adhesives systems. Am J Orthod Dentofacial Orthop. 2005;128(1):99-102.
9. Cacciafesta V, Sfondrini MF, Calvi D, Scribante A. Effect of fluoride application on shear bond strength of brackets bonded with a resin-modified glass-ionomer. Am J Orthod Dentofacial Orthop. 2005;127(5):580-3.
10. Cacciafesta V, Sfondrini MF, Scribante A, De Angelis M, Klersy C. Effect of blood contamination on shear bond strength of brackets bonded with a self-etching primer combined with a resin-modified glass ionomer. Am J Orthod Dentofacial Orthop. 2004;126(6):703-8.
11. Campos MIC, Campos CN, Vitral RWF. O uso de dentes bovinos como substitutos em dentes humanos em pesquisas odontológicas: uma revisão de literatura. Pesq Brasil Odontop Clin Odontol. 2008;8(1):127-32.
12. Correr Sobrinho L, Correr GM, Consani S, Sinhoreti MAC, Consani RLX. Influência do tempo pós-fixação na resistência ao cisalhamento de bráquetes colados com diferentes materiais. Pesqui Odontol Bras. 2002;16(1):43-9.
13. Dominguez GC, Tortamato A, Carvalho PAL, Bomfim RA, Horliana RF, Vigorito JW. Self-etching primer: resistência confiável na colagem de acessórios ortodônticos? Estudo clínico. Ortodontia SPO. 2005;38(1):10-5.
14. Dorminey JC, Dunn WJ, Taloumis LJ. Shear bond strength of orthodontic brackets bonded with a modified 1-step etchand-and-primer technique. Am J Orthod Dentofacial Orthop. 2003;124(4):410-3.
15. Dutra GAA, Rocha JM, Fraga MR, Vitral RWF. Avaliação comparativa in vitro da resistência à força de cisalhamento apresentada pelo bráquete ceramico InVu. Pesq Bras Odontoped Clin Integr. 2009;9(2):173-9.
16. Eliades T, Eliades G, Brantley WA, Johnston WM. Polymerization efficiency of chemically cured and visible light-cured orthodontic adhesives: degree of cure. Am J Orthod Dentofacial Orthop. 1995;108(3):294-301.
17. Fonseca RB, Haiter-Neto F, Fernandes-Neto AJ, Barbosa GA, Soares CJ. Radiosensity of enamel and dentin of human, bovine and swine teeth. Arch Oral Biol. 2004;19(11):912-22.
18. Onofre NML, Retamoso LB, Marchioro EM, Berthold TB. Atuação da luz halógena e do LED (light emitting diode) na resistência de união de brackets colados no esmalte dentário humano. Rev Odonto Ciênc. 2007;22(57):238-42.
19. Owens BM, Rodriguez KH. Radiometric and spectrophotometric analysis of third generation light-emitting diode (LED) light-curing units. J Contemp Dent Pract. 2007;8(2):43-51.
20. Rueggeberg FA. State-of-the-art: Dental photocuring – A review. Dent Mater. 2011;27(1):39-52.
21. Sayinsu K, Isik F, Sezen S, Aydemir B. Effect of blood and saliva contamination on bond strength of brackets bonded with a protective liquid polish and a light-cured adhesive. Am J Orthod Dentofacial Orthop. 2007;131(3):391-4.
22. Saleh F, Taymour N. Validity of using bovine teeth as a substitute for human counterparts in adhesive tests. East Mediterr Health J. 2003; 9(1-2):201-7.
23. Talbot TQ, Blankenau RJ, Zobitz ME, Weaver AL, Lohse CM, Rebellato J. Effect of argon laser irradiation on shear bond strength of orthodontic brackets: an in vitro study. Am J Orthod Dentofacial Orthop. 2000;118(3):274-9.
24. Thind BS, Stirrups DR, Lloyd CH. A comparison of tungsten-quartz-halogen, plasma arc and light-emitting diode light sources for the polymerization of an orthodontic adhesive. Eur J Orthod. 2006;28(1):78-82.

25

Welding strength of NiTi wires

Tatyane Ribeiro Mesquita[1], Lídia Parsekian Martins[1], Renato Parsekian Martins[1]

Objective: To identify the appropriate power level for electric welding of three commercial brands of nickel-titanium (NiTi) wires. **Methods:** Ninety pairs of 0.018-in and 0.017 × 0.025-in NiTi wires were divided into three groups according to their manufacturers — GI (Orthometric, Marília, Brazil), GII (3M OralCare, St. Paul, CA) and GIII (GAC,York, PA) — and welded by electrical resistance. Each group was divided into subgroups of 5 pairs of wires, in which welding was done with different power levels. In GI and GII, power levels of 2.5, 3, 3.5, 4, 4.5 and 5 were used, while in GIII 2.5, 3, 3.5 and 4 were used (each unit of power of the welding machine representing 500W). The pairs of welded wires underwent a tensile strength test on an universal testing machine until rupture and the maximum forces were recorded. Analysis of variance (ANOVA) and *post-hoc* tests were conducted to determine which subgroup within each brand group had the greatest resistance to rupture. **Results:** The 2.5 power exhibited the lowest resistance to rupture in all groups (43.75N for GI, 28.41N for GII and 47.57N for GIII) while the 4.0 power provided the highest resistance in GI and GII (97.90N and 99.61N, respectively), while in GIII (79.28N) the highest resistance was achieved with a 3.5 power welding. **Conclusions:** The most appropriate power for welding varied for each brand, being 4.0 for Orthometric and 3M, and 3.5 for GAC NiTi wires.

Keywords: Welding. Orthodontic wire. Tensile strength.

[1] Universidade Estadual Paulista, Faculdade de Odontologia de Araraquara, Departamento de Clínica Infantil (Araraquara/SP, Brazil).

Renato Parsekian Martins
Rua Humaitá, 1680, Centro, Araraquara/SP, Brasil – CEP:14.801-903
E-mail: dr_renatopmartins@hotmail.com

» The authors report no commercial, proprietary or financial interest in the products or companies described in this article.

INTRODUCTION

Electric resistance spot welding allows two or more metallic surfaces to be joined by the heat produced from an electric current conducted by two electrodes that hold both surfaces in tight contact.[1,2] This procedure is routinely in orthodontics with stainless steel and beta-titanium wires, but has not been used with nickel-titanium (NiTi) alloys. The reason for that might be associated to orthodontic literature reports that NiTi wires cannot be welded,[3-6] even though this information diverges from evidences on the field of materials engineering.[7]

NiTi wires could be further explored if welding is used. Short pieces of NiTi wires could be welded to the NiTi leveling wire, acting as hooks, allowing early use of elastics, and also as stops, decreasing cost in the orthodontic office. Moreover, springs made of NiTi could also be welded to the main wires, allowing use of superelasticity, shape-memory and low deformation of NiTi in nonconventional clinical situations. Thus, an approximate weld of round wires, usually used as initial leveling wires, to rectangular wires might he used for the mentioned situations.

Even though four papers on electrical resistance welding of NiTi wires have been published,[8-11] two of them did not compare the resistance to rupture among the welding power used.[8,9] Moreover, none of them tested the welding configuration of round to rectangular wires and did not use more than one commercial brand of NiTi. If assumed that different wires might exhibit different responses to heat, incorrect power levels used for welding may damage the wires.

Therefore, the present study aims to test the weld resistance of NiTi wires, in order to identify the most appropriate power level to be used in wires manufactured by three different trademarks.

MATERIALS AND METHODS

Ninety pairs of round 0.018-in and 0.017 × 0.025-in NiTi wires were divided into three groups according to their manufacturers: Group I (GI) was made with wires from Orthometric (Marília, São Paulo, Brazil), Group II (GII), from 3M (3M OralCare, St. Paul, CA); and Group III (GIII), from GAC International (GAC, York, PA, United States).

The thinner surface of the rectangular wire of each group was welded by electrical resistance to a respective round wire (Fig 1), using a modified spot welding machine (Pontomatic NiTi - Electronic Automatic, Kernit, Indaiatuba, São Paulo, Brazil). Subgroups were created within each group, according to the power levels used for the welding. Groups I and II were divided into six subgroups, which were welded with power levels of 2.5, 3, 3.5, 4, 4.5 and 5 (each power level of the welding machine represents 500W), while Group III wires were divided into four subgroups, welded with power levels of 2.5, 3, 3.5 and 4. The tests started at a power level of 2.5 because this was the smallest power capable of welding wires, while higher values than the ones tested damaged the wires during welding. The welding machine was calibrated to apply an electric current for 3 milliseconds between two flat electrodes, producing a force of 12N when joining the wires. All the welding procedures were performed by the same calibrated operator.

For the tension test, the welded wires were secured at a distance of 4 cm from the weld, with clamps specially made for the study, and subjected to the tensile strength tests using a universal testing machine (EMIC, São José dos Pinhais, Paraná, Brazil), with a 5 kN load cell. The tests were performed with a crosshead speed of 0.5 mm per minute until the rupture of the wires.

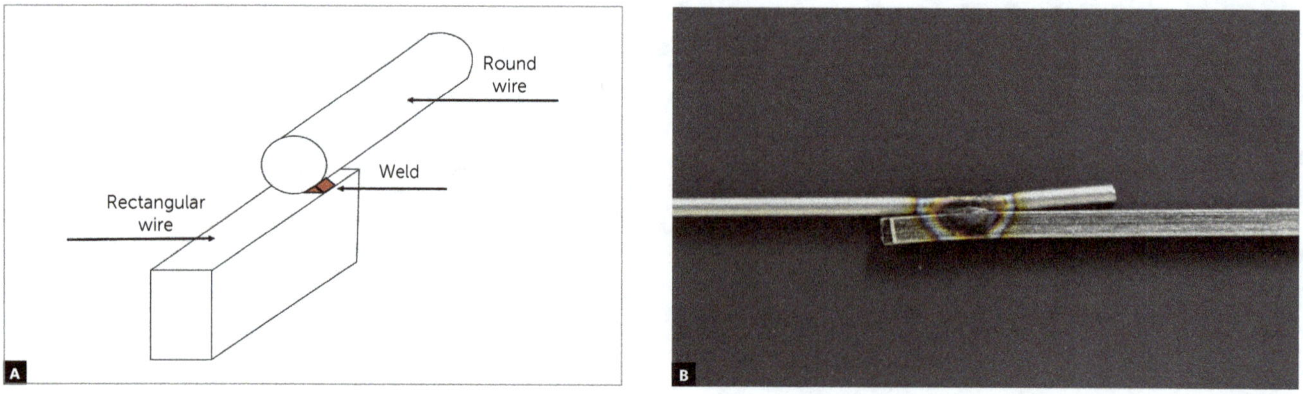

Figure 1 - **A)** Schematic drawings of the electric resistance weld. **B)** Image of a weld analyzed in this study.

The dedicated software of the machine recorded the breaking-point force, in Newtons (N).

Statistical analysis was performed using SPSS software, version 16.0. (SPSS Inc., Chicago, IL, USA). The data distribution was normal and subgroups were compared using an analysis of variance with a significance level of 0.05, to identify subgroup differences while Tukey *post-hoc* test ($p = 0{,}05$) was used to determine which groups were different.

RESULTS

All the wire ruptures were very close to the weld. There was a difference between the forces registered in the GI subgroups ($p < 0.001$) (Table 1). The power levels of 2.5, 3, 3.5 and 5 produced similar forces of rupture, with values of 43.75N, 61.69N, 65.00N and 53.76N, respectively. The power levels 4 and 4.5 were statistically similar to each other, but different from the remaining levels, with forces of 97.90N and 92.11N, respectively (Fig 2).

There was also a difference between the force values of GII ($p < 0.001$). The power level 2.5 resulted in a maximum force (28.41N) different to the other power levels. The power levels 5 and 3 (58.79N and 79.66N, respectively) produced similar forces, which were different from the remaining levels. The levels 3, 3.5, 4 and 4.5 were statistically similar and produced forces of 79.66N, 89.75N, 99.61N and 93.61N, respectively (Fig 2).

GIII also showed a difference between the registered forces ($p = 0.004$). The weld with a power level of 2.5 produced a maximum force of 47.57N, which was similar to the power levels 3 (67.96N) and 4 (67.69N). The power level 3.5 produced a maximum force of 79.28N, which was statistically similar to the power levels 3 and 4. The power levels 4.5 and 5 were not tested as the wires were destroyed during welding (Fig 2).

Table 1 - Average and standard deviations of the tensile strength (in Newtons) of NiTi wires welded at different power levels.

Power level	GI (N)	GIII (N)	GIII (N)
2.5	43.75 ± 6.10 [a]	28.41 ± 12.36 [a]	47.57 ± 4.39 [a]
3	61.69 ± 9.41 [a]	79.66 ± 7.64 [b,c]	67.96 ± 4.77 [a,b]
3.5	64.99 ± 11.11 [a]	89.75 ± 12.48 [c]	79.28 ± 12.62 [b]
4	97.90 ± 11.59 [b]	99.61 ± 10.14 [c]	67.69 ± 18.14 [a,b]
4.5	92.11 ± 17.51 [b]	93.61 ± 15.74 [c]	...
5	53.74 ± 14.39 [a]	58.79 ± 18.29 [b]	...
Sig.	<.001	<.001	.004

Each unit of power level of the welding machine represents 500W. Equal letters: absence of statistically significant difference ($p > 0.05$, ANOVA).

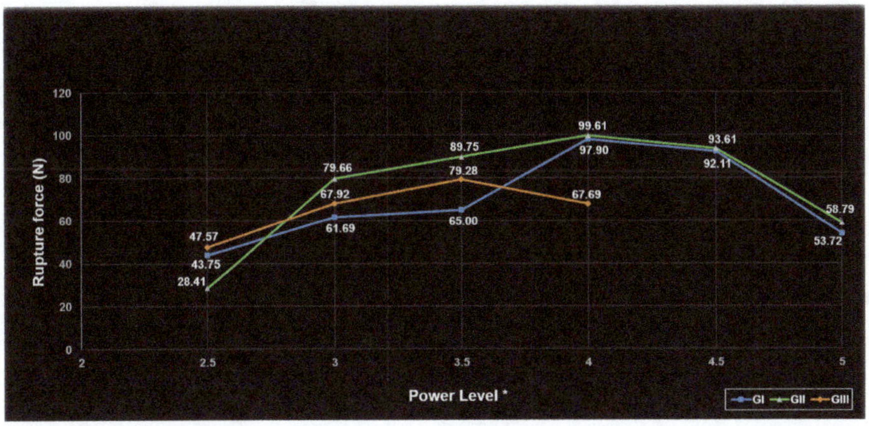

Figure 2 - Graph of maximum tensile strength of the welds performed in NiTi wires of the tested groups, according to the used power levels. * One unit of power level of the welding machine represents 500W.

DISCUSSION

The power that produced the strongest weld in the NiTi wires was identified for each tested brands. Although there are only four articles in the literature related to electric resistance welding in NiTi wires,[8-11] none of them tested wires of different commercial brands, which is very important, according to the present results. Moreover, none of them tested which power was more appropriate to be used according to the resistance of the weld.

The most appropriate power level for each brand was defined as the one that produced a weld with the highest tensile strength. The tests started at a power level of 2.5 —since lower levels did not weld the NiTi wires—, and these power levels were increased in steps of 0.5 until the heat produced by the weld broke the wires during the welding process. Present results show that the maximum tensile strength of the welded wires increased with the power levels up to a certain point, after which the resistance began to decrease. These peaks of resistance (Fig 2) were at the power 4 for the GI and GII groups, and 3.5 for GIII group. The resistance decrease with higher power levels occurred because the heat produced by the weld causes annealing of the wire[10], which is sufficient to significantly alter its mechanical properties and sometimes even break the wire, as occurred in the wires of the GIII group when welded at power levels higher than 4 (and therefore were not used in this study). The difference of power levels that obtained the highest resistance for each group can be explained by variations in the manufacturing process of the wires, which may be due to its composition, as the nickel percentage can vary,[12] or due to the tested welding machine setting and cooking processes.

The rupture of the wires never occurred at the weld but very close to it. This was probably due to the heat produced around the weld, which anneals the wire making it less resistant. Welded wires show less maximum resistance to tension than solid wires,[8,13-15] however, it need to be strong enough to tolerate orthodontic forces. In this report, it were found values ranging from 8 to 10 kilograms-force, which are high enough to support orthodontic forces. Even though the objective of this paper was not to compare the tensile forces of NiTi and stainless steel (SS) wires, a tension test was performed on same dimension SS wires (3M OralCare, St. Paul, CA) for discussion purposes. This comparison was not present in the objectives of this study, since SS wires need a higher power to produce adequate weld than NiTi wires, due to its higher melting point. Nonetheless, necessarily using a higher power level (5), the SS wires showed an average force of resistance to rupture of 134.3 ± 6.96 N, which was approximately 35, 37 and 69% higher than for the GII, GI and GIII groups, respectively.

This results are lower than the results reported in the literature[8-10] because the wires used in this work had smaller diameters. The clinical implications of welded NiTi orthodontic wires are of great importance as they allow a combination of the advantages of this alloy, such as high flexibility, shape memory, superelasticity, the possibility of using hooks for attaching elastics, and the use of omega loops or stops (Fig 3). Additionally, springs

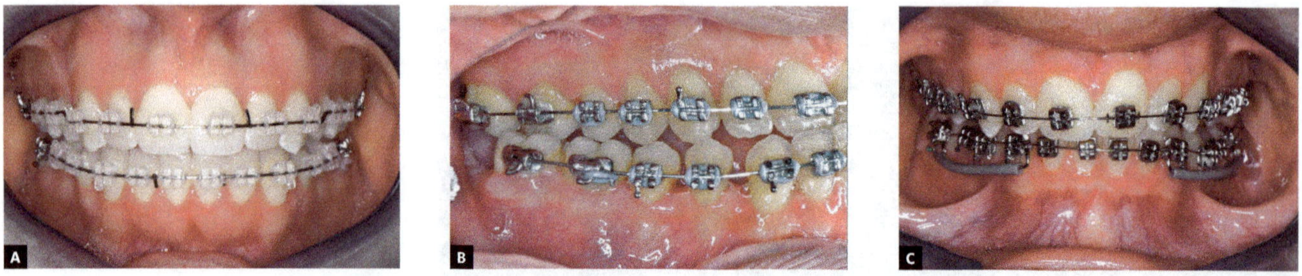

Figure 3 - A) Welded NiTi hooks for vertical elastic use. B) Welded stop for tying the archwire. C) Stops to keep wire from sliding distally.

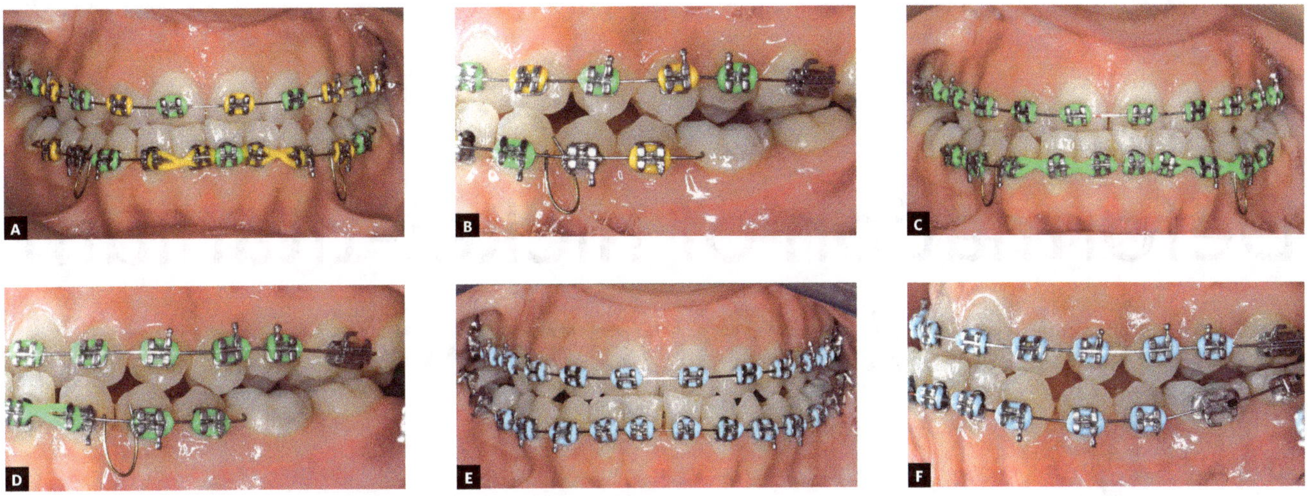

Figure 4 - 0.014-in NiTi proclining loops welded to the main wire, initial stage: **A)** frontal view and **B)** lateral view. Same patient, 30 days after: **C)** frontal view and **D)** lateral view. Same patient, after 30 more days: **E)** frontal view and **F)** lateral view.

may also be welded to alignment wires, to assist in that phase of treatment (Fig 4).

Although these results open up new possibilities for the use of NiTi alloys in orthodontics, further studies should be made to evaluate these welded wires in the long term within the oral cavity, where they are subjected to factors such as corrosion by saliva as well as thermal and mechanical cycling. Additionally, it would be of great value to develop, if possible, a type of weld in which there is no annealing of the wire around the weld point, both for NiTi wires and steel wires, which are usually reinforced with a silver alloy weld.

CONCLUSIONS

The most suitable power levels for electric resistance welding of NiTi wires varied for the different brands.

The most appropriate power level to weld the wires with the parameters given by the used welding machine was identified as being 4 (2000W) for the Orthometric and 3M brands, and 3.5 (1750W) for GAC.

REFERENCES

1. Darwish S, Ghanya A. Critical assessment of weld-bonded technologies. J Mater Process Technol. 2000;105(3):221-9.
2. Wu K. Resistance spot welding of high contact resistance for weld-bonding. Weld J. 1975;54:436s-43s.
3. Kapila S, Sachdeva R. Mechanical properties and clinical applications of orthodontic wires. Am J Orthod Dentofacial Orthop. 1989 Aug;96(2):100-9.
4. Iijima M, Brantley WA, Yuasa T, Muguruma T, Kawashima I, Mizoguchi I. Joining characteristics of orthodontic wires with laser welding. J Biomed Mater Res B Appl Biomater. 2008 Jan;84(1):147-53.
5. Blackman R, Baez R, Barghi N. Marginal accuracy and geometry of cast titanium copings. J Prosthet Dent. 1992 Apr;67(4):435-40.
6. Burstone CJ. Welding of TMA wire. Clinical applications. J Clin Orthod. 1987 Sept;21(9):609-15.
7. Duerig P. TiNi Shape Memory Alloys. In: Collings EW, Welsch G, editors. Material Properties Handbook Titanium Alloys. Materials Park, OH: ASM International; 1994. p. 1047.
8. Matsunaga J, Watanabe I, Nakao N, Watanabe E, Elshahawy W, Yoshida N. Joining characteristics of titanium-based orthodontic wires connected by laser and electrical welding methods. J Mater Sci Mater Med. 2015 Jan;26(1):5391.
9. Nascimento LE, Santos RL, Pithon MM, Araújo MT, Nojima MG, LI. N. The effect of electric spot-welding on the mechanical properties of different orthodontic wire alloys. Mat Res. 2012 May-June;15(3):409-14.
10. Tam B, Pequegnat A, Khan MI, Zhou Y. Resistance Microwelding of Ti-55.8 wt pct Ni Nitinol Wires and the Effects of Pseudoelasticity. Metall Mater Trans A. 2012 Aug;43(8):2969-78.
11. Fukumoto S, Morikawa SAY. Small-scale resistance welding of crossed TiNi fine wire. Mater Sci Forum. 2008;580-582:225-8.
12. Kararia V, Jain P, Chaudhary S, Kararia N. Estimation of changes in nickel and chromium content in nickel-titanium and stainless steel orthodontic wires used during orthodontic treatment: an analytical and scanning electron microscopic study. Contemp Clin Dent. 2015;6(1):44-50.
13. Sevilla P, Martorell F, Libenson C, Planell JA, Gil FJ. Laser welding of NiTi orthodontic archwires for selective force application. J Mater Sci Mater Med. 2008;19(2):525-9.
14. Bock JJ, Fraenzel W, Bailly J, Gernhardt CR, Fuhrmann RA. Influence of different brazing and welding methods on tensile strength and microhardness of orthodontic stainless steel wire. Eur J Orthod. 2008 Aug;30(4):396-400.
15. Gugel H, Schuermann A, Theisen W. Laser welding of NiTi wires. Mater Sci Eng A. 2008;481-482:668-71.

26

Deformation of nickel-titanium closed coil springs: An *in vitro* study

Camilla Ivini Viana Vieira[1], José Maurício dos Santos Nunes Reis[2], Luiz Geraldo Vaz[3], Lídia Parsekian Martins[4], Renato Parsekian Martins[5]

Objective: The aim of this paper was to determine the amount of deformation in four commercial brands of nickel-titanium closed springs. **Methods:** A total of 130 springs were divided into 13 subgroups, according to their features and manufacturers (Morelli, Orthometric, Ormco and GAC) and activated from 100% to 1000% of the effective length of the nickel-titanium portion present at the spring, at 37 °C. Deactivation data were plotted and deformation was found graphically. The values were compared by analysis of variance and Tukey's *post-hoc* test. **Results:** Springs manufactured by Morelli had the same amount of deformation when they were activated up to 700% of Y activation; springs by Orthometric had the same amount of deformation up to 600-700% of Y; springs by Ormco had the same amount of deformation up to 700-800% of Y; and finally, the majority of springs by GAC had similar deformation up to 800%-1000% of activation. All springs tested could be activated up to 700% without rupture. **Conclusions:** Most subgroups were similarly deformed up to 700% of activation, without rupture of springs. Subgroups 4B, 4C, 4D and 4E showed the same amount of deformation up to 1000% of activation without any rupture at all.

Keywords: NiTi. Deformation. Biomechanics.

[1] MSc, Universidade Estadual Paulista (UNESP), Department of Pediatric Dentistry, School of Dentistry, Araraquara, São Paulo, Brazil.

[2] Assistant Professor, Universidade Estadual Paulista (UNESP), Department of Dental Material, School of Dentistry, Araraquara, São Paulo, Brazil.

[3] Full Professor, Universidade Estadual Paulista (UNESP), Department of Dental Material, School of Dentistry, Araraquara, São Paulo, Brazil.

[4] Assistant Professor, Universidade Estadual Paulista (UNESP), Department of Pediatric Dentistry, School of Dentistry, Araraquara, São Paulo, Brazil.

[5] Private practice and part-time Faculty, Universidade Estadual Paulista (UNESP), Department of Pediatric Dentistry, School of Dentistry, Araraquara, São Paulo, Brazil.

» The authors report no commercial, proprietary or financial interest in the products or companies described in this article.

Renato Parsekian Martins
E-mail: dr_renatopmartins@hotmail.com

INTRODUCTION

In the late 1960s, the U.S. Navy developed a nickel-titanium alloy known as Nitinol,[1] which had the property of returning to its original shape after being heated above a certain temperature. This property was called "shape memory." Nitinol was introduced in Orthodontics in the 1970s,[2] due to its low elastic modulus and good elastic recovery. In the following decade, two new nickel-titanium alloys[3,4] were introduced in Orthodontics, bringing up a new property to orthodontic therapy: superelasticity (SE).

SE is characterized by a near-to-constant force (during unloading) depicted on the alloy's load/deflection graph, caused by a stress-induced transformation from austenitic to martensitic phase (SIMT), which are two different crystallographic structures that can exist within the same alloy. The image of this near-to-constant force on the graph is referred to as a plateau because of its shape, but it will be termed pseudo-plateau in this paper because it is not completely flat. Each of those two phases has a different elastic modulus, which makes this alloy unique.[5,6,7] In Orthodontics, it is often desired for nickel-titanium springs to work in its SE plateau, but a high stress is needed to induce SIMT. However, the literature is not clear on how much these springs need to be activated without suffering any significant permanent deformation. There are reports in the literature, without presenting any evidence, of activations of 500% the spring's original length without permanent deformation,[8,9,10] although imposing no limits to a higher activation. Only one paper[11] mentions ruptures in nickel-titanium springs excessively activated, but it does not correlate the rupture to the effective length of the nickel-titanium portion in the spring.

Currently, springs are available in different sizes and several martensitic plateaus, as informed by the manufacturer. This makes the choice for the ideal device for each situation very difficult, especially regarding the size of orthodontic space, force produced, amount of activation and the limit that each device allows for activation without permanent deformation.

Therefore, the aim of this study was to determine the percentage of deformation of four commercially available nickel-titanium closed coil springs subjected to several activations.

MATERIAL AND METHODS

Four groups of springs were established according to the manufacturer: Group 1, Morelli Ortodontia (Sorocaba/SP, Brazil); Group 2, Orthometric (Orthometric Importadora Exportadora Ltda, Marília/ SP, Brazil); Group 3, Ormco Co. (Glendora, Ca, USA); and Group 4, Dentsply GAC Int. (Bohemia, NY, USA). Within each group, subgroups of ten springs were determined according to length and force plateau provided by the manufacturer. All ten springs from each subgroup were from the same batch, totaling 130 springs (Table 1).

An EMIC DL2000 (São José dos Pinhais, Paraná, Brazil) universal testing machine equipped with load cell of 0.1kN was used for testing. The entire system was submerged in distilled water at $37 \pm 1°C$,[12] controlled with a 30-W heater (Termodelfim, São Paulo, Brazil) and a thermostat (Alife, São Paulo, Brazil).

The size of the springs in each group was measured with a digital caliper (Mitutoyo SC-6, Suzano, São Paulo, Brazil) and the averages were calculated to determine the total size of the spring (X), as well as the effective length of the nickel-titanium portion (Y) (Fig 1).

Previously to testing, each spring was adjusted with the aid of a digital indicator of extension and force in order to avoid any looseness of the spring, compromising the true activation of the spring in the test.

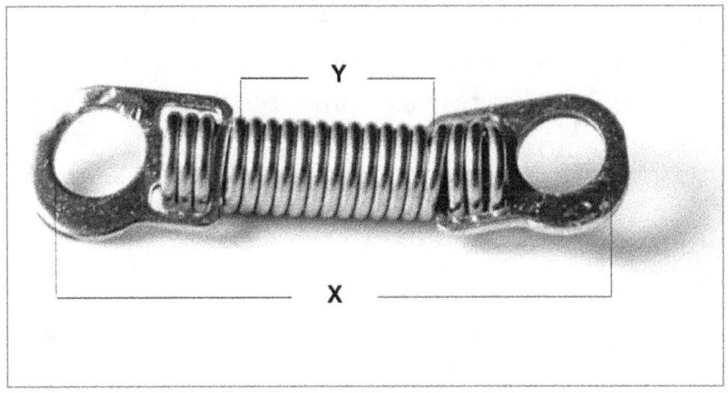

Figure 1 - Nickel-titanium closed coil spring, the X dimension corresponds to the total length of the spring and the Y dimension corresponds to the length of the nickel-titanium portion.

Table 1 - Commercial brands and groups division.

Commercial brand	Specification	Length (mm)*	X (mm)	Y (mm)	Force plateau (gf)*	Subgroup	n
Group 1		7	8.6	2.3	250	1A	10
(Morelli Ortodontia, Brazil)		9	10.3	3.9	250	1B	10
Group 2		7	6.8	2.1	175	2A	10
(Orthometric, Brazil)		9	8.9	4.1	250	2B	10
Group 3	Light	9	8.85	3.25	80	3A	10
(Ormco, USA)	Heavy	9	9	3.1	150	3B	10
Group 4 (GAC, USA)	Sentalloy 25g	10	8.5	3.2	25	4A	10
	Sentalloy 50g	10	8.5	3.2	50	4B	10
	Sentalloy 100g	10	8.5	3.2	100	4C	10
	Sentalloy 150g	10	8.5	3.2	150	4D	10
	Sentalloy 200g	10	8.5	3.2	200	4E	10
	Sentalloy 250g	10	8.5	3.2	250	4F	10
	Sentalloy 300g	10	8.5	3.2	300	4G	10

* information supplied by manufacturer.

The springs were activated to 100% of Y, and then returned to their original position. The test continued to 200%, 300%, 400%, 500%, 600%, 700%, 800%, 900%, 1000% of Y. A dedicated software (EMIC - Equipamentos e Sistemas de Ensaio Ltda, São José dos Pinhais, PR, Brazil) registered, in raw format, the force values obtained throughout the trial. The test was performed at 20 mm/min.

The data obtained were exported to Microsoft Office Excel 2007 (Microsoft, Redmond, USA) in which the amount of deformation was graphically identified at each activation. Deformations were only assessed in the subgroups at the activation that presented SE behavior, as determined according to the methods described in the literature.[13]

Deformation values were transferred to SPSS™ software, v. 16.0 (Chicago, Illinois, USA) in which analysis of variance was carried out in order to identify differences between groups, followed by Tukey's *post-hoc* test to compare subgroups, since data were normally distributed.

RESULTS

Deformations of subgroup 1A springs from 400% to 700% of activation of Y were similar; deformations at 800% of activation were larger than the activations from 400 to 600%, but similar to 700%; while deformations at 900% and 1000% of activation were the same, but different from all others activations; there was no rupture to these springs. In subgroup 1B, deformations at 400% to 800% of activation were the same; deformation at 800% of activation was the same as 900% of activation, which was equal to 1000% of activation; in this subgroup, one spring ruptured at 1000% activation (Table 2).

Deformations of subgroup 2A springs occurring from 400% to 700% of activation were similar; deformations at 800% were different from those that occurred from 400 to 600% of activation, but similar to those at 700% of activation; above 800% of activation deformations were similar; one spring ruptured at 800% of activation, two at 900%, and three at 1000%. In subgroup 2B, from 400% to 600% of activation, deformations were the same; deformation caused at 600% was equal to the one caused at 700%; at 800% of activation, deformation was equal to 700% of activation; five springs ruptured at 800% of activation, four at 900%, and one at 1000% of activation (Table 3).

Deformations caused at 400% to 700% of activation in subgroup 3A were equal, but different from deformations that occurred at 800% to 1000% of activation, which were equal to each other; five springs ruptured at 900% of activation; from the five springs remaining, two ruptured at 1000% of activation and tree remained intact. Subgroup 3B did not show SE behavior, so no comparison was performed. In subgroup 3C, deformations that occurred at 600% to 800% of activation were equal, with deformation at 800% being the same as the deformation at 900% of activation, which was the same deformation that occurred at 1000% of activation; four springs of this subgroup ruptured at 1000% of activation (Table 4).

In subgroup 4A, deformations that occurred at 400% to 800% of activation were equal to each other and different from deformations occurring at 900% and at 1000% of activation, which were equal. In subgroups 4B, 4D, 4C, and 4E, all deformations were the same at 400% to 1000% of activation for the first two subgroups, at 300% to 1000% of activation for subgroup 4C, and at 500% to 1000% of activation for 4E. In subgroup 4F, deformations were equal at 400% to 800% of activation, but different at 900% and 1000%. In subgroup 4G, deformations were equal at 500% to 800% and different at 900% and 1000%. None of the springs in subgroups 4A, 4B, 4C, 4D, 4E, and 4F ruptured. Only one spring in subgroup 4G ruptured at 900% of activation and two springs at 1000% (Table 5).

Table 2 - Average deformation in millimeters (SD in parenthesis) and in percentage values of the total length of group 1 springs.

Activation	Subgroup 1A			Subgroup 1B		
		Deformation			Deformation	
	n	%	mm	n	%	mm
400%	10	2.6%	0.06 (0.05)^{A}	10	1.3%	0.05 (0.07)^{A}
500%	10	3.9%	0.09 (0.05)^{A}	10	3.1%	0.12 (0.08)^{A}
600%	10	3.9%	0.09 (0.11)^{A}	10	5.6%	0.22 (0.18)^{A}
700%	10	9.1%	0.21 (0.09)^{AB}	10	7.7%	0.30 (0.33)^{A}
800%	10	17.4%	0.40 (0.18)^{B}	10	16.4%	0.64 (0.50)^{AB}
900%	10	29.6%	0.68 (0.26)^{C}	10	36.4%	1.42 (0.68)^{BC}
1000%	10	35.2%	0.81 (0.36)^{C}	9	55.9%	2.18 (1.28)^{C}
p		< 0.001			< 0.001	

Table 3 - Average deformation in millimeters (SD in parenthesis) and in percentage values of group 2 springs.

Activation (%)	Subgroup 2A			Subgroup 2B		
		Deformation			Deformation	
	n	%	mm	n	%	mm
400%	10	10.0%	0.21 (0.18)^{A}	10	6.6%	0.27 (0.18)^{A}
500%	10	13.8%	0.29 (0.24)^{A}	10	14.4%	0.59 (0.26)^{A}
600%	10	15.7%	0.33 (0.28)^{A}	10	22.4%	0.92 (0.37)^{AB}
700%	10	36.2%	0.76 (0.38)^{AB}	10	36.8%	1.51 (0.84)^{BC}
800%	9	66.2%	1.39 (0.68)^{BC}	5	44.1%	1.81 (0.63)^{C}
900%	7	96.7%	2.03 (0.84)^{C}	1	81.2%	3.33
1000%	4	102.4%	2.15 (1.74)^{C}	0	-	-
p		< 0.001			< 0.001	

Table 4 - Average deformation in millimeters (SD in parenthesis) and in percentage values of the total length of group 3 springs.

Activation (%)	Subgroup 3A Deformation			Subgroup 3C Deformation		
	n	%	mm	n	%	mm
300%	10	3.7%	0.12 (0.08)^{A}	-	-	-
400%	10	6.5%	0.21 (0.10)^{A}	-	-	-
500%	10	9.5%	0.31 (0.16)^{A}	-	-	-
600%	10	17.5%	0.57 (0.23)^{A}	10	17.7%	0.55 (0.24)^{A}
700%	10	42.1%	1.37 (0.37)^{A}	10	31.6%	0.98 (0.39)^{A}
800%	10	107.1%	3.48 (1.58)^{B}	10	66.1%	2.05 (1.05)^{A}
900%	5	147.1%	4.78 (0.98)^{B}	10	120.0%	3.72 (1.81)^{B}
1000%	3	137.5%	4.47 (3.67)^{B}	6	154.5%	4.79 (1.38)^{B}
p		< 0.001			< 0.001	

- Non SE.

Table 5 - Average deformation in millimeters (SD in parenthesis) and in percentage values of the total length of group 4 springs.

Activation	Subgroup 4A Deformation			Subgroup 4B Deformation			Subgroup 4C Deformation			Subgroup 4D Deformation		
	n	%	mm	n	%	mm	n	%	mm	n	%	mm
300%	-	-	-	-	-	-	10	2.2%	0.07 (0.05)	-	-	-
400%	10	3.4%	0.11 (0.09)^{A}	10	2.2%	0.07 (0.05)	10	2.2%	0.07 (0.06)	10	3.4%	0.10 (0.07)
500%	10	2.5%	0.08 (0.05)^{A}	10	2.2%	0.07 (0.06)	10	2.5%	0.08 (0.05)	10	4.1%	0.13 (0.13)
600%	10	3.4%	0.10 (0.12)^{A}	10	2.2%	0.07 (0.06)	10	2.5%	0.08 (0.06)	10	4.1%	0.13 (0.13)
700%	10	2.8%	0.11 (0.08)^{A}	10	2.2%	0.07 (0.06)	10	2.5%	0.08 (0.06)	10	3.4%	0.10 (0.12)
800%	10	14.0%	0.45 (0.29)^{A}	10	1.6%	0.05 (0.05)	10	2.5%	0.08 (0.04)	10	3.4%	0.10 (0.12)
900%	10	59.7%	1.91 (1.02)^{B}	10	1.3%	0.04 (0.04)	10	1.3%	0.04* (0.07)	10	3.8%	0.12 (0.19)
1000%	10	44.1%	1.41 (0.96)^{B}	10	-0.6%	-0.02 (0.14)	10	1.3%	0.04* (0.25)	10	2.8%	0.09* (0.19)
p		< 0.001			0.076			0.965			0.981	

Activation	Subgroup 4E Deformation			Subgroup 4F Deformation			Subgroup 4G Deformation		
	n	%	mm	n	%	mm	n	%	mm
300%	-	-	-	-	-	-	-	-	-
400%	-	-	-	10	4.1%	0.13 (0.05)^{A}	-	-	-
500%	10	1.6%	0.05 (0.04)	10	4.1%	0.13 (0.07)^{A}	10	3.4%	0.10 (0.09)^{A}
600%	10	0.6%	0.02 (0.03)	10	3.8%	0.12 (0.08)^{A}	10	3.4%	0.10 (0.08)^{A}
700%	10	0.9%	0.03 (0.03)	10	3.4%	0.11 (0.06)^{A}	10	1.6%	0.05 (0.05)^{A}
800%	10	-0.01	-0.02* (0.18)	10	0.9%	0.03* (0.07)^{A}	10	0.9%	0.03* (0.86)^{A}
900%	10	1.6%	0.05* (0.27)	10	12.5%	- 0.4 (0.23)^{B}	9	38.1%	1.22 (1.41)^{B}
1000%	10	1.6%	0.05* (0.38)	10	72.5%	2.32 (0.66)^{C}	7	89.7%	2.87 (1.11)^{C}
p		0.975			< 0.001			< 0.001	

* Non significant values.
- Non SE.

DISCUSSION

All springs tested could be activated up to 700% without rupturing, some subgroups however, showed more resistance to rupture. Springs in subgroups 1A, 4A, 4B, 4C, 4D, 4E, and 4F did not rupture up to the length tested, while the ones in subgroups 1B, 3B, and 4G only ruptured at 1000% of activation. Springs of subgroup 3A began to rupture at 900%, and the ones in Group 2 began to rupture at 800% of activation. Comparison of these values is difficult because the literature mentions activations only up to 500%,[8,9,10] and only one study[11] tested springs until they ruptured. In this last study, however, activations were not correlated to the percentage of activation in relation to Y. Despite the risk of rupture being one of the determinant factors to how much a spring can be activated, there are other more important factors, such as deformation.

In most springs of Groups 1, 2, and 3, there was no difference between deformation up to 700% of activation. From that percentage of activation on, deformations increased (except for subgroups 2B and 3C). Even at the smallest activations where SIMT occurred (mostly at 400%), there was already a small deformation that remained stable until 700% of activation, which could be due to stress relaxation of the springs. An interesting fact is that all springs in groups 1 and 2 showed resistance to rupture up to approximately 36% of deformation, and started to rupture above that amount. Deformations measured by this research in nickel-titanium springs may have happened partially because of stress relaxation, residual permanent deformation,[14] and reversible martensitic deformation, which is reversible upon heating above a certain temperature, due to shape memory (Fig 2).

Springs in group 4 ruptured and deformed less than in other groups. In subgroups 4B, 4C, 4D, and 4E, deformation was the same in all activations, even at 1000% of activation, deformations were not clinically significant and were smaller than 2.8%. Subgroups 4A, 4F, and 4G showed the same amount of deformation up to 800% of activation, with maximum deformations of 14%, 0.9%, and 0.9%, respectively. It is clear that, even with a subjective assessment, springs in group 4 were superior when compared to the ones in other groups in relation to deformation and resistance. Similarly to springs of groups 1 and 2, springs of subgroup 4G started to rupture above 38% of deformation.

From a clinical standpoint, even with significant deformations of about 30%, some springs could still be efficient depending on the situation they are used. When closing pre-molars spaces (Fig 3), nickel-titanium springs are normally attached from hooks on the first molars to hooks on the canines (around 23 mm of distance),[15] and after a 7 mm space closure, they would still be active over the 16-mm space left. Thus, if a spring of subgroup 1A (8.6 mm in total length) is attached to the molar hook, stretched to 900% and then engaged over the hook of the archwire during deactivation, it would be effectively activated 14.4 mm and it would remain active up to 7.4 mm of activation with constant force. With a slight difference, one spring from subgroup 1B (10.3 mm) would be active from 12.7 to 5.7 mm (Fig 4). In those two clinical situations, deformations smaller than 7.4 mm and 5.7 mm, respective to each situation, would be considered clinically irrelevant. However, there are two other variables that should be considered when using nickel-titanium springs: one is the desired force, since the force plateau decreases with increased activation;[11,16] and the second is the relationship between the spring's clinical work range (Fig 3) and the SE plateau length, because even at a SIMT, the dimensions that are clinically used in Orthodontics could make the spring work outside its SE plateau (Fig 4), thus acting in a SE way only after some space is closed or even never acting in a SE way at all.

The decrease of inclination and increase of length in force plateau with activation occurs because stress in not evenly distributed throughout the spring with activation. As activation is gradually increased, there is a tendency for more areas of the spring to be stressed enough to produce a SIMT; thus, with more areas going through reverse transformation, more "superelastic" the spring becomes. For that reason, limiting nickel-titanium springs activation with the purpose of maintaining forces at a low level is illogical. Moreover, it appears to be a good idea to overactivate those springs upon affixation, in order to improve the springs ability to produce constant and relatively lower forces.[17] That directly connects to the fact that the vast majority of nickel-titanium materials does not behave in a superelastic manner when used in Orthodontics, due to the fact that they are not activated enough to produce SIMT. Large springs will not work properly since not enough stress is produced (Fig 5);[17] thus, a pseudo-pla-

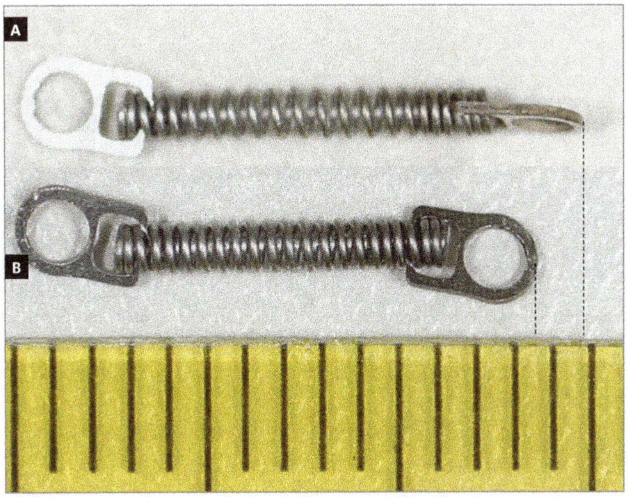

Figure 2 - Nickel-titanium closed coil spring, before activation (B) and after 900% of activation (A). After heating it above a certain temperature (Af), the martensitic deformation will resume due to the shape memory effect.

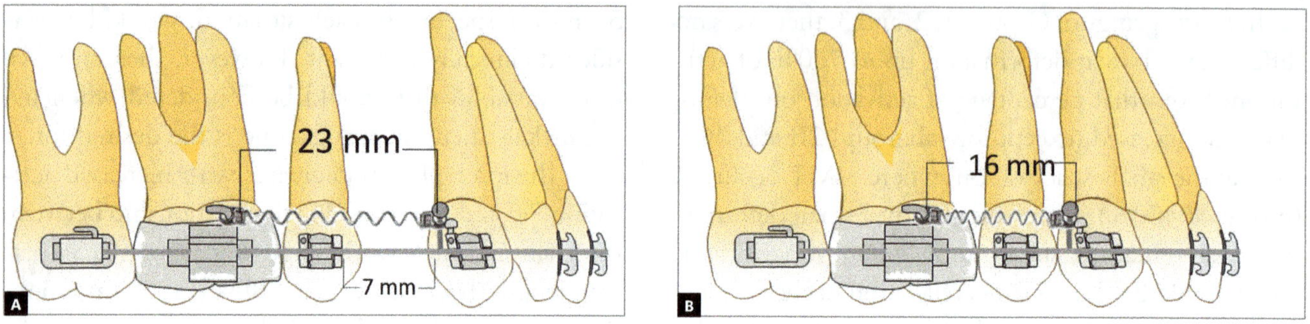

Figure 3 - Space closure after extraction of first premolars where a nickel titanium spring was attached to a hook from the first molar to a hook distal to the canine (23mm distance), remaining active even after space closure (minus 7mm of pre-molar space).

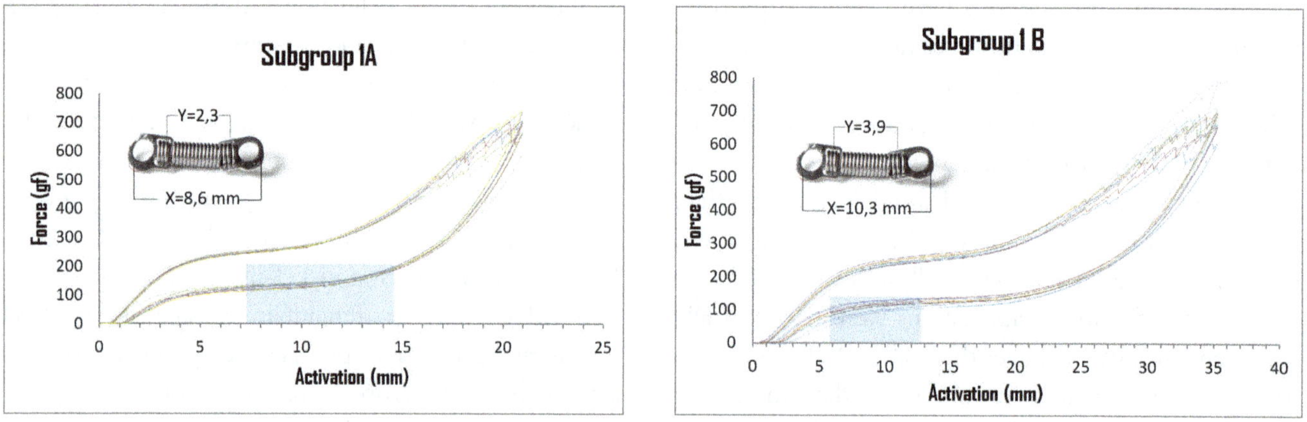

Figure 4 - **A)** Load/deflection graph for the springs of the subgroup 1A activated at 900% of Y (20.7mm of activation or 29.3mm if the size of the spring is accounted). The blue box corresponds to the distance between the hook of the first molar and a hook distal to the upper canine (minus size of the spring), as in Figure 3 (23mm minus X). Note that to take full advantage of the springs' SE properties, an increase of approximately 3mm in the eyelets (not in nickel titanium portion) would be required in order to maintain the force in the SE plateau. That would shift the blue box to the left the same 3mm. **B)** Same situation on the subgroup 1B, however, full SE capability would not be achieved in last 2mm or so of space closure, since the force would start to decrease due to lack of stress.

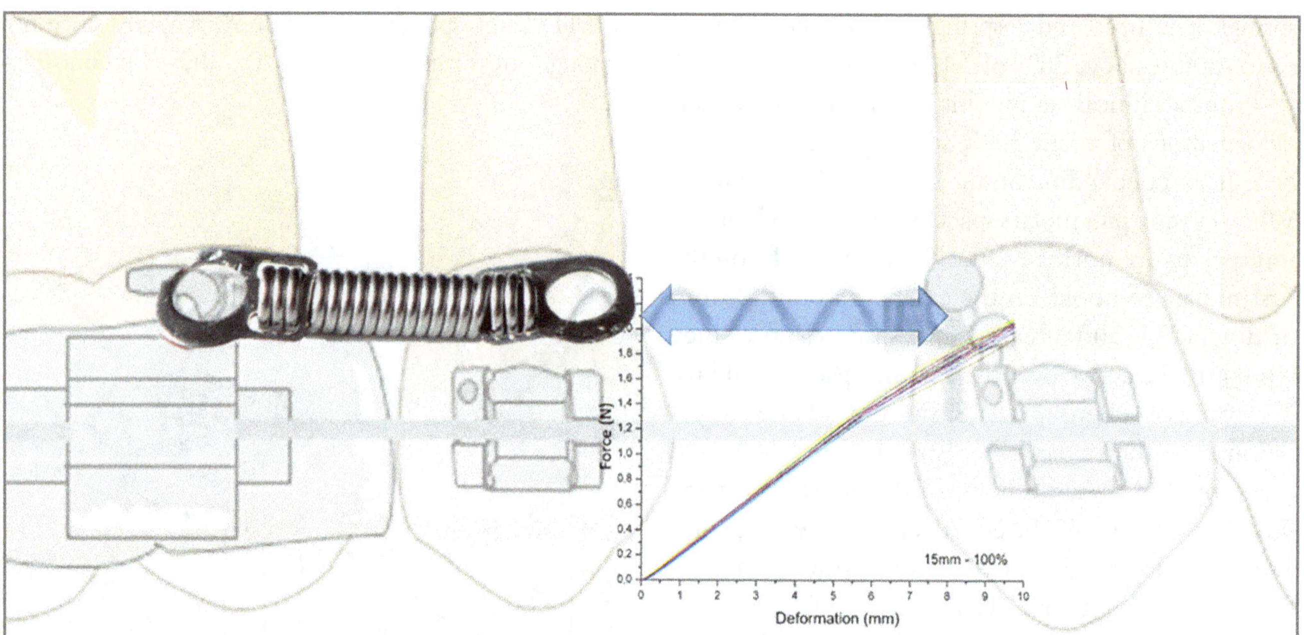

Figure 5 - A 15-mm long nickel-titanium spring (nickel-titanium portion with 9.8mm), activated 9.8mm. A spam of activation from the hook of a first molar to the canine, from 23mm to 16mm (similar to Figure 3), is shown by the blue arrow. In this case, due to the springs length, that activation would account 8mm, deactivating to 1mm after space closure. Note that no superelasticity will not exist in this spring at this activation.

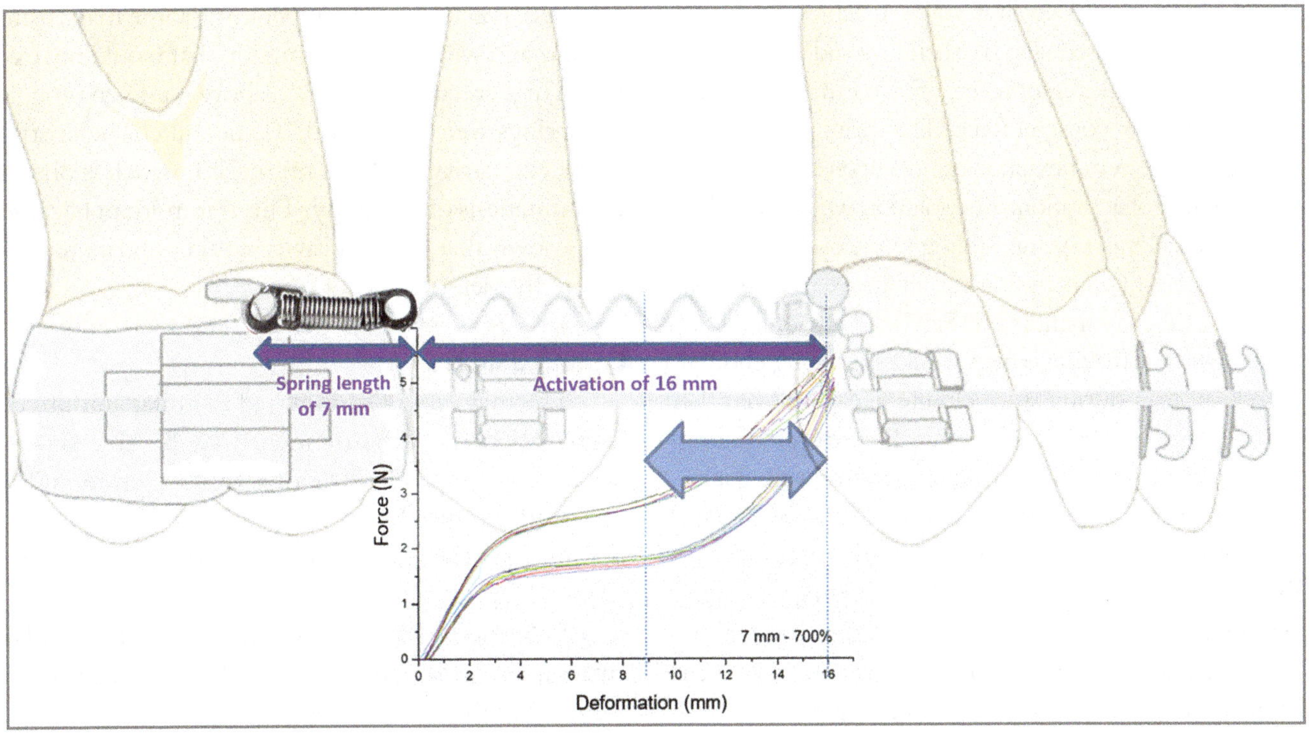

Figure 6 - A 7-mm long nickel-titanium spring (2.3mm of nickel-titanium portion) activated approximately 16mm, which would result in an activation of 23mm. It can be observed that due to the shape of the load-deflection graph, the pseudo-plateau area, or the near-to-constant force, of the spring would not be used during a 7mm space closure.

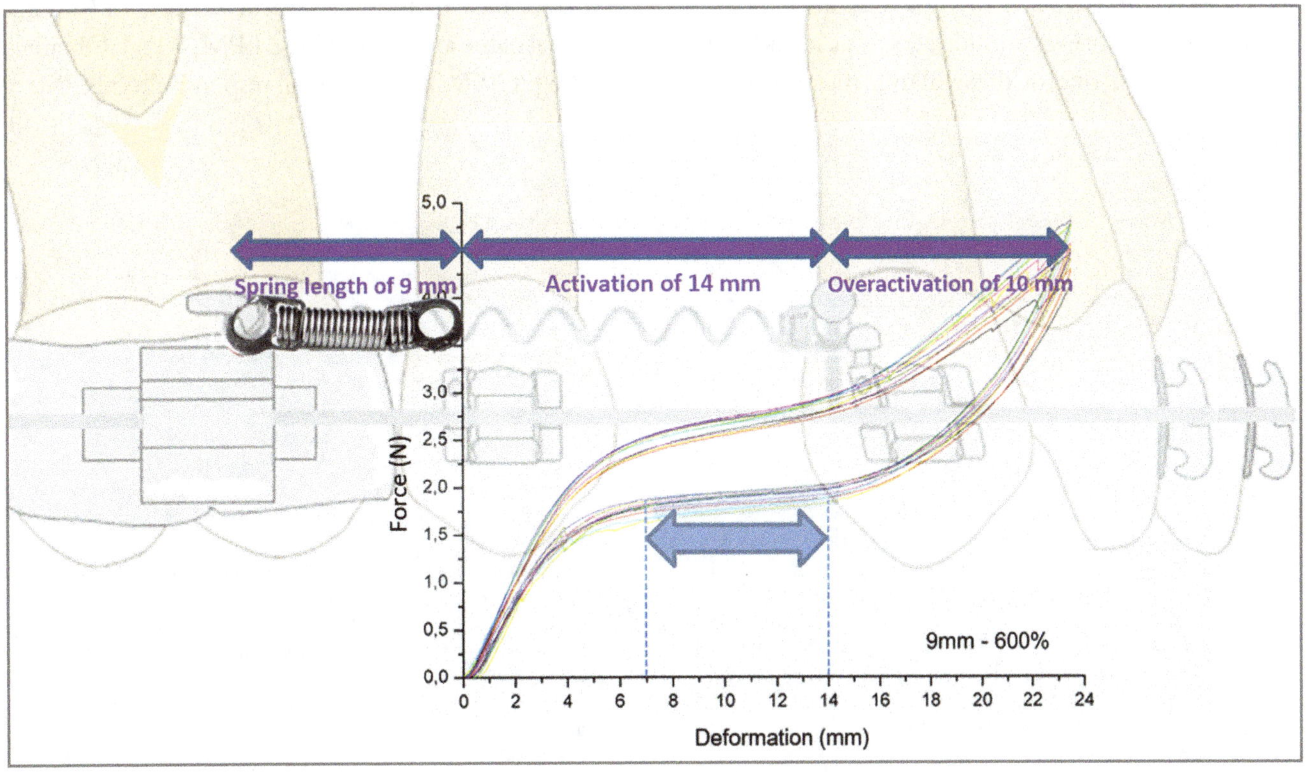

Figure 7 - A 9-mm long nickel-titanium spring (3.9mm of nickel-titanium portion) activated 23.4mm, or 600% the length of its SE material. A spam of activation from 14mm to 7mm is shown by the blue arrow. Note that a pseudo-plateau can be used in this situation only if the spring is overactivated 10mm beyond its affixation. The amount of overactivation will depend on the spring's total length, the length of nickel-titanium portion, and the interbracket distance.

teau is not produced. Even if SIMT is achieved when a shorter spring is used (Fig 6), there is a sudden drop of force in the beginning of reverse transformation, which would not allow constant force. The spring in this situation could be very flexible, but not superelastic on that 7-mm range of activation. The solution would be either to produce a longer spring, adding to the eyelets and not to the nickel-titanium portion,[17] or to overactivate the springs, as already mentioned (Fig 7). That would allow a window of activation which would use a long enough pseudo-plateau during space closure, escaping from the sudden drop of force, as depicted by Figure 6. Activating the spring only up to 14 mm, and not overactivating it on this particular situation (Fig 7), would include the sudden drop of force characteristically seen in the beginning of the reverse SIMT up to 7 mm of deactivation spam, similar to what is shown in Figure 6. The force, therefore, would not be as continuous as the one produced when overactivating the spring during space closure.

All springs were tested at 37°C, as mentioned in the Methods section, according to the American Dental Association specification of 2006.[12] That was necessary because shape-memory alloys respond differently to a given temperature[14,18] and, therefore, it was the objective of this paper to know how nickel-titanium closed coil springs would deform at mouth temperature. When one of those alloys, nickel-titanium included, is below its Af temperature, some martensite is stable and will allow deformation that would not exist at a higher temperature; i.e., above Af. Even though the springs were tested at 37°C, not all characteristics of the oral cavity could be mimicked, which is one of the limitations of this study. This is important because it is known that the oral cavity could contribute further to the deformation of springs.[19]

CONCLUSIONS

» The majority of springs had a similar amount of deformation from the moment they became superelastic, from around 400% of activation up to 700% of activation, in relation to the length of the nickel-titanium portion present in the closed coil springs, without rupturing.

» Subgroups 4B, 4C, 4D, and 4E had a similar amount of deformation up to 1000% of activation (32 mm) without rupturing.

Author contributions

Conception or design of the study: JMSNR, LGV, LPM. Data acquisition, analysis or interpretation: CIVV, JMSNR, LGV. Writing the article: CIVV, RPM. Critical revision of the article: LGV, LPM. Final approval of the article: JMSNR, LPM, RPM. Obtained funding: CIVV, LPM. Overall responsibility: RPM.

REFERENCES

1. Buehler WJ, Wiley RC. TiNi-Ductile intermetallic compound. Trans ASM. 1962;55:269-76.
2. Andreasen GF, Hilleman TB. An evaluation of 55 cobalt substituted Nitinol wire for use in orthodontics. J Am Dent Assoc. 1971 June;82(6):1373-5.
3. Burstone CJ, Qin B, Morton JY. Chinese NiTi wire--a new orthodontic alloy. Am J Orthod. 1985 Jun;87(6):445-52.
4. Miura F, Mogi M, Ohura Y, Hamanaka H. The super-elastic property of the Japanese NiTi alloy wire for use in orthodontics. Am J Orthod Dentofacial Orthop. 1986 July;90(1):1-10.
5. Miura F, Mogi M, Ohura Y. Japanese NiTi alloy wire: use of the direct electric resistance heat treatment method. Eur J Orthod. 1988 Aug;10(3):187-91.
6. Khier SE, Brantley WA, Fournelle RA. Bending properties of superelastic and nonsuperelastic nickel-titanium orthodontic wires. Am J Orthod Dentofacial Orthop. 1991;99(4):310-8.
7. Gangbing KB, Agrawal BN, Lam PC, Srivatsan TS. Application of shape memory alloy wire actuator for precision position control of a composite beam. J Mat Eng Perf. 2000;9(3):330-3.
8. Miura F, Mogi M, Ohura Y, Karibe M. The super-elastic Japanese NiTi alloy wire for use in orthodontics. Part III. Studies on the Japanese NiTi alloy coil springs. Am J Orthod Dentofacial Orthop. 1988 Aug;94(2):89-96.
9. Manhartsberger C, Seidenbusch W. Force delivery of Ni-Ti coil springs. Am J Orthod Dentofacial Orthop. 1996 Jan;109(1):8-21.
10. Tripolt H, Burstone CJ, Bantleon P, Manschiebel W. Force characteristics of nickel-titanium tension coil springs. Am J Orthod Dentofacial Orthop. 1999 May;115(5):498-507.
11. Wichelhaus A, Brauchli L, Ball J, Mertmann M. Mechanical behavior and clinical application of nickel-titanium closed-coil springs under different stress levels and mechanical loading cycles. Am J Orthod Dentofacial Orthop. 2010 May;137(5):671-8.
12. American National Standards Institute. American Dental Association. Orthodontic wires not containing precious metals specification 32. New Work: ANSI; 2006.
13. Segner D, Ibe D. Properties of superelastic wires and their relevance to orthodontic treatment. Eur J Orthod. 1995 Oct;17(5):395-402.
14. Duerig TW, Melton KN, Stockel D, Wayman CM. Engineering aspects of shape memory alloys. London: Butterworth-Heinimann; 1990.
15. Martins RP, Buschang PH, Gandini LG Jr. Group A T-loop for differential moment mechanics: an implant study. Am J Orthod Dentofacial Orthop. 2009 Feb;135(2):182-9.
16. Maganzini AL, Wong AM, Ahmed MK. Forces of various nickel titanium closed coil springs. Angle Orthod. 2010 Jan;80(1):182-7.
17. Vieira CI, Caldas SG, Martins LP, Martins RP. Superelasticity and force plateau of nickel-titanium springs: an in vitro study. Dental Press J Orthod. 2016 June;21(3):46-55.
18. Tonner RI, Waters NE. The characteristics of super-elastic Ni-Ti wires in three-point bending. Part I: The effect of temperature. Eur J Orthod. 1994 Oct;16(5):409-19.
19. Magno AF, Monini Ada C, Capela MV, Martins LP, Martins RP. Effect of clinical use of nickel-titanium springs. Am J Orthod Dentofacial Orthop. 2015 July;148(1):76-82.

Superelasticity and force plateau of nickel-titanium springs: An *in vitro* study

Camila Ivini Viana Vieira[1], Sergei Godeiro Fernandes Rabelo Caldas[2], Lídia Parsekian Martins[3], Renato Parsekian Martins[4]

Objective: This paper analyzed whether nickel-titanium closed coil springs (NTCCS) have a different superelastic (SE) behavior according to activation and whether their force plateau corresponds to that informed by the manufacturer. **Methods:** A total of 160 springs were divided into 16 subgroups according to their features and activated proportionally to the length of the extensible part (NiTi) of the spring (Y). The force values measured were analyzed to determine SE rates and force plateaus, which were mathematically calculated. These plateaus were compared to those informed by the manufacturer. Analysis of variance was accomplished followed by Tukey post-hoc test to detect and analyze differences between groups. **Results:** All subgroups were SE at the activation of 400% of Y length, except for: subgroups 4B and 3A, which were SE at 300%; subgroups 4E and 4G, which were SE at 500%; and subgroup 3C, which was SE at 600%. Subgroup 3B did not show a SE behavior. Force plateaus depended on activation and, in some subgroups and some activations, were similar to the force informed. **Conclusions:** Most of the springs showed SE behavior at 400% of activation. Force plateaus are difficult to compare due to lack of information provided by manufacturers.

Keywords: NiTi. Superelasticity. Force plateau.

[1] Private practice, Aracaju, Sergipe, Brazil.
[2] Assistant professor, Universidade Federal do Rio Grande do Norte (UFRN), Natal, Rio Grande do Norte, Brazil.
[3] Assistant professor, Director of Orthodontics program, Universidade Estadual Paulista Julio de Mesquita Filho (UNESP), School of Dentistry, Araraquara, São Paulo, Brazil.
[4] Adjunct professor, Universidade Estadual Paulista Julio de Mesquita Filho (UNESP), School of Dentistry, Department of Orthodontics, Araraquara, São Paulo, Brazil.

» The authors report no commercial, proprietary or financial interest in the products or companies described in this article.

Renato Parsekian Martins
E-mail: dr_renatopmartins@hotmail.com

INTRODUCTION

In the 1980's, two new nickel-titanium alloys were suggested for orthodontic use, the "Chinese NiTi"[1] and the "Japanese NiTi".[2] These alloys had some advantages over the already existing nickel-titanium alloy used at the time, termed Nitinol;[3] one was the fact that they did not obey Hooke's Law which determines proportionality between load and deflection of metals.

This is due to a transformation in the crystallographic structure from a martensitic to an austenitic phase, which can be induced by changes in temperature and/or stress.[4,5,6] Since each of these two phases presents an inherent load-deflection rate, these alloys will behave differently depending on at which phase they are. Below a particular temperature termed "austenitic start" (A_s), inherent to each alloy, the structure is completely martensitic; whereas above a second temperature termed "austenitic final" (A_f) the structure is completely austenitic. At a given temperature above A_s, a phase transformation could be induced by stress, transforming part of the alloy which is in austenitic phase into martensitic phase, e.g., when a nickel-titanium spring is activated,[2] changing the alloy's properties.

When this transformation occurs, producing different load/deflection rates, and, when upon removal of stress, a reverse transformation takes place, producing a plateau in the curve of load/deflection, it is said that superelasticity (SE) occurred.

In Orthodontics, it is desired for a nickel-titanium closed coil spring (NTCCS) to be SE, in which the elastic modulus is low and the force is mostly constant. In this context, several manufacturers have produced NTCCS of different lengths and plateaus, but they need enough activation to produce sufficient stress to induce transformation or they will not be SE. Even though there is plenty of articles on NTCCSs,[7-11] they lack information on how much activation is needed to induce SE.

Therefore, the aim of the present study is to determine the minimal activation for NTCCSs to be SE and to verify if the force plateaus measured are consistent with those informed by manufacturers.

MATERIAL AND METHODS

Four groups of NTCCSs were created, according to the manufacturer, and further divided into 16 subgroups of ten NTCCS from the same batch, according to the length and plateau informed (Table 1).

The size of each spring was measured with a digital caliper (Mitutoyo model SC-6, Suzano, São Paulo, Brazil), in order to obtain the total length of the spring (from eyelet to eyelet, made of stainless steel) (X), as well as the length of the extensible part (NiTi) of the spring (Y) (Fig 1).

Hooks adapted to a mechanical testing machine (EMIC DL2000, São José dos Pinhais, Brazil) were submerged in water at 37 ± 1°C (Fig 3),[12] controlled with a heater (Termodelfim, São Paulo, Brazil) and a thermostat (Alife, São Paulo, Brazil).

Previously to each test, NTCCSs were adjusted at every 0.1 mm, so as to avoid any looseness that could compromise correct activation measurements.

The NTCCSs were activated to 100% of Y, deactivated and reactivated to increments of 100% until 1000% of Y. Tesc Software (EMIC, São José dos Pinhais, Brazil) registered deactivation forces at 20 mm/min in *.raw* format.

The plateau was the segment determined by two inflexion points calculated in the deactivation curve of the force data obtained (Fig 2). The value of the plateau was determined by the segment's midpoint[13] and averages were compared to the information provided by the manufacturers, which were considered similar within a variation of 10%.

The first and second derivatives of force in relation to deformation were calculated in MATLAB R12™ software (The MathWorks Inc., Massachusetts, USA). The first derivative was located in the beginning of the deactivation curve, while the second one was located in the plateau — being determined in ± 20% of the plateau to minimize errors (Fig 2).[13] These values were exported to Microcal Origin 8.0™ software (OriginLab, Northampton, USA) in which SE rates were calculated by dividing the first by the second derivative. NTCCSs were considered SE when the rate was above eight.

Since data were normally distributed, averages were calculated for SE rates and ANOVA with Tukey or Tamhane's T2 post hoc tests were used for comparison, performed with the aid of SPSS Software v.16.0 (SPSS Inc., Chicago, IL, USA).

Table 1 - Commercial brands and groups division.

Commercial brand	Length*	X	Y	Force plateau (gf)	Subgroup	n
Group 1 (Morelli Ortodontia, Sorocaba, Brazil)	7 mm	8.6 mm	2.3 mm	250	1A	10
	9 mm	10.3 mm	3.9 mm	250	1B	10
	12 mm	13.3 mm	6.8 mm	250	1C	10
	15 mm	16.3 mm	9.8 mm	250	1D	10
Group 2 (Orthometric Imp. Exp. Ltda., Marília, Brazil)	7 mm	6.8 mm	2.1 mm	175	2A	10
	9 mm	8.9 mm	4.1 mm	250	2B	10
Group 3 (Ormco Co., Glendora, USA)	9 mm	8.9 mm	3.25 mm	80	3A	10
	9 mm	9.0 mm	3.1 mm	200	3B	10
	12 mm	12.0 mm	6.0 mm	150	3C	10
Group 4 (GAC International Inc., Bohemia, NY, USA)	10 mm	8.5 mm	3.2 mm	25	4A	10
	10 mm	8.5 mm	3.2 mm	50	4B	10
	10 mm	8.5 mm	3.2 mm	100	4C	10
	10 mm	8.5 mm	3.2 mm	150	4D	10
	10 mm	8.5 mm	3.2 mm	200	4E	10
	10 mm	8.5 mm	3.2 mm	250	4F	10
	10 mm	8.5 mm	3.2 mm	300	4G	10

X = total length of the spring (from eyelet to eyelet); Y = length of the extensible part of the spring; * = length informed by the manufacturer.

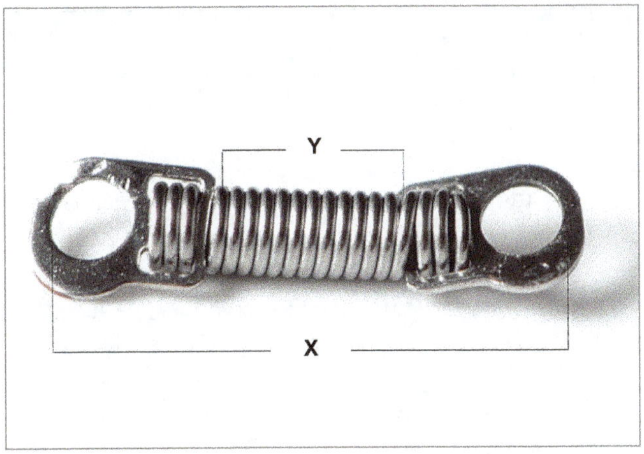

Figure 1 - Nickel-titanium coil spring, the X dimension corresponds to the total length of the spring (from eyelet to eyelet, made os stainless steel) and the Y dimension is the length of the extensible part (NiTi) of the spring.

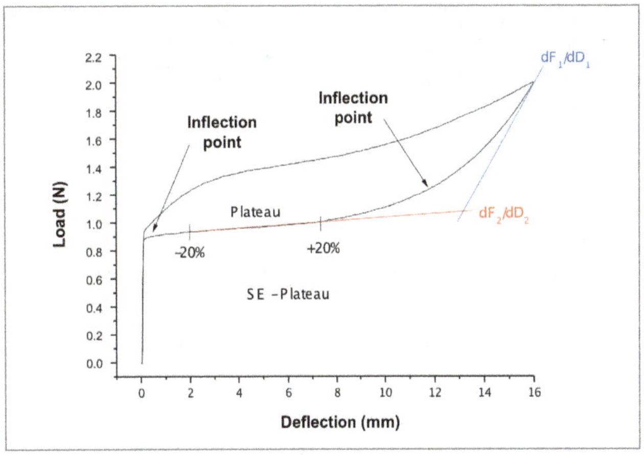

Figure 2 - General load/deflection graph of a superelastic (SE) alloy. Indication of the inflection points and SE plateau (± 20%) and the first and second derivative (dF_1/dD_1 and dF_2/dD_2, respectively). Source: adapted from Segner et al,[13] 1995.

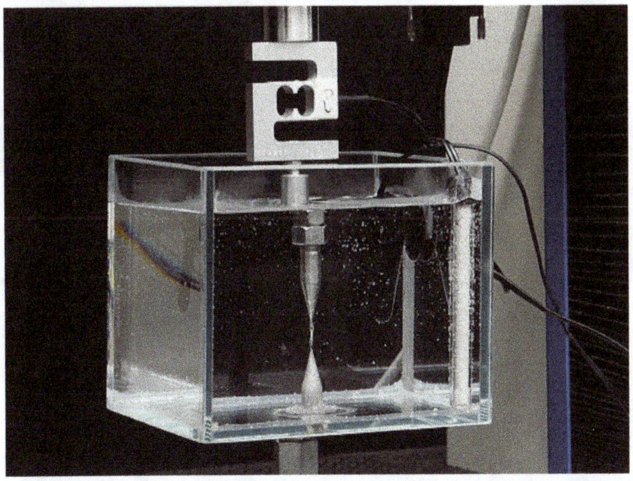

Figure 3 - Glass aquarium attached to the testing machine.

RESULTS

Only at 400% of Y activation (9.3 mm; 15.7 mm; 27.4 mm; 39.1 mm for subgroups 1A, 1B, 1C, and 1D, respectively) the NTCCSs of Group 1 were SE. They maintained that behavior up to 1000% of Y (Table 2 and Fig 4).

In Group 2, NTCCSs were SE at 400% of activation (8.4 mm and 16.6 mm in subgroups 2A and 2B, respectively) and above that activation (Table 3 and Fig 5).

NTCCSs of Group 3 behaved very differently. While in subgroup 3A they were SE at 300% of activation (9.7 mm), in subgroup 3C, a minimum of 600% of activation (18.5 mm) was required. NTCCSs in subgroup 3B were not SE (Table 4 and Fig 6).

NTCCSs in subgroup 4C were SE at 300% of Y (9.6 mm) and above, while in subgroups 4A, 4B, 4D, and 4F SE started at 400% of Y (12.8 mm). Subgroups 4E and 4G were SE from 500% of activation on (16.0 mm) (Table 5 and Fig 7).

In general, SE rate increased with activation, but in subgroup 1A, it decreased at 1000%; in subgroup 1C it decreased at 900%, and in subgroup 1B, the rate decreased at 900% and increased at 1000%. In subgroup 2A, SE rate began to decrease at 900%, and in subgroup 2B at 700%. In subgroup 3B, SE rate did not decrease, while in subgroup 3C it began to decrease at 900%. In subgroup 3A, the rate showed a different behavior, in which it decreased from 800% and increased again at 1000%. In subgroups 4A, 4D, 4E, and 4G, the SE rate decreased at 1000%, while in subgroup 4C, it did not decrease. In subgroup 4B, the SE rate decreased at 900% and increased again

Table 2 - SE rate and force plateau values, mean (SD), of Group 1. Comparisons were only made for SE behavior.

Activation	Subgroup 1A		Subgroup 1B		Subgroup 1C		Subgroup 1D	
	SE rate	Force plateau (gf)	SE rate	Force plateau (gf)	SE rate	Force plateau (gf)	SE rate	Force plateau (gf)
100%	0.7*	214.1 (4.1)	0.8*	193.7 (4.1)	0.8*	188.6 (4.1)	0.8*	188.6 (5.1)
200%	2.2**	216.2 (5.1)	1.9*	214.1 (4.1)	2.1**	209.0 (4.1)	2.1**	209.0 (5.1)
300%	4.1**	211.1 (4.1)	5.4**	214.1 (4.1)	4.0**	209.0 (4.1)	3.5**	216.1 (4.1)
400%	8.9***	209.0 (3.0)^{A}	9.1***	212.1 (4.1)^{A}	10.5***	214.1 (5.1)^{A}	10.6***	216.1 (5.1)^{A}
500%	19.1***	199.9 (3.0)^{B}	16.8***	206.0 (5.1)^{A}	20.0***	206.0 (4.1)^{B}	13.9***	206.0 (4.1)^{B}
600%	21.7***	190.7 (5.1)^{C}	25.9***	189.7 (5.1)^{B}	23.9***	204.0 (4.1)^{B}	30.9***	191.7 (3.1)^{C}
700%	24.1***	171.3 (5.1)^{D}	27.9***	176.4 (4.1)^{C}	29.8***	186.6 (4.1)^{C}	32.7***	176.4 (4.1)^{D}
800%	26.3***	150.9 (4.1)^{E}	22.4***	144.8 (5.1)^{D}	36.1***	154.0 (5.1)^{D}	34.3***	153.0 (4.1)^{E}
900%	33.7***	128.5 (3.0)^{F}	19.2***	127.5 (4.1)^{E}	28.95***	128.5 (4.1)^{E}	41.1***	123.4 (5.1)^{F}
1000%	30.0***	110.1 (4.2)^{G}	28.1***	107.1 (4.1)^{F}	23.2***	107.1 (5.1)^{F}	40.9***	93.8 (5.1)^{G}
p-value	< 0.001		< 0.001		< 0.001		< 0.001	

*Non-SE behavior; ** Tendency to SE behavior; ***SE behavior. Similar groups show similar superscript letters

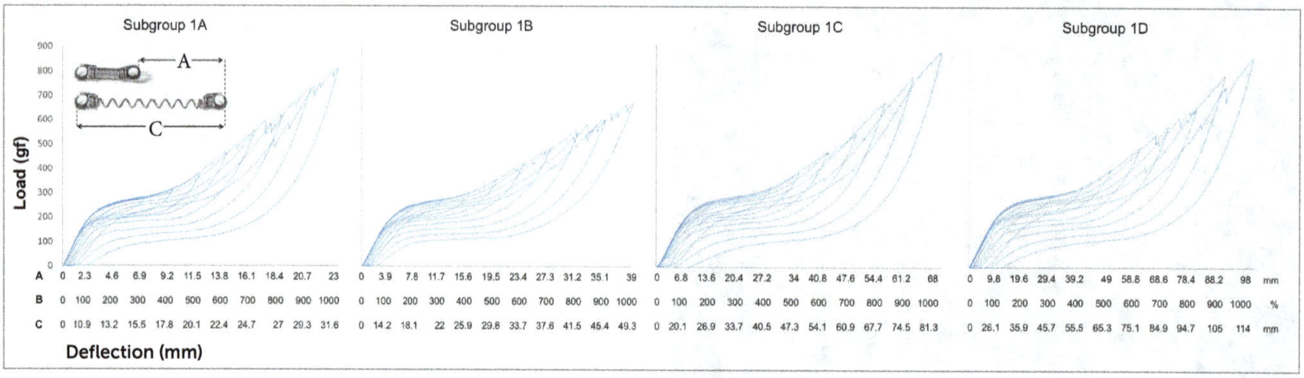

Figure 4 - Load/deflection graph of one average spring of Group 1 (100 to 1000% of activation). On the axis of deflection, the amount of activation of the springs (mm) can be seen on the first line (**A**), the amount of activation corresponding to Y's percentage is on the second one (**B**), and the amount of activation of the springs added to its size is on the third line (**C**).

at 1000%; while in subgroup 4F, the SE rate started to decrease at 700% and increased again at 800% and 1000% (Tables 2, 3, 4 and 5).

During 800% of activation, one NTCCS ruptured in subgroup 2A, two in subgroup 1D, and five in subgroup 2B. At 900% of activation, one NTCCS in subgroup 4G, two in subgroups 2A and 1D, four in subgroup 2B, five in subgroup 3A and eight in 3B ruptured. At 1000%, one NTCCS ruptured in subgroups 1D, 1B, 2B, and 3B, two in subgroups 3A and 4G, three in subgroup 2A, four springs in subgroup 3C, and five springs in subgroup 1C.

There were differences between all SE plateaus in Group 1 (Table 2). In subgroup 2A, the plateaus showed similar forces when activated at 400%, 500% and 600% of Y; at 600%, 700% and 800%, the plateaus were also similar, and at 900% and 1000%, the plateaus were different from themselves and from the other activations (Table 3). In subgroup 2B, the plateaus were the same from 400% to 600% of activation and from 500% to 800% of activation; and in subgroup 3A, the plateaus systematically decreased (subgroup 3B was not compared, since it was not SE) (Table 4). In Group 4, nearly all activations produced similar SE plateaus in lower activations and different SE plateaus in higher activations (Table 5).

Table 3 - SE rate and force plateau values, mean (SD), of Group 2. Comparisons were only made for SE behavior.

Activation	Subgroup 2A		Subgroup 2B	
	SE rate	Force plateau (gf)	SE rate	Force plateau (gf)
100%	1.0*	123.4 (10.2)	0.9*	134.6 (10.2)
200%	1.6*	209.0 (15.3)	2.6**	255.9 (20.3)
300%	2.37**	217.2 (18.3)	6.8**	244.7 (20.3)
400%	12.4***	210.0 (15.3)^{A}	19.2***	240.6 (18.3)^{A}
500%	29.1***	196.8 (12.2)^{A}	19.5***	229.4 (15.3)^{AB}
600%	33.4***	188.6 (15.3)^{AB}	27.6***	219.2 (15.3)^{AB}
700%	45.9***	176.4 (10.2)^{BC}	21.3***	210.1 (15.3)^{B}
800%	46.7***	160.1 (10.2)^{C}	19.3***	206.0 (20.3)^{B}
900%	39.1***	137.7 (12.2)^{D}	24.9***	144.8 (1.0)$^{\#}$
1000%	27.9***	130.5 (10.2)^{D}	X	X
p-value	< 0.001		< 0.001	

*Non-SE behavior; ** Tendency to SE behavior; ***SE behavior. X = all springs ruptured, # not included on statistic due to n < 2.
Similar groups show similar superscript letters.

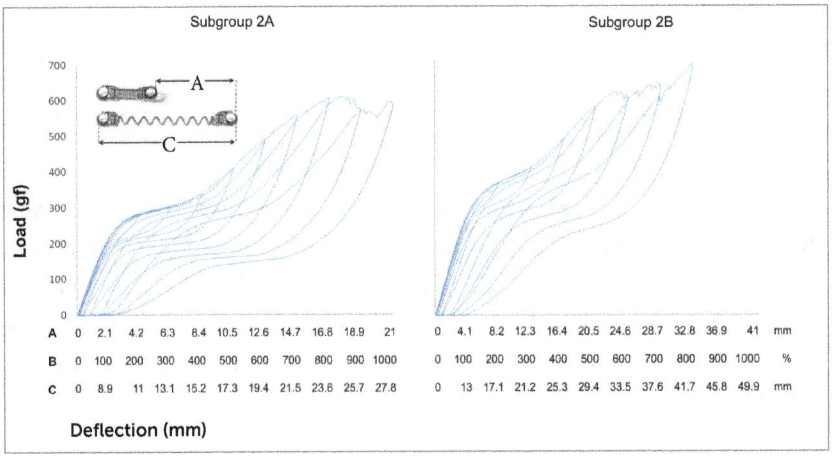

Figure 5 - Load/deflection graph of one average spring of subgroup 2A (100 to 1000% of activation) and of subgroup 2B (100 to 900% of activation). On the axis of deflection, the amount of activation of the springs (mm) can be seen on the first line (**A**), the amount of activation corresponding to Y's percentage is on the second one (**B**), and the amount of activation of the springs added to its size is on the third line (**C**).

Table 4 - SE rate and force plateau values, mean (SD), of Group 3. Comparisons were made only among activations that induced superelasticity (according to the SE ratio) – subgroup 3B was not analyzed because NTCCSs did not show high enough SE rates.

Activation	Subgroup 3A		Subgroup 3B		Subgroup 3C	
	SE rate	Force plateau (gf)	SE rate	Force plateau (gf)	SE rate	Force plateau (gf)
100%	1.6*	127.5 (10.2)	0.9*	173.3 (8.1)	0.8*	150.9 (15.3)
200%	3.8**	124.4 (10.2)	0.9*	203.9 (8.1)	1.1*	156.0 (15.3)
300%	12.7***	122.4 (8.1)^{A}	1.4*	287.5 (10.2)	1.8*	172.3 (15.3)
400%	32.0***	109.1 (15.3)^{AB}	1.8*	254.9 (10.2)	3.7**	184.6 (15.3)
500%	41.4***	92.8 (15.3)^{BC}	3.1**	249.8 (8.1)	6.8**	173.3 (10.2)
600%	62.4***	79.5 (15.3)^{CD}	4.5**	249.8 (10.2)	8.3***	167.2 (10.2)^{A}
700%	82.1***	59.1 (15.7)^{DE}	5.2**	239.6 (8.1)	14.7***	157.0 (15.3)^{AB}
800%	58.9***	48.9 (12.2)^{EF}	5.3**	222.3 (15.3)	17.2***	143.8 (15.3)^{BC}
900%	59.5***	27.5 (12.2)^{F}	6.9**	234.5 (10.2)	16.4***	130.5 (15.3)^{C}
1000%	88.5***	18.3 (10.2)^{EF}	7.9**	238.6 (2.0)	16.5***	112.2 (15.3)^{C}
p-value	< 0.001				< 0.001	

*Non-SE behavior; ** Tendency to SE behavior; ***SE behavior. Similar groups show similar superscript letters.

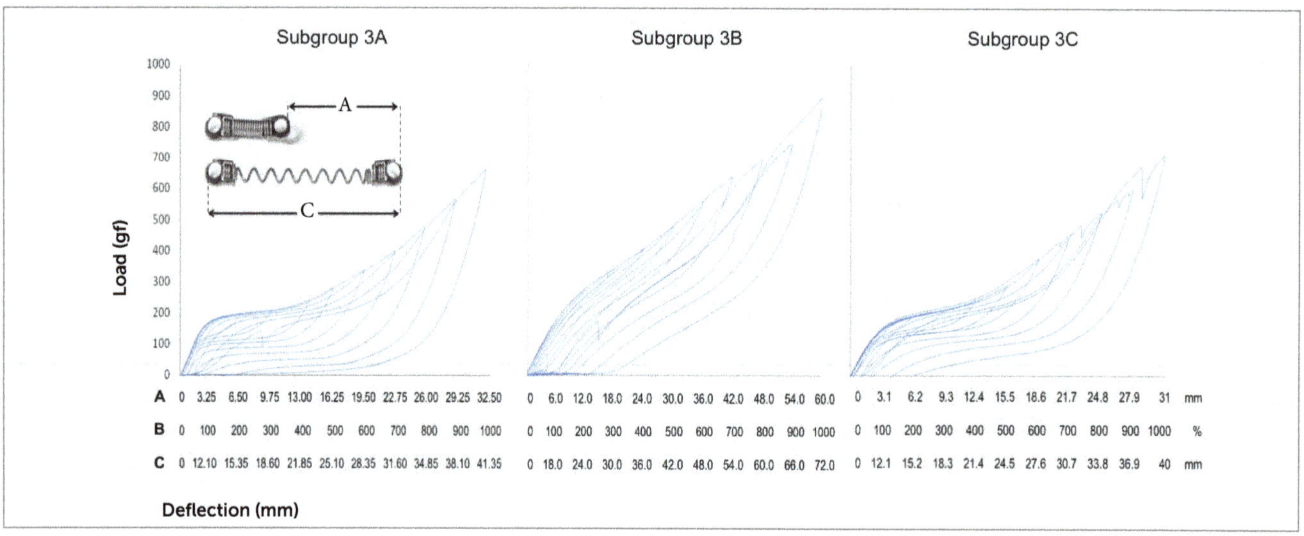

Figure 6 - Load/deflection graph of one average spring of each of the subgroups of Group 3 (100 to 1000% of activation). On the axis of deflection, the amount of activation of the springs (mm) can be seen on the first line (**A**), the amount of activation corresponding to Y's percentage is on the second one (**B**), and the amount of activation of the springs added to its size is on the third line (**C**).

The SE plateaus informed by the manufacturers (Table 1) of Group 1 and subgroup 3C did not correspond to the values observed in this study. For subgroups 3A, 4E, and 4A, NTCCSs produced a similar plateau to the informed one at 600%, 500%, and 400% of activation, respectively. In subgroups 2A, 2B, 4B, 4C, 4D, 4F, and 4G, the plateaus corresponded to the values provided by the manufacturer from 600% to 800%, 400% to 500%, from 600% to 800%, from 400% to 700%, 400% to 600%, from 400% to 600%, and from 500% to 700% of initial activation, respectively.

Table 5 - SE rate and force plateau values, mean (SD), of Group 4. Comparisons were only made for SE behavior.

Activation	Subgroup 4A		Subgroup 4B		Subgroup 4C		Subgroup 4D		Subgroup 4E		Subgroup 4F		Subgroup 4G	
	SE rate	Force plateau (gf)	SE rate	Force plateau (gf)	SE rate	Force plateau (gf)	SE rate	Force plateau (gf)	SE rate	Force plateau (gf)	SE rate	Force plateau (gf)	SE rate	Force plateau (gf)
100%	1.9*	40.8 (3.0)	1.6*	77.5 (3.0)	2.4*	114.2 (2.0)	2.2*	168.2 (5.1)	2.0*	212.1 (5.1)	2.2**	287.5 (4.1)	1.4*	378.3 (6.1)
200%	4.7**	32.6 (2.0)	5.6**	66.3 (3.0)	6.2**	107.1 (2.0)	4.5**	163.1 (5.1)	3.6**	209.0 (5.1)	4.0**	284.5 (4.1)	2.8**	358.0 (5.1)
300%	7.4**	28.5 (2.0)	6.9**	63.2 (2.0)	9.8***	105.0 (2.0)^{A}	6.4**	158.0 (5.1)	7.1**	206.0 (4.1)	6.7**	282.4 (4.1)	2.8**	346.7 (5.1)
400%	15.7***	21.4 (3.0)^{A}	11.1***	59.1 (3.0)^{A}	16.0***	102.0 (4.1)^{AB}	9.9***	157.0 (5.1)^{A}	7.0**	206.0 (4.1)	9.3***	270.2 (4.1)^{A}	6.6**	336.5 (4.1)
500%	18.0***	18.3 (2.0)^{AB}	21.8***	58.1 (2.0)^{A}	24.9***	99.9 (2.0)^{B}	20.9***	149.9 (6.1)^{AB}	14.1***	188.6 (3.0)^{A}	15.5***	251.9 (4.1)^{B}	10.3***	290.6 (4.1)^{A}
600%	41.4***	16.3 (2.0)^{B}	30.3***	54.0 (2.0)^{B}	30.2***	96.9 (2.0)^{B}	29.8***	142.7 (5.1)^{B}	16.9***	176.4 (3.0)^{B}	20.3***	231.5 (2.0)^{C}	11.6***	279.4 (5.1)^{B}
700%	43.6***	12.2 (3.0)^{C}	41.9***	48.9 (4.1)^{C}	34.1***	91.8 (2.0)^{C}	31.5***	131.5 (5.1)^{C}	25.3***	162.1 (4.1)^{C}	19.7***	209.0 (4.1)^{D}	16.1***	236.6 (4.1)^{C}
800%	47.1***	6.1 (1.0)^{D}	70.4***	44.9 (3.0)^{D}	37.2***	89.7 (1.0)^{C}	38.8***	117.3 (5.1)^{D}	27.5***	139.7 (5.1)^{D}	21.8***	160.1 (3.0)^{E}	19.0***	168.2 (5.1)^{D}
900%	136.8***	2.0 (1.0)^{E}	62.1***	36.7 (2.0)^{E}	51.3***	71.4 (2.0)^{D}	41.0***	99.9 (5.1)^{E}	29.3***	127.5 (5.1)^{E}	17.5***	115.2 (5.1)^{F}	21.2***	132.6 (5.1)^{E}
1000%	103.8***	1.0 (1.0)^{E}	105.5***	29.6 (2.0)^{F}	55.8***	57.1 (2.0)^{E}	33.4***	84.6 (6.1)^{F}	27.9***	96.9 (4.1)^{F}	29.0***	84.6 (5.1)^{G}	19.4***	104.0 (4.1)^{F}
p-value	< 0.001		< 0.001		< 0.001		< 0.001		< 0.001		< 0.001		< 0.001	

*Non-SE behavior; ** Tendency to SE behavior; ***SE behavior; X = all springs ruptured. Similar groups show similar superscript letters.

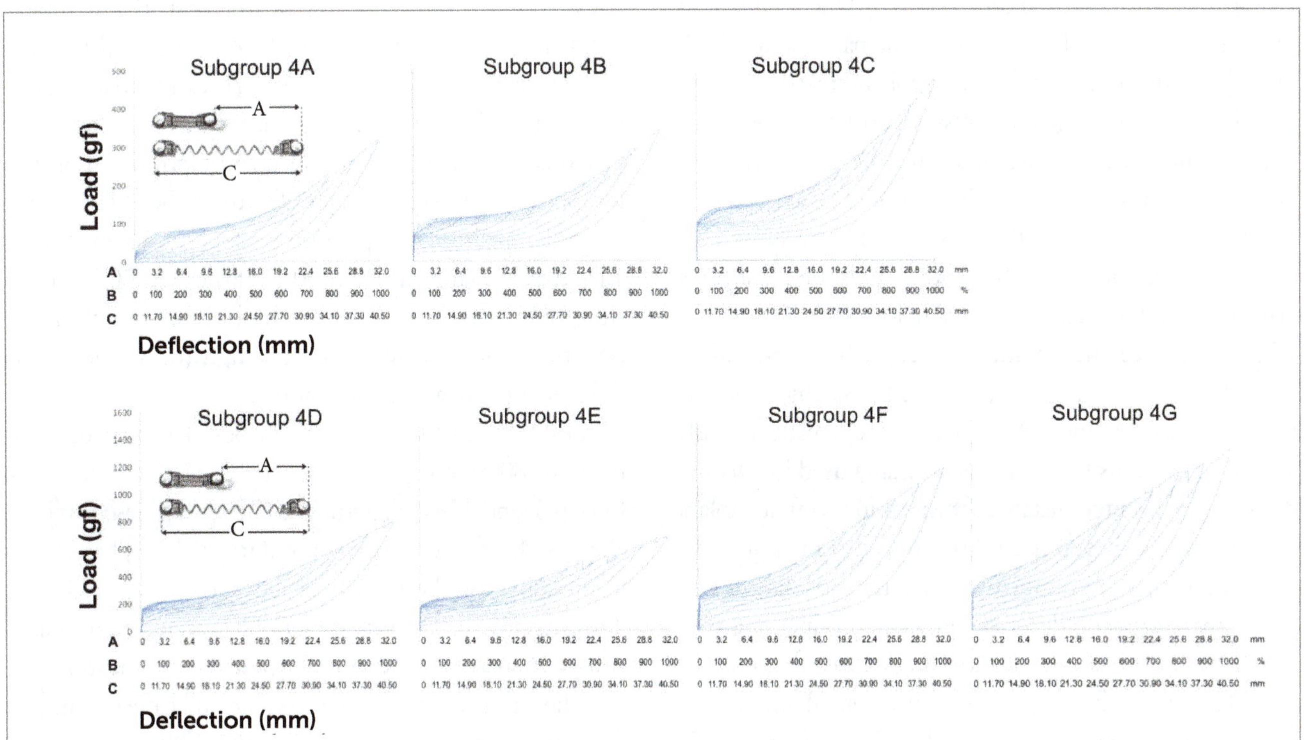

Figure 7 - Load/deflection graph of one average spring of each of the subgroups of Group 4 (100 to 1000% of activation). On the axis of deflection, the amount of activation of the springs (mm) can be seen on the first line (**A**), the amount of activation corresponding to Y's percentage is on the second one (**B**), and the amount of activation of the springs added to its size is on the third line (**C**).

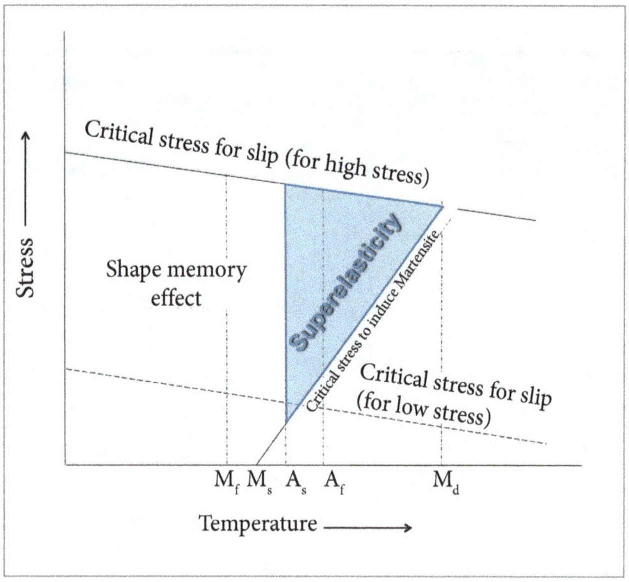

Figure 8 - Graph of stress/temperature of SE alloys. M_f = martensitic final temperature, M_s = martensitic initial temperature, A_s = austenitic initial temperature, A_f = austenitic final temperature, M_d = temperature in which it is not possible for martensitic transformation to occur through stress. Source: adapted from Otsuka, Wayman, 1998.[20]

DISCUSSION

In most subgroups (10/16), the springs were SE above 400% of activation. It should be reminded that the percentage of activation used does not regard the total length of the NTCCSs, as the majority of the papers published, but regards the length of the extensible part of the spring. Despite the knowledge that stress is a critical factor in using and measuring nickel-titanium, the literature does not describe how much NTCCSs should be activated in order to induce martensitic transformation by stress and, consequently, obtain a SE behavior.[11] This information is critical, since low activation may not induce SE,[7-10,14,15,16] which is in agreement with the present findings. Clinically, this is very important, since small springs, such as in subgroups 1A and 2A, will produce a plateau with smaller activations than what is normally used in Orthodontics (the average distance from canine to first molars is 23 mm),[17] and even if a 1000% of activation equals to 23 mm, as in subgroup 1A, reverse transformation occurs only after some deactivation, only producing a plateau after 10 mm of deactivation (Fig 4). For that reason, NTCCS should be longer, but with non-SE materials, i.e., increasing the size of the eyelets. In medium length NTCCSs, such as subgroups 1B, 2B, 3A, 3C and all of Group 4, they should be overactivated as they are being engaged, returning to a smaller activation and securing them in place. On the same given example, a Group 4E NTCCS should be engaged, overactivated to 32 mm, returned to 23 mm and secured in place. Even then, some NTCCS would not produce a clear plateau and should be increased in size with non-SE materials, because 23 mm might fall a little short of the plateau, as in subgroup 3C at 1000% of activation. Long springs, such as subgroups 1C and 1D, should be hard to manipulate; in the same situation, they should be activated around 500-600% and upon return to 23 mm, engaged on the wire. Large activations would make the plateau end too soon, i.e., before the 7-mm space closure, while smaller activations would not produce SE. Since the NTCCS tested is very different, manufacturers should supply SE plateaus lengths, starts and finishes related to the amount of activation.

NTCCSs in subgroup 3B were not SE. This was possibly due to the fact that their alloy has transition temperatures higher than 37 °C. Since nickel-titanium martensitic transformation is a thermo/stress dependent phenomenon,[11,18-19] whenever it cannot be induced, it is possible that either activation was insufficient to induce transformation (present results show SE rates increasing with activation), or that the temperature was lower than the required for a transformation to be stress-induced (M_s) and also lower than the temperatures in which SE may be induced by transformation (A_s)[20] (Fig 8). Even with the American Dentistry Association (ADA) regulating that all SE material should be tested at 37 °C,[7,9,11] NTCCS may not exhibit SE at this temperature. Therefore, manufacturers should be able to control transition temperatures properly. Even though an activation larger than 1000% of the NTCCSs of this subgroup (3B) could induce phase transformation, the possibility of rupture would be high (only one spring did not rupture at that activation).

Only 4% of the springs in Group 4 ruptured, compared to 80% of rupture in Group 2, 67% of rupture in Group 3, and 17% of rupture in Group 1. These findings, along with the activation required to produce phase transformation, limit the amount of activation of the NTCCSs. This has not been reported by the literature, even though rupture may not be the only factor limiting activation.

The minimum percentage values that create enough stress to cause stress-induced martensitic transformation can be calculated back into NTCCSs length and round to the next millimeter, if clinicians want to use those values clinically in order to use the springs' SE properties. It should be reminded that those values are the least amount that NTCCSs need in order to be activated, and that they should also be overactivated in order to avoid the fast drop of force that occurs upon the start of the reverse transformation from martensite back to austenite just before the plateau starts (Fig 2). Subgroup 1A NTCCSs (7 mm in length) should be activated at least 9.2 mm; subgroup 1B (9 mm), 15.6 mm; subgroup 1C (12 mm), 27.2 mm; and subgroup 1D (15 mm), 39.2 mm. Subgroup 2A (7 mm) should be activated at least 8.4 mm and subgroup 2B (9 mm) at least 16.4 mm. Subgroup 3A (9 mm) should be activated at least 9.75 mm and subgroup 3B (12 mm), 36 mm. Finally, Group 4 (10 mm) should be activated at least 12.8 mm on subgroups 4A, 4B, 4D and 4F, 9.6 mm on subgroup 4C and 16 mm on subgroups 4E and 4G. It should be noted that longer NTCCSs will need activations that will be too large for the orthodontic parameters and will not have superelastic behavior in the oral cavity.

SE rate increased with activation in all subgroups, but above certain activations in few subgroups, it either maintained itself or decreased (Table 3). When analyzing this table along with the load/deflection plots of average NTCCSs from each group (Figs 4, 5, 6 and 7), it can be observed that the lighter NTCCSs in Groups 3 and 4 showed higher rates with very smaller activations. That is probably due to thermal treatment which is commonly used to increase M_s.[21,22] This procedure will decrease the stress required to start martensitic transformation,[23] thereby producing a lower SE plateau.[14,21,22]

SE plateaus varied with activation and, while these values did not correspond to the information supplied by manufacturer in some groups, in other groups it corresponded only at specific activations. This could be a problem when using nickel-titanium because, as demonstrated (Tables 2, 3, 4, and 5), plateaus change at different activations and the manufacturers do not provide the information of which activation will produce the plateau informed. The need for this information was suggested in the literature[8] and is essential, so that orthodontists and researchers could select the most adequate NTCCS.

CONCLUSIONS

1) Most subgroups showed a SE behavior above 400% of activation, except for subgroups 4B and 3A which exhibited it above 300%. Subgroups 4E and G, and subgroups 3C were SE above 500% and 600% of activation, respectively.

2) Subgroup 3B was not SE.

3) SE rates increased with activation, while force plateaus decreased.

4) Force plateaus provided by the manufacturers are difficult to compare, since initial activation alters it. Manufacturers should provide more specific information on their nickel-titanium CCSs.

5) NTCCSs are not always superelastic, especially at low activations. If SE is desired, NTCCSs must be activated at least 5 to 6 times the length of active part of the spring.

REFERENCES

1. Burstone CJ, Qin B, Morton JY. Chinese NiTi wire--a new orthodontic alloy. Am J Orthod. 1985 Jun;87(6):445-52.
2. Miura F, Mogi M, Ohura Y, Hamanaka H. The super-elastic property of the Japanese NiTi alloy wire for use in orthodontics. Am J Orthod Dentofacial Orthop. 1986 July;90(1):1-10.
3. Andreasen GF, Hilleman TB. An evaluation of 55 cobalt substituted Nitinol wire for use in orthodontics. J Am Dent Assoc. 1971 Jun;82(6):1373-5.
4. Gangbing S, Lam PC, Srivatsan TS, Kelly B, Agrawa BN. Application of shape memory alloy wire actuator for precision position control of a composite beam. J Mat Eng Perf. 2000;9:330-3.
5. Khier SE, Brantley WA, Fournelle RA. Bending properties of superelastic and nonsuperelastic nickel-titanium orthodontic wires. Am J Orthod Dentofacial Orthop. 1991 Apr;99(4):310-8.
6. Santoro M, Beshers DN. Nickel-titanium alloys: stress-related temperature transitional range. Am J Orthod Dentofacial Orthop. 2000 Dec;118(6):685-92.
7. Maganzini AL, Wong AM, Ahmed MK. Forces of various nickel titanium closed coil springs. Angle Orthod. 2010 Jan;80(1):182-7.
8. Melsen B, Topp LF, Melsen HM, Terp S. Force system developed from closed coil springs. Eur J Orthod. 1994 Dec;16(6):531-9.
9. Santos ACS, Tortamano A, Naccarato SRF, Rodriguez GCD, Vigorito JW. An in vitro comparison of the force decay generated by different commercially available elastomeric chains and NiTi closed coil springs. Braz Oral Res. 2007;21(1):51-7.
10. Vidoni G, Perinetti G, Antoniolli F, Castaldo A, Contardo L. Combined aging effects of strain and thermocycling on unload deflection modes of nickel-titanium closed-coil springs: an in-vitro comparative study. Am J Orthod Dentofacial Orthop. 2010 Oct;138(4):451-7.
11. Wichelhaus A, Brauchli L, Ball J, Mertmann M. Mechanical behavior and clinical application of nickel-titanium closed-coil springs under different stress levels and mechanical loading cycles. Am J Orthod Dentofacial Orthop. 2010 May;137(5):671-8.
12. American National Standards Institute. American Dental Association. Orthodontic Wires Not Containing Precious Metals Specification 32. 2006.
13. Segner D, Ibe D. Properties of superelastic wires and their relevance to orthodontic treatment. Eur J Orthod. 1995 Oct;17(5):395-402.
14. Barwart O. The effect of temperature change on the load value of Japanese NiTi coil springs in the superelastic range. Am J Orthod Dentofacial Orthop. 1996 Nov;110(5):553-8.

15. von Fraunhofer JA, Bonds PW, Johnson BE. Force generation by orthodontic coil springs. Angle Orthod. 1993 Summer;63(2):145-8.
16. Han S, Quick DC. Nickel-titanium spring properties in a simulated oral environment. Angle Orthod. 1993 Spring;63(1):67-72.
17. Martins RP, Buschang PH, Gandini LG Jr. Group A T-loop for differential moment mechanics: an implant study. Am J Orthod Dentofacial Orthop. 2009 Feb;135(2):182-9.
18. Santoro M, Nicolay OF, Canglalosi TJ. Pseudoelasticity and thermoelasticity of nickel-titanium alloys: a clinically oriented review. Part I: Temperature transitional ranges. Am J Orthod Dentofacial Orthop. 2001 Jun;119(6):587-93.
19. Santoro M, Nicolay OF, Cangialosi TJ. Pseudoelasticity and thermoelasticity of nickel-titanium alloys: a clinically oriented review. Part II: Deactivation forces. Am J Orthod Dentofacial Orthop. 2001 Jun;119(6):594-603.
20. Otsuka K, Wayman C. Shape memory materials. 1st ed. Cambridge: Cambridge University Press; 1998.
21. Miura F, Mogi M, Ohura Y. Japanese NiTi alloy wire: use of the direct electric resistance heat treatment method. Eur J Orthod. 1988 Aug;10(3):187-91.
22. Miura F, Mogi M, Ohura Y, Karibe M. The super-elastic Japanese NiTi alloy wire for use in orthodontics. Part III. Studies on the Japanese NiTi alloy coil springs. Am J Orthod Dentofacial Orthop. 1988 Aug;94(2):89-96.
23. Duerig TW, Melton KN, Stockel D, Wayman CM. Engineering aspects of shape memory alloys. London: Butterworth-Heinimann; 1990.

28

Translucency and color match with a shade guide of esthetic brackets with the aid of a spectroradiometer

Yong-Keun Lee[1], Yu Bin[2]

Objective: Since the color of esthetic brackets should match that of teeth, the aims of this study were to determine the color and translucency of esthetic brackets by means of the clinically relevant use of a spectroradiometer, and to compare the color of brackets with that of a commercial shade guide. **Methods:** The color of central and tie-wing regions of four plastic and four ceramic brackets was measured according to the CIE L★a★b★ color scale over white and black backgrounds. Brackets were classified into five groups based on their composition. The color of Vitapan Classical Shade Guide tabs was also measured. Translucency parameter (TP) and contrast ratio (CR) were calculated to determine translucency. **Results:** Color differences between brackets and the shade guide tabs were 10.4–34.5 $\Delta E^{\star}_{ab}$ units. TP and CR values for the central region were 16.4–27.7 and 0.38–0.58, whereas for the tie-wings they were 24.0–39.9 and 0.25–0.45, respectively. The color coordinates, TP and CR values were significantly influenced by bracket composition and brand ($p < 0.05$). **Conclusions:** Esthetic brackets investigated herein showed unacceptable color differences ($\Delta E^{\star}_{ab} > 5.5$) compared with the shade guide tabs. Differences in the translucency of brackets by brand were within the visually perceptible range ($\Delta CR > 0.07$). Therefore, brackets showing the best matching performance for each case should be selected considering esthetic and functional demands.

Keywords: Orthodontic bracket. Color compatibility. Translucency. Esthetic performance. Spectroradiometer.

[1] Director, Institute for Clinical Performance of Biomaterials (ICPB) and ETN Dental Clinic, Seoul, Korea.
[2] Associate Professor, Chinese Academy of Sciences, State Key Laboratory of Multiphase Complex Systems, Institute of Process Engineering, Beijing, China.

» The authors report no commercial, proprietary or financial interest in the products or companies described in this article.

Yong-Keun Lee
E-mail: ykleedm@gmail.com

INTRODUCTION

The increasing need for esthetic orthodontic treatment has led to the development of acceptable esthetic appliances, such as those with plastic and ceramic brackets.[1,2,3] Initially, plastic brackets were made of acrylic resin and polycarbonate;[2,4] later on, polyurethane brackets reinforced with ceramic or glass fillers were introduced.[1,2] These improved brackets showed significantly better clinical performance;[1,2] however, even improved plastic brackets showed clinically unacceptable color stability in the long-term.[5] Ceramic brackets provide better color stability than plastic ones.[1,2,6] Although the term "ceramic" encompasses a variety of compounds, most ceramic brackets are composed of either polycrystalline or monocrystalline aluminium oxide.[7,8]

Color and translucency of esthetic brackets have several clinical considerations.[1,9,10] Firstly, bracket color should either match the color of teeth or bracket should be translucent enough to allow the underlying color to shine through. Secondly, since light-curing orthodontic adhesives are light-cured through brackets, polymerization of adhesives is influenced by the translucency of brackets.[11]

Quantitative color match performance of esthetic material is usually determined by the Commission Internationale de L'Eclairage (CIE) L★a★b★ color difference ($\Delta E^\star_{ab}$) value. Physical meanings of color difference values have been provided,[12,13,14] and 2.6 $\Delta E^\star_{ab}$ units was considered as a clinically perceptible threshold, while 5.5 $\Delta E^\star_{ab}$ units was considered as an acceptable threshold, based on spectroradiometer readings.[12] Translucency of dental material has been usually determined with the aid of parameters, such as light transmittance, translucency parameter (TP) and/or contrast ratio (CR).[11,13,15] The higher the TP value or the lower the CR value, the higher the translucency. TP and CR values correspond directly to common visual assessments of translucency.[13] As to the relationship between instrumental translucency measurement and subjective visual assessment, the mean translucency perception threshold (ΔCR) was 0.07, while 50% of participants could perceive 0.06 ΔCR between specimens.[16]

A few studies directly measured the color and translucency of esthetic brackets,[9,10,17] mainly because contact type spectrophotometers are designed to measure the color of a big object flat surface.[9] Nowadays, noncontact type spectroradiometer has been introduced in Dentistry.[18,19] Spectroradiometers were used to measure the color of ceramics,[18,19] teeth,[20] shade guide tabs[21] and esthetic brackets,[22] as well as the translucency of resin composites.[23] Color and translucency values of irregularly shaped objects, measured by means of a spectroradiometer, have several strengths. A spectroradiometer provides clinically relevant values because this measurement can eliminate the edge-loss effect,[20-23] closely simulate clinical viewing conditions,[18,24,25] and also provide optical values of a specified area, such as wings or body of a bracket. According to a spectroradiometer-based bracket color study,[22] color blending of brackets placed on less chromatic or lighter shade guide tabs was better than that on more chromatic or darker tabs; however, color and translucency ranges of esthetic brackets by composition or brand were not provided.

The aims of this study were to determine the color and translucency of esthetic brackets with a noncontact type spectroradiometer and to compare the color of brackets with that of a commercial shade guide. The null hypothesis assumed in the present study was that the color and translucency of esthetic brackets would not be different by the composition and brand of brackets based on noncontact type color measurements.

MATERIAL AND METHODS

Material

Four plastic and four ceramic bracket brands were investigated (n = 5 for each brand; Table 1). All brackets were Roth prescription for maxillary central incisors with 0.018-in slot. Two plastic (ES-P and SP-P) and one ceramic (CL-C) bracket had a metal-lined archwire slot. According to the composition, the brackets were classified into five groups.

Methods

A spectroradiometer equipped with Macro-Spectar MS-75 lens (PR 670, Photo Research, Chatsworth, CA, USA) was fixed vertically in a light-tight box (Color Sense II, Sungjin Hi-Tech, Gunpo, Korea), 450 mm above the specimen. The measuring geometry was d/0 (i.e. diffuse illumination/0° viewing angle). Two F20T12/65 6500K lamps (standard illuminant D65 simulator; GretagMacbeth, New Windsor, NY, USA) were fixed to the inner top surface of the light-tight box parallely (Fig 1).[18,19] The color of a 3-mm diameter area in the central region of the bracket and 1-mm diameter region in three out of four tie-wings was measured according to the CIE L★a★b★ color scale

Table 1 - Brackets investigated.

Material	Composition	Code	Brand name	Batch number	Manufacturer
Plastic	Hybrid polymer	ES-P	Esther II	197-101R	Tomy Orthodontics, Tokyo, Japan.
	Glass-reinforced plastic	IM-P	Image	IM-11-45	Gestenco International, Gothenburg, Sweden.
	Ceramic-reinforced plastic	SI-P	Silkon Plus	002922M	American Orthodontics, Sheboygan, WI, USA.
		SP-P	Spirit MB	494-0110	Ormco, Orange, CA, USA.
Ceramic	Polycrystalline	CL-C	Clarity	6400-601	3M Unitek, Monrovia, CA, USA.
		CR-C	Crystalline V	165-101R	Tomy Orthodontics, Tokyo, Japan.
		SI-C	Signature III	KQ9042	RMO, Denver, CO, USA.
	Monocrystalline	IN-C	Inspire ICE	443-0110	Ormco, Orange, CA, USA.

* The size of all brackets was 0.018-in, Roth for UR1.

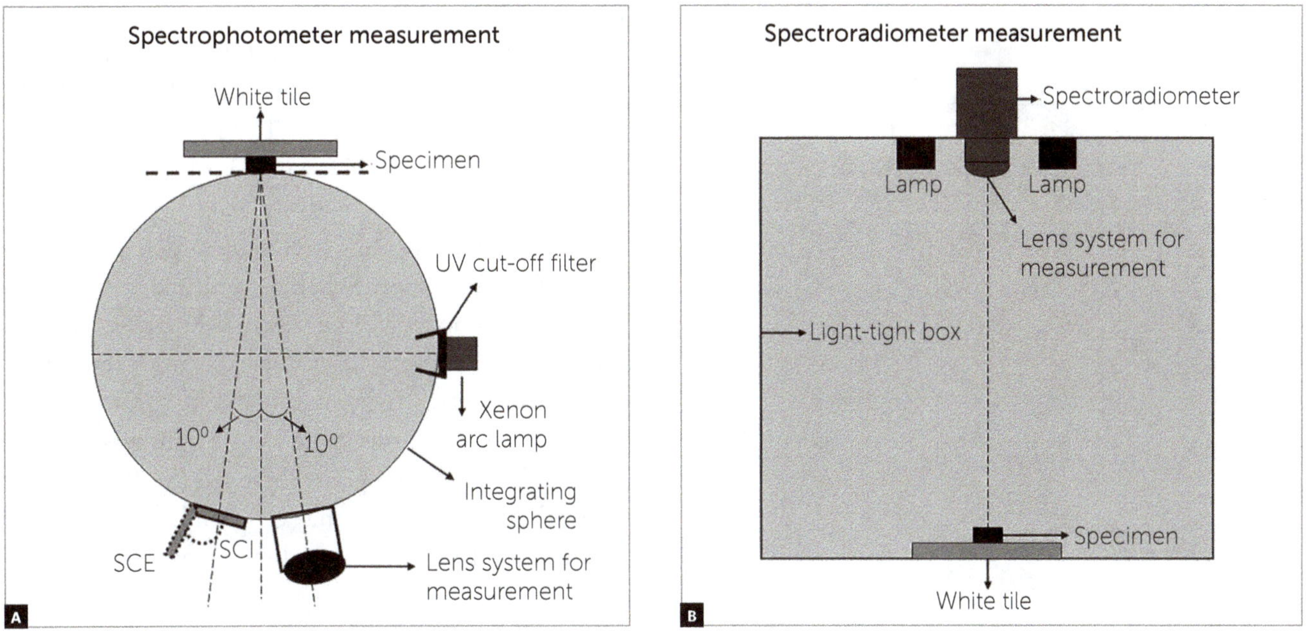

Figure 1 - Color measurement geometries for the spectrophotometer (**A**) and spectroradiometer (**B**).[18,19]

over a white (CIE L★ = 94.4, a★ = -0.1 and b★ = -0.6) and a black background (CIE L★ = 5.3, a★ = -0.4 and b★ = -1.4). Measurements were repeated three times for the central region and once for each one of the three tie-wings. The color of the tie-wing with the color-coded ID dot was not measured. 1-mm area was measured in tie-wings because of the limited size of this region. To simulate clinical situations, a stainless steel wire (0.016 x 0.022-in; Ormco, Glendora, CA, USA) was placed into the slot of each bracket during the color measurement procedure (Fig 2).[22] The color of a 3-mm diameter area in the central region of 16 Vitapan Classical Shade Guide (VITA Zahnfabrik, Bad Sackingen, Germany) tabs was also measured.

In the CIE $L^\star a^\star b^\star$ color space, CIE $L^\star$ is a measure of lightness. The CIE $a^\star$ value is a measure of redness or greenness and CIE $b^\star$ is a measure of yellowness or blueness. Chroma was calculated[26] as $C^\star_{ab} = (a^{\star 2} + b^{\star 2})^{1/2}$. TP was calculated as: $TP = [(L_W^\star - L_B^\star)^2 + (a_W^\star - a_B^\star)^2 + (b_W^\star - b_B^\star)^2]^{1/2}$, in which the subscripts W and B refer to color coordinates over white and black backgrounds, respectively.[22] CR was calculated as the ratio of bracket reflectance when it was placed on the black background (Y_b) to that of the same specimen when it was placed over the white background (Y_w): $CR = Y_b/Y_w$. The CIE $L^\star a^\star b^\star$ color difference between brackets and shade guide tabs was calculated with the equation: $\Delta E^\star_{ab} = [(\Delta L^\star)^2 + (\Delta a^\star)^2 + (\Delta b^\star)^2]^{1/2}$, based on the color coordinates at the central region of brackets measured over the white background.

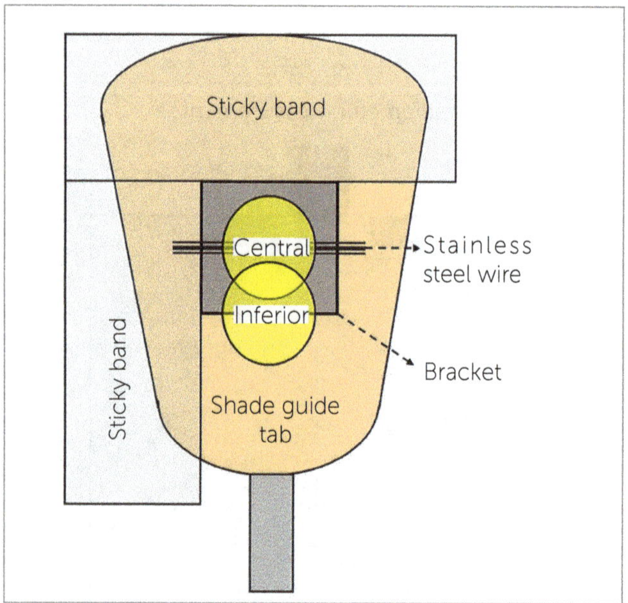

Figure 2 - Experimental set up.[22]

Statistical analysis

To determine the differences in color coordinates and translucency, two-way analysis of variance (ANOVA), was used according to bracket composition and brand (SPSS 16.0, Chicago, IL, USA). The means, representing bracket composition and brand, were compared by means of Scheffe's multiple comparison test ($\alpha = 0.05$). Pearson correlations between TP and CR, and between TP values of the central region and the tie-wings, were determined.

RESULTS

CIE $L^\star$ and $C^\star_{ab}$, as well as CIE $a^\star$ and $b^\star$ values in the central region of brackets over the white background are given in Table 2. The ranges for CIE $L^\star$, $a^\star$, $b^\star$ and $C^\star_{ab}$ were 75.8 to 98.3, -1.4 to 0.3, 2.6 to 8.0, and 2.6 to 8.1, respectively. All color coordinates were influenced by bracket composition and brand ($p < 0.05$). Based on Scheffe's multiple comparison test, the monocrystalline ceramic bracket (IN-C) showed the highest $L^\star$ value. Ceramic-reinforced plastic brackets (SI-P) and ceramic policrystaline brackets (CL-C) showed the lowest lightness, whereas ceramic-reinforced plastic brackets (SI-P and SP-P) showed the highest chroma ($C^\star_{ab}$) and polycrystalline ceramic bracket (CL-C) the lowest chroma.

Table 2 - CIE $L^\star$, $C^\star_{ab}$, $a^\star$ and $b^\star$ values in the central region of brackets over a white background.

Code	CIE $L^\star$	CIE $C^\star_{ab}$	CIE $a^\star$	CIE $b^\star$
ES-P	80.7 (1.1)^{c}	4.6 (0.5)^{C}	-0.2 (0.1)^{de}	4.6 (0.5)^{C}
IM-P	82.0 (0.5)^{cd}	5.0 (0.4)^{CD}	-0.5 (0.2)^{c}	5.0 (0.4)^{CD}
SI-P	77.6 (0.6)^{ab}	8.1 (0.2)^{E}	-1.4 (0.1)^{a}	8.0 (0.2)^{E}
SP-P	78.0 (0.5)^{b}	5.8 (0.3)^{D}	-1.0 (0.1)^{b}	5.7 (0.3)^{D}
CL-C	75.8 (0.5)^{a}	2.6 (0.1)^{A}	0.1 (0.1)^{ef}	2.6 (0.1)^{A}
CR-C	83.1 (0.7)^{d}	4.8 (0.4)^{C}	-0.5 (0.1)^{c}	4.8 (0.4)^{C}
IN-C	98.3 (0.7)^{f}	2.7 (0.3)^{AB}	-0.4 (0.2)^{cd}	2.7 (0.4)^{AB}
SI-C	86.7 (1.0)^{e}	3.6 (0.3)^{B}	0.3 (0.1)f	3.5 (0.3)^{B}

Standard deviations are within parentheses. There were no significant differences by brand marked with the same lowercase (CIE $L^\star$ and CIE $a^\star$) or uppercase ($C^\star_{ab}$ and CIE $b^\star$) letters ($p > 0.05$).

Color differences ($\Delta E^{\star}_{ab}$) between brackets and Vitapan Classical Shade Guide tabs were within the range of 10.4 to 34.5 $\Delta E^{\star}_{ab}$ units. CL-C bracket showed the smallest color differences with the shade tabs, while SI-C bracket showed the largest color differences (Fig 3). B1 tab always showed the smallest color difference with brackets. Ratios for color differences between brackets and the shade tabs, compared with that of the B1 tab, are shown in Figure 3. More chromatic tabs always showed higher color difference ratios as compared to less chromatic tabs in the same hue series, such as A, B, C and D.

TP and CR values of brackets are given in Table 3 for the central region and the tie-wings. TP and CR values were 16.4 to 27.7 and 0.38 to 0.58 for the central region, and 24.0 to 39.9 and 0.25 to 0.45 for the tie-wings, respectively. TP values of the central region and tie-wings showed significant correlation (coefficient of determination; $r^2 = 0.48$, $p < 0.01$). TP and CR values were significantly influenced by bracket composition and brand based on two-way ANOVA ($p < 0.05$). Based on Scheffe's tests, the following order was obtained for TP of the central region ($p < 0.05$): polycrystalline ceramic (mean: 18.4); ceramic-reinforced plastic (20.5); ceramic-reinforced plastic and hybrid polymer (21.7); monocrystalline ceramic (27.2) and glass-reinforced plastic (27.7). The correlation between TP and CR values is shown in Figure 4. CR values were negatively correlated with TP values ($r^2 = 0.955$, $p < 0.05$).

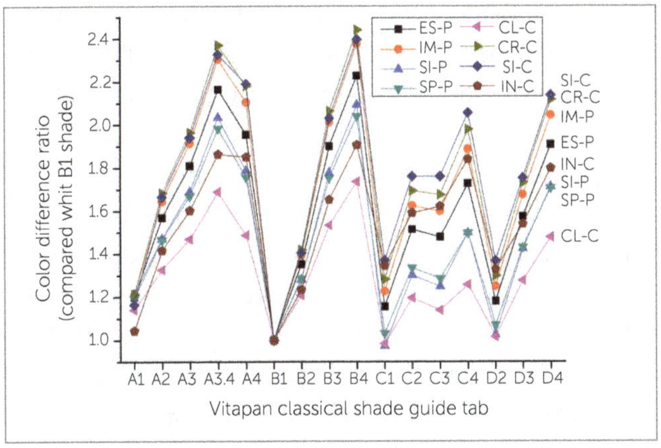

Figure 3 - Ratios for the color differences between brackets and shade tabs as compared with the B1 shade tab. All color difference values were based on the color of the central region of brackets over a white background.

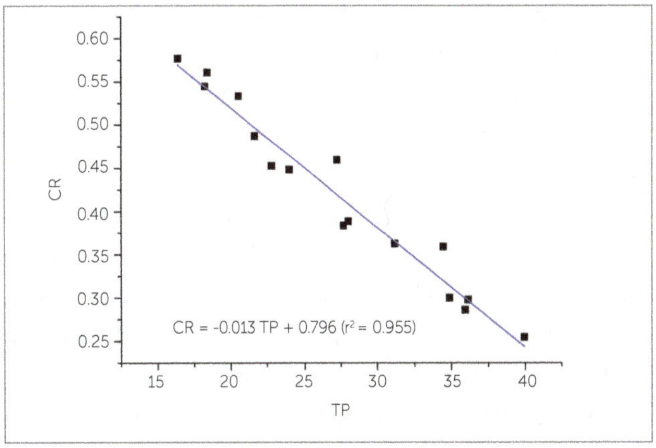

Figure 4 - Correlation between TP and CR values of brackets.

Table 3 - TP and CR values at central and tie-wing regions of brackets.

Code	TP		CR	
	Central	Tie-wings	Central	Tie-wings
ES-P	21.7 (2.1)^{*c}	34.9 (2.9)^{cd}	0.49 (0.04)^{B}	0.30 (0.03)^{AB}
IM-P	27.7 (0.9)^{d}	39.9 (4.0)^{d}	0.38 (0.02)^{A}	0.25 (0.03)^{A}
SI-P	22.8 (1.0)^{c}	35.9 (1.8)^{cd}	0.45 (0.02)^{B}	0.29 (0.02)^{AB}
SP-P	18.2 (1.5)^{ab}	28.0 (0.8)^{ab}	0.54 (0.03)^{CD}	0.39 (0.01)^{CD}
CL-C	16.4 (1.2)^{a}	24.0 (1.4)^{a}	0.58 (0.03)^{D}	0.45 (0.02)^{D}
CR-C	18.4 (0.6)^{ab}	36.1 (3.1)^{cd}	0.56 (0.01)^{CD}	0.30 (0.04)^{AB}
SI-C	20.5 (0.6)^{bc}	31.2 (1.4)^{bc}	0.53 (0.01)^{C}	0.36 (0.02)^{BC}
IN-C	27.2 (1.2)^{d}	34.5 (1.1)^{d}	0.46 (0.02)^{B}	0.36 (0.01)^{BC}

* Standard deviations are within parentheses.
There were no significant differences by brand marked with the same lowercase (TP) or uppercase (CR) letters ($p > 0.05$).

DISCUSSION

The null hypotheses of this study was rejected because all color coordinates and translucency of the investigated brackets were influenced by bracket composition and brand ($p < 0.05$). This *in vitro* study also found that the color of esthetic brackets was unacceptably different from that of any tab of Vitapan Classical Shade Guide ($\Delta E^{\star}_{ab}$>5.5).[12] Ideally, esthetic brackets should match the color of natural teeth. Since the color coordinates of natural teeth vary by race, sex and age,[27] shade guide tabs, which are regarded to represent the color ranges of natural teeth, were used in this study. However, the color of brackets was measured over a white background with light reflectance of nearly 100%, whereas shade tabs themselves had their original color; therefore, the measuring conditions for brackets and shade tabs were not identical. Therefore, color difference ratios to that of B1 tab were compared in the present study (Fig 3). All brackets showed similar trends in color difference ratios with the shade tabs.

Recently, acceptability and perceptibility thresholds for color differences in Dentistry were reviewed and concluded that more than half of studies defined perceptibility threshold as $\Delta E^{\star}_{ab}= 1$, and one third of studies referred to $\Delta E^{\star}_{ab}= 3.7$ as the threshold at which 50% of observers accepted the color difference.[14] However, threshold values of 2.6 and 5.5, respectively, were used in the present study because these values were based on spectroradiometer measurements.[12] It is clear that color difference values are influenced by the measuring instrument.[20]

In a previous study, color of esthetic brackets was measured with a spectrophotometer over a zero calibration cylinder, and it was reported that all color coordinates were influenced by the brand of bracket.[10] In the present study, the central region of brackets was measured over a white background and color coordinates were found to be significantly influenced by bracket brand, even in the same composition group (Table 2). Significantly higher $L^{\star}$ values, in the present study, were attributed to the difference in backgrounds used in two studies. The white background had light reflectance of nearly 100%, whereas the zero calibration cylinder had light reflectance of nearly 0.[10] Among the brackets investigated, monocrystalline ceramic bracket (IN-C) showed the highest lightness and the lowest chroma, which would make it suitable for use on bleached teeth.

Because the color of esthetic brackets and natural teeth is hard to be matched, translucency is an important optical attribute of esthetic brackets. Highly translucent brackets would allow the underlying tooth color to shine through them. In the present study, it was found that translucency was significantly influenced by bracket composition and brand. As to the discrepancies in color and translucency of brackets made of the same material, differences in thickness and geometry of brackets, especially in the tie-wings, might be the main reason.

Based on the TP value of the central region, glass-reinforced plastic and monocrystalline ceramic brackets were significantly more translucent than the other brackets, which might be attributed to their different microstructures (Table 3). Transparency of glass fillers in the glass-reinforced plastic bracket and lack of grain boundaries in the monocrystalline ceramic bracket could account for the high translucency of these brackets.[1] These results are in agreement with a previous study[10] which measured diffuse light transmittance value with a spectrophotometer to describe the translucency of esthetic brackets. Translucency at the tie-wing of the glass-reinforced plastic bracket was significantly greater than other bracket types, and the hybrid polymer plastic bracket was more translucent than the polycrystalline ceramic brackets (Table 3). Due to different thicknesses and geometries of the brackets, a weak, but statistically significant correlation was observed between TP values of the central region and the tie-wings ($r^2 = 0.48$).

Based on the results of the present study, CR and TP values were significantly and negatively correlated, which was in agreement with previous studies based on other types of material.[15,28] As the coefficient of determination between CR and TP was 0.955, TP and CR values may be used interchangeably. However, the clinical implications of these findings require further study. Since the mean CR value of eight brackets was 0.50, and the range was 0.38 to 0.58 (Table 3), the translucency difference was perceptible in many pairs of brackets compared, based on the translucency perception threshold (ΔCR) of 0.07.[16]

The strengths of this study included that the color and translucency of esthetic brackets were directly determined by means of a noncontact color measuring instrument. Additionally, this study proved quantitatively that the color of esthetic brackets and natural teeth (shade guide tabs in this study) rarely match, hence it highlighted the importance of translucency of esthetic brackets.

There were also several weaknesses. Firstly, the shade guide tabs as substitutes for natural teeth might have not represented the true color range of natural teeth. Secondly, only limited brands of esthetic brackets were examined. Thirdly, color and translucency of esthetic brackets might change with use, but only new brackets were investigated in the present study. Lastly, although the numerical data of the present study indicated that color differences between brackets and the shade guide tabs were higher than the acceptable limit, there have been several limitations in experimental methods of the present study. Therefore, clinical color matching performance might be better than that extrapolated from the *in vitro* numerical values.

The clinical implications of the present study were that orthodontists have to consider not only the color and translucency of brackets when choosing the most esthetic appliance, but also the shade of patient's teeth. In addition to color and translucency, the shape and thickness of brackets varied by bracket brand, which would also influence the esthetic performance.

CONCLUSIONS

Color coordinates and translucency of brackets investigated with a spectroradiometer were significantly influenced by composition and brand. Translucency difference by bracket brand was perceptible ($\Delta CR > 0.07$). All investigated brackets showed unacceptable color differences compared with all of Vitapan Classical Shade Guide tabs, based on *in vitro* experimental results. Therefore, brackets with the best matching performance for each case should be selected considering esthetic and functional demands.

Acknowledgements

This work was supported by the National Natural Science Foundation of China (#51102237).

REFERENCES

1. Eliades T. Orthodontic materials research and applications: Part 2. Current status and projected future developments in materials and biocompatibility. Am J Orthod Dentofacial Orthop. 2007 Feb;131(2):253-62.
2. Russell JS. Aesthetic orthodontic brackets. J Orthod. 2005 Jun;32(2):146-63.
3. Walton DK, Fields HW, Johnston WM, Rosenstiel SF, Firestone AR, Christensen JC. Orthodontic appliance preferences of children and adolescents. Am J Orthod Dentofacial Orthop. 2010 Dec;138(6):698.e1-12; discussion 698-9.
4. Kusy RP, Whitley JQ. Degradation of plastic polyoxymethylene brackets and the subsequent release of toxic formaldehyde. Am J Orthod Dentofacial Orthop. 2005 Apr;127(4):420-7.
5. Faltermeier A, Behr M, Müssig D. In vitro colour stability of aesthetic brackets. Eur J Orthod. 2007 Aug;29(4):354-8.
6. Bishara SE, Fehr DE. Ceramic brackets: something old, something new, a review. Semin Orthod. 1997 Sept;3(3):178-88.
7. Jena AK, Duggal R, Mehrotra AK. Physical properties and clinical characteristics of ceramic brackets: a comprehensive review. Trends Biomater Artif Organs. 2007 Jan;20(2):101-15.
8. Karamouzos A, Athanasiou AE, Papadopoulos MA. Clinical characteristics and properties of ceramic brackets: A comprehensive review. Am J Orthod Dentofacial Orthop. 1997 July;112(1):34-40.
9. Lopes Filho H, Maia LE, Araújo MV, Ruellas AC. Influence of optical properties of esthetic brackets (color, translucence, and fluorescence) on visual perception. Am J Orthod Dentofacial Orthop. 2012 Apr;141(4):460-7.
10. Lee YK. Color and translucency of tooth-colored orthodontic brackets. Eur J Orthod. 2008 Apr;30(2):205-10.
11. Johnston WM. Review of translucency determinations and applications to dental materials. J Esthet Restor Dent. 2014 July-Aug;26(4):217-23.
12. Douglas RD, Steinhauer TJ, Wee AG. Intraoral determination of the tolerance of dentists for perceptibility and acceptability of shade mismatch. J Prosthet Dent. 2007 Apr;97(4):200-8.
13. Johnston WM, Ma T, Kienle BH. Translucency parameter of colorants for maxillofacial prostheses. Int J Prosthodont. 1995 Jan-Feb;8(1):79-86.
14. Khashayar G, Bain PA, Salari S, Dozic A, Kleverlaan CJ, Feilzer AJ. Perceptibility and acceptability thresholds for color differences in dentistry. J Dent. 2014 Jun;42(6):637-44.
15. Yu B, Ahn JS, Lee YK. Measurement of translucency of tooth enamel and dentin. Acta Odontol Scand. 2009 Jan;67(1):57-64.
16. Liu MC, Aquilino SA, Lund PS, Vargas MA, Diaz-Arnold AM, Gratton DG, et al. Human perception of dental porcelain translucency correlated to spectrophotometric measurements. J Prosthodont. 2010 Apr;19(3):187-93.
17. Lee YK. Changes in the reflected and transmitted color of esthetic brackets after thermal cycling. Am J Orthod Dentofacial Orthop. 2008 May;133(5):641.e1-6.
18. Lim HN, Yu B, Lim JI, Lee YK. Correlations between spectroradiometric and spectrophotometric colors of all-ceramic materials. Dent Mater. 2010 Nov;26(11):1052-8.
19. Lee YK, Yu B, Lim HN. Lightness, chroma, and hue distributions of a shade guide as measured by a spectroradiometer. J Prosthet Dent. 2010 Sept;104(3):173-81.
20. Krikken JB, Zijp JR, Huysmans MC. Monitoring dental erosion by color measurement: an in vitro study. J Dent. 2008 Sept;36(9):731-5.
21. Bayindir F, Kuo S, Johnston WM, Wee AG. Coverage error of three conceptually different shade guide systems to vital unrestored dentition. J Prosthet Dent. 2007 Sept;98(3):175-85.
22. Yu B, Lee YK. Aesthetic colour performance of plastic and ceramic brackets: an in vitro study. J Orthod. 2010 Sept;38(3):167-74.
23. del Mar Pérez M, Saleh A, Pulgar R, Paravina RD. Light polymerization-dependent changes in color and translucency of resin composites. Am J Dent. 2009 Apr;22(2):97-101.
24. Lim HN, Yu B, Lee YK. Spectroradiometric and spectrophotometric translucency of ceramic materials. J Prosthet Dent. 2010 Oct;104(4):239-46.
25. Bolt RA, Bosch JJ, Coops JC. Influence of window size in small-window colour measurement, particularly of teeth. Phys Med Biol. 1994 July;39(7):1133-42.
26. Commission Internationale de l´Eclairage. Colorimetry - Technical Report. CIE Pub. no. 15. 3 edn. Vienna, Austria: Bureau Central de la CIE; 2004. p. 30-6.
27. Li Y. Tooth color measurement using Chroma Meter: techniques, advantages, and disadvantages. J Esthet Restor Dent. 2003;15 Suppl 1:S33-41.
28. Yu B, Lee YK. Translucency of varied brand and shade of resin composites. Am J Dent. 2008 Aug;21(4):229-32.

Assessment of the dimensions and surface characteristics of orthodontic wires and bracket slots

Gabriel Schmidt Dolci[1], Ana Maria Spohr[2], Eduardo Rigon Zimmer[3], Ernani Menezes Marchioro[4]

Objective: The purpose of this study was to evaluate the dimensions and surface characteristics of orthodontic wires and bracket slots of different commercial brands. **Methods:** Thirty metallic brackets (0.022 x 0.028-in and 0.022 x 0.030-in) were divided in three groups: DYN/3M group = Dyna-Lock, 3M/Unitek (stainless steel, or SS); STD/MO group = Slim Morelli (SS); and Ni-Free/MO group = Slim Morelli (Ni-Free). The stainless steel wires (0.019 x 0.025-in) were divided into two groups: MO group = Morelli; and 3M group = 3M/Unitek. The bracket and wire measurements were done by two methods: (a) Surface Electron Microscopy (SEM), and (b) Profile projection. The surface analysis was done qualitatively, based on SEM images and/or by a rugosimeter. The quantitative results were analyzed by ANOVA with Tukey's test ($p < 0.05$) and Student's *t* test. **Results:** A significant difference in the dimensions of slots was observed, and the NiFree/MO group showed the greatest changes when compared to the other groups. The analysis of surface topography of the brackets indicated greater homogeneity of the metallic matrix for DYN/3M and STD/MO groups. As for the dimensions of the wires, groups showed statistically different mean heights. **Conclusions:** It was concluded that wires and brackets slots can present altered dimensions, which might directly and unintentionally affect the planned tooth movement.

Keywords: Orthodontic brackets. Orthodontic wires. Friction.

[1] Associate Professor, Department of Orthodontics, Brazilian Association of Dental Surgeons.
[2] Associate Professor, Department of Dental Materials, PUC-RS.
[3] PhD student, Department of Biochemistry, McGill University.
[4] Head, Department of Orthodontics, Brazilian Association of Dental Surgeons.

» The author reports no commercial, proprietary or financial interest in the products or companies described in this article.

Gabriel Schmidt Dolci
Rua Múcio Teixeira, 1380 – Menino Deus
CEP: 90.150-090 – Porto Alegre/RS, Brazil

E-mail: gabriel@sorrirfazbem.com

INTRODUCTION

Among the adverse effects of brackets and wires with altered size and geometry, the reduction of dental movements control and increasing friction in the bracket/wire interface stands out.[1,2,26] Undesirable effects such as torque loss of upper and lower incisors (5 – 10°) during space closure mechanics can be attributed to changes in the bracket slot size.[1] The lack of standardization in the wire and bracket slots dimensions will also directly influence on the frictional resistance, hindering the sliding mechanics.[2] It must be observed that with the best combination between bracket and wires, at least 40 g of friction should be included in the force applied to the tooth to start its movement.[3]

Other factors have been linked to the force of friction between brackets and wires during tooth movement; among them, the surface texture of bracket slots and orthodontic wires.[5] Preliminary studies indicate that less homogenous surface characteristics of orthodontic wires are those that have greater surface roughness, which generates more friction in the bracket/wire interface.[5] In addition, orthodontic accessories with less homogenous surfaces tend to be more susceptible to corrosion,[6] which increases the risk of tissue damage, esthetic changes (staining of the tooth by corrosive products) and loss of metal properties.

Companies responsible for the manufacture of orthodontic accessories do not usually indicate their possible size variations; however these variations exist and they are associated to the bracket/wire manufacturing process. Studies point to the need for the introduction of regulatory standards of orthodontic products[24] and therefore technical standards of orthodontic wires and brackets manufacturing were described.[25] Since most orthodontic devices are directly associated with the relationship between size and prescription of brackets and with the section and size of wires, it is important that professionals know more about the materials used in their daily clinical practice. This study aimed to measure the size of rectangular wires and metal bracket slots of different trademarks, *in vitro*. The null hypothesis is the similarity between measures specified by the manufacturers and the actual size of orthodontic brackets and wires. In addition, roughness and surface characteristics of these orthodontic wires and brackets were analyzed.

MATERIAL AND METHODS

a) Analysis of brackets size

Thirty metal edgewise upper right premolar brackets of two different trademarks (3M/Unitek, Monrovia, CA, USA and Dental Morelli, Sorocaba, SP, Brazil) were used. The accessories were divided into three groups of 10 brackets each, as described in Table 1. Two different methods were used to evaluate the slot sizes (height and depth) by one trained operator:

a1) Scanning Electron Microscopy (SEM, Philips XL2000, Holland) – The preparation of brackets consisted of cleaning with acetone by ultrasound (Equipal USC700) for six minutes. After cleaning, the brackets were dried with a nitrogen jet and mounted on metal supports properly identified for SEM observation. After bracket placement, they were pressed against the supports with the aid of a dental probe number 5, so that the bracket bases were parallel to the horizontal plane.

Three frontal images of the brackets were taken: The first was enlarged by 50x, for a general view of the slot conformation (Fig 1); the two others, enlarged by 230x, were taken for a detailed view of each half of the brackets. Thus, for each image at 230x magnification, three measures of the vertical dimension (height) of the slot were analyzed, totaling six measures for each bracket (Fig 1). The average of these values was estimated for each accessory and, finally, for each group.

a2) Profile Projection (PP) – After cleaning the accessories, a profile projector (Nikkon V16, Japan) was used for measuring the vertical and horizontal dimensions of the bracket slots (height and depth). The accessories were fixed to a glass plate using dental wax, so that the slots remained perpendicular to the horizontal plane. The set brackets/glass plate was taken to a projector table, obtaining the shadow projection of the slots. Then, the height and depth of the bracket slot sizes were measured (Fig 2).

Table 1 - Description of studied brackets.

Manufacturer	Bracket	Dimension	Alloy
3M/Unitek	Dyna-Lock; Edgewise Standard (DYN/3M)	0.022 x 0.028-in	Stainless steel (Fe, Ni, Cr)*
Dental Morelli	Slim; Edgewise Standard (STD/MO)	0.022 x 0.030-in	Stainless steel (Fe, Ni, Cr)*
	Slim; Edgewise Standard (Ni-Free/MO)	0.022 x 0.030-in	Stainless steel (nickel free) (chromium, manganese, molybdenum and nitrogen)

* Composition of Stainless Steel Source: Anusavice[7] (1996).

b) Analysis of the wire dimensions

Four rectangular wire segments (0.019 x 0.025-in) of two different commercial brands (3M/Unitek, Monrovia, CA, USA and Dental Morelli, Sorocaba, SP, BR) were used. Each segment was sectioned into six pieces of approximately 1.97 inches each. The samples were divided into two groups according to the wire trademark (Table 2).

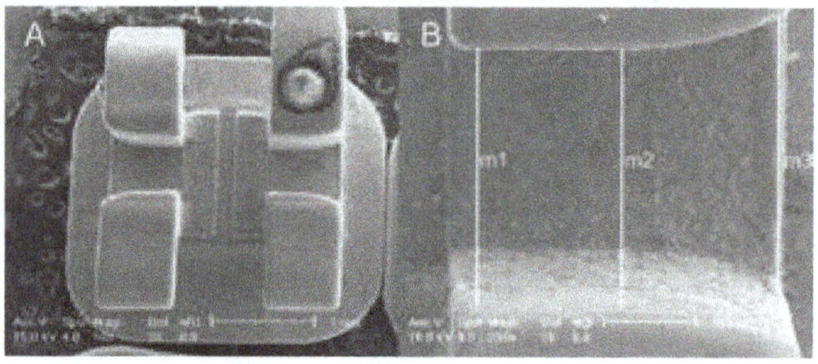

Figure 1 - Scanning Electron Microscopy image of a bracket pertaining to Group III – (**A**) magnification at 50x and (**B**) 230x. The lines m1, m2 and m3 are the regions were the measurements were done to calculate slot height. The large variation of bracket dimensions can be observed, especially on mesial and distal ends.

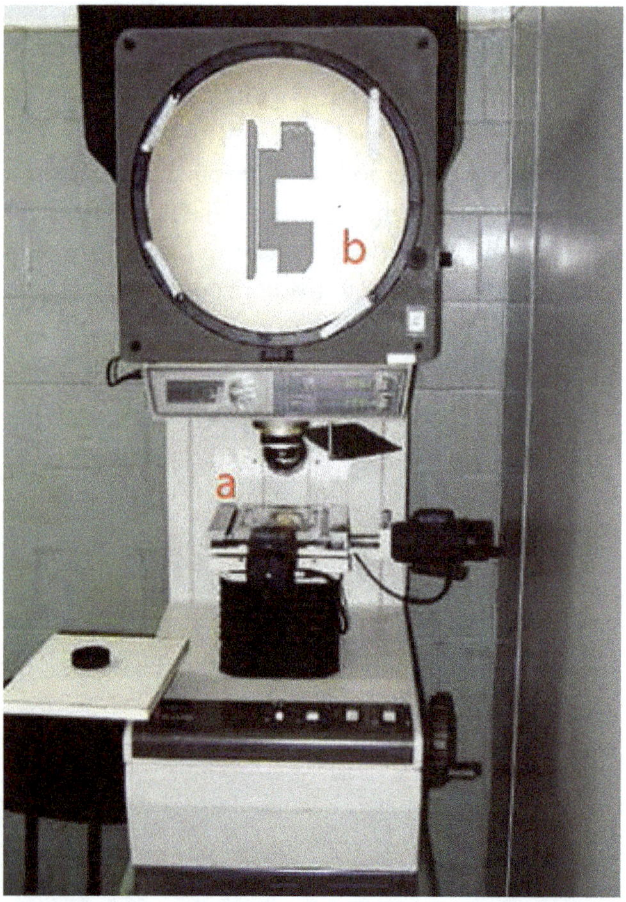

Figure 2 - Profile projector. (**a**) Once the brackets were correctly positioned on this device, their shadows were projected with a substantial magnification. (**b**) Bracket height and depth were measured.

The analysis of the wire dimensions was performed using a profile projector (Nikkon V16, Japan). For the measurement of both sections of the wire, the segments were observed in frontal and profile views. After projection of the wire shadows, their height and depth were measured.

c) Surface characteristics analysis of brackets and wires

Bracket and wires surface characteristic analysis was performed by SEM at a magnification of 1000x (Fig 3). Initially, a point above the mesial gingival tie-wing of the bracket slot and a point in the center of the wire segment were pre-determined. The images taken were recorded, identified and randomly distributed in the Microsoft Office Power Point 2010 software,. Subsequently, the images were analyzed by two examiners, using a discrete scale quantitative classification containing four scores: 0 – very rough surface; 1 – rough surface; 2 – smooth surface; and 3 – very smooth surface. Twenty per cent of samples from each group were re-evaluated, in order to verify conformity between examiners.

Table 2 - Description of studied wires.

Manufacturer	Dimension	Alloy
3M/Unitek (3M)	0.019 x 0.025-in	Stainless steel (Fe, Ni, Cr)*
Dental Morelli (MO)	0.019 x 0.025-in	

* Composition of stainless steel. Source: Anusavice[7] (1996).

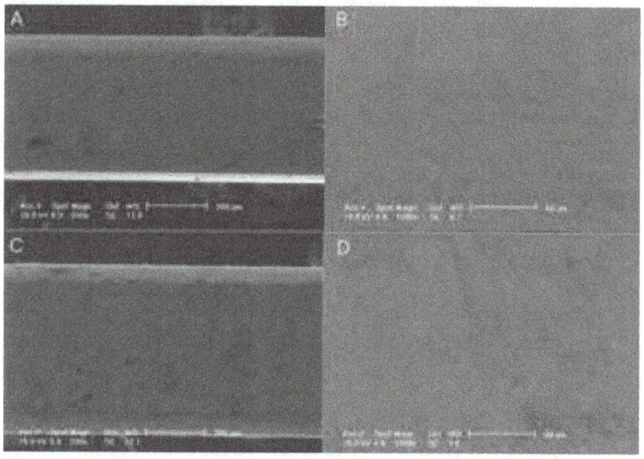

Figure 3 - Scanning Electron Microscopy of wires. (**A**) 3M-Unitek wires - Group IV –at a magnification of 230x and (**B**) 1000x; (**C**) Morelli wires at a magnification of 230x and (**D**) 1000x.

d) Wire surface roughness analysis

Roughness of wires was evaluated with a surface roughness tester (Mitotoyo SJ201, USA). After cleaning, the wire segments were stuck to a flat table using dental wax, where the roughness tests were carried out. Each wire was rated five times in different regions. Finally, the average values for each wire and different groups were calculated.

All tests were conducted in a climate-controlled environment and with controlled relative air humidity, avoiding any size change of the metal used for manufacturing orthodontic accessories.

e) Statistical analysis

Data normality was confirmed by the Kolmogorov-Smirnov test ($p > 0.05$) and the homogeneity of variances was tested by Levene's test ($p > 0.01$).The results associated with the sizes of the bracket slots were subjected to analysis of variance (ANOVA) followed by Tukey's test ($p > 0.05$). Student's *t* test was used for comparison between heights, depths and surface roughness of wires. The null hypothesis was tested by one-way ANOVA. The analysis of surface characteristics was performed descriptively. Inter-examiners agreement was evaluated by Kappa test and it was considered excellent (Kappa = 0.867). All tests were conducted with the Statistical Package for the Social Sciences, version 17.0 for Windows (SPSS, Chicago, IL, USA).

RESULTS

According to the SEM evaluation (Table 3), DYN/3M, STD/MO and Ni-Free/MO brackets showed slots with heights larger than those specified by the manufacturers ($p < 0.05$). The Ni-Free/MO bracket slots showed larger size, followed by DYN/3M and STD/MO brackets, respectively (Table 3). According to the PP method, there was no statistical difference between the slot heights measured in this study and the standard dimension specified by manufacturer, except for the Ni-Free/MO group (Table 3). On the other hand, regarding the slot depth, DYN/3M and Ni-Free/MO groups showed larger dimensions than those specified by the manufacturers. The comparison between groups did not indicate statistical differences (Table 4).

For the wire dimensions (SEM and PP), the DYN/3M group showed greater heights than that specified by the manufacturers, which was statistically different from the MO groups. With regard to the wire depth, there were no statistical differences (Table 5).

The analysis of surface characteristics of the bracket slots (SEM) showed a better metal polishing for the accessories of the DYN/3M group: 90% of the sample scored 3 and 10% scored 2; followed by the STD/MO group, which showed that 80% scored 1, 10% scored 2, and 10% scored 0. With a more irregular surface characteristic, Ni-Free/MO accessories showed that 40% scored 0 and 60% scored 1.

For the wire segments, the visual surface analysis (SEM) indicated that the MO groups showed 17% scoring 3 and 83% scoring 2. The 3M group showed 33% scoring 3 and 67% scoring 2. The surface roughness of wires indicated no significant differences between groups (Table 6).

DISCUSSION

SEM analysis indicated that the brackets of all groups presented slot height larger than 0.022-in (Table 3). It is important to emphasize that in the Ni-Free/MO group, the presence of changes in the slot conformation was observed, i.e., the height of the slots in the mesial and distal extremities showed greater sizes than those heights in internal extremities (medial), as can be seen in Figure 1.

Table 3 - Statistical analysis of the bracket slot heights (results in inches).

Method	Group	Mean	Median	SD	SE	MIN.	MAX.
MEV	DYN/3M*#	0.02396	0.02371	8.10×10^{-4}	2.8×10^{-4}	0.02251	0.02534
	STD/MO*#	0.02251	0.02252	4.3×10^{-4}	1.3×10^{-4}	0.02199	0.02335
	Ni-Free/MO*#	0.02570	0.02554	9.1×10^{-4}	2.8×10^{-4}	0.02438	0.02697
PP	DYN/3M	0.0223	0.0225	1.0×10^{-3}	3.3×10^{-4}	0.0210	0.0240
	STD/MO	0.02169	0.02185	6.9×10^{-4}	2.2×10^{-4}	0.0200	0.0225
	Ni-Free/MO*	0.02247	0.0223	5.2×10^{-4}	1.6×10^{-4}	0.0220	0.0232

n = 10 brackets (each group);
* = difference between slots dimension obtained (SEM and PP) and the manufacturer specified dimension (One sample t test, $p < 0.05$).
# = Statistical differences between groups (one way ANOVA,followed by Tukey test, $p < 0.05$).

Table 4 - Statistical analysis of bracket slot depth (results in inches).

Method	Group	Mean	Median	SD	SE	MIN.	MAX.
PP	DYN/3M*	0.0308	0.0310	1.3×10^{-3}	4.1×10^{-4}	0.0290	0.0330
	STD/MO	0.02892	0.02935	3.1×10^{-3}	9.9×10^{-4}	0.0250	0.0350
	Ni-Free/MO*	0.0290	0.0290	9.4×10^{-4}	2.9×10^{-4}	0.0280	0.0310

* = difference between bracket dimension obtained (PP) and the manufacturer specified dimension (One sample *t* test, $p < 0.05$).
# = Statistical differences between groups (one way ANOVA, followed by Tukey test, $p < 0.05$).

Table 5 - Height and depth comparison between studied wires (results in inches).

	Manufacturer	Mean	Median	SD	SE	MIN.	MAX.
Wires' height	3M*#	0.01967	0.02200	5.1×10^{-4}	2.1×10^{-4}	0.0190	0.0240
	MO#	0.02072	0.02200	1.8×10^{-3}	7.4×10^{-4}	0.0190	0.0240
	Brand	**Mean**	**Median**	**SD**	**SE**	**MIN.**	**MAX.**
Wires' depth	3M	0.0250	0.0250	6.3×10^{-4}	2.5×10^{-4}	0.0240	0.0260
	MO	0.02457	0.0245	9.4×10^{-4}	3.8×10^{-4}	0.0234	0.0260

* = difference between wire dimension obtained and the manufacturer specified dimension (One Sample *t* test, $p < 0.05$).
# = Statistical differences between Groups (one way ANOVA, followed by Tukey test, $p < 0.05$).

Table 6 -Statistical analysis of wire roughness (results in micrometers).

Manufacturer	Mean	Median	SD	SE	MIN.	MAX.
3M	0.0360	0.0330	1.1×10^{-2}	3.3×10^{-3}	0.0200	0.0640
MO	0.04483	0.0390	1.5×10^{-2}	4.6×10^{-3}	0.0320	0.0880

Thus, the Ni-Free/MO group showed a vertical size of the slots statistically larger than the other groups, followed by the accessories of DYN/3M and STD/MO groups, respectively. Assad-Loss et al[8] also observed rounding of the exterior angle of the brackets slots. Cash et al,[9] when assessing the size and geometry of bracket slots that belonged to 11 different trademarks, concluded that all analyzed accessories showed greater slots than those specified by the manufacturers, confirming the findings of this study.

On the other hand, when the profile projector was used to measure the slot height in this study, no statistical differences were found between the groups. Only accessories from the Ni-Free/MO group showed a significant greater height than that specified by the manufacturers. It should be noted that this method is based on linear measurements from the projection of the shadow of a piece (Fig 2). Therefore, a superimposition of the shadow of the middle region of the slot on the shadow of the lateral region is unavoidable, which can mask the conformation change of the slots observed by SEM from a front view (Fig 1). In this way, it must be considered that the PP methodology does not take into account possible variations in the vertical size of the slots, i.e., the measurement value obtained expresses the smaller vertical size of the bracket slots. This fact makes PP results found for the Ni-Free/MO group more relevant, since accessories of this group showed slot height significantly larger than that specified by the manufacturers (Table 3).

The analysis of the slot depth (PP) did not indicate differences between groups, as the DYN/3M group presented the highest average, followed by the Ni-Free/MO and STD/MO groups respectively. It should be noted that the Ni-Free/MO and DYN/3M groups showed slot depth greater than that specified by the manufacturers. This lack of standardization of size and geometry of bracket slots has been reported by several authors.[3,8,9,26] Kusy and Whitley[2] assessed 24 brackets of different trademarks and found that three brackets had slots that were smaller than specified, while 20 others had slots larger than specified.

Assad-Loss et al[8] studied nine types of brackets of five different trademarks, concluding that there were differences between the slot height and depth when compared with the standard announced by the manufacturer. Onthe other hand, Astrid et al[26] analyzed the sizes of brackets and wires of different trademarks and concluded that the brackets studied showed standardized sizes, while some wires were outside the expected standard.

Regarding the size of the wires, statistical differences between the 3M and MO groups were observed in this study (Table 5). It is interesting to note that the 3M group showed an average height statistically different from that specified by the manufacturers. Regarding the MO group, a wide variety of wire sizes was observed, which indicates a smaller standardization of wires belonging to this group. Professionals must be aware of the possible clinical disadvantages that represent these results. Several authors confirm the direct relationship between the diameter/section of wires and frictional force.[2,10-15] Nanda and Ghosh[2] state that the size and shape of wires and the height and depth of the slots of the brackets are factors that can affect the friction force during sliding mechanics. Kapur, Sinha and Nanda[15] observed that the frictional resistance of stainless steel brackets was higher with increasing diameter/section of the wire.

The qualitative analysis of slot surface characteristics obtained in this study points to the fact that DYN/3M brackets have greater homogeneity of the metal matrix, followed by brackets from STD/MOR and Ni-Free/MOR groups, which confirm previous studies.[17,19] Some authors have reported minor frictional forces during the sliding mechanics on accessories that have slots with smoother surface[18,19] and this fact is an area of controversial discussion.[20] Also, it should be noted that the superficial homogeneity of metal alloy constituent of orthodontic accessories is an important factor in the prevention of the corrosive process, which has become a topic of interest in orthodontic literature.[6]

The qualitative analysis of surface characteristics of wires showed no significant differences between the groups studied (Fig 3), which is a result that was confirmed by the analysis of roughness (Table 6). This consistency between the results obtained by the two different methodologies (SEM and the Roughness Tester) confirms the effectiveness of visual analysis regarding surface characteristics by means of Scanning Electron Microscopy, in accordance with the findings of Menezes et al[17] and Chappard et al.[23]

The standardization of bracket slot sizes seems essential to consolidate certain technological advances, such as the clinical option of using the straight wire technique. Such decision is usually based on angular values that vary according to the chosen prescription and, theoretically, manufacturers should establish such values with precision. This research considers the evident lack of standardization of these accessories during manufacturing process, which may be clinically associated with undesirable changes in tooth positioning and movement. Therefore, it is suggested to conduct studies that investigate this lack of standardization of torque and angulations as specified by the manufacturers for straight-wire brackets with different prescriptions. In addition, it is necessary to understand possible determining factors of this remarkable lack of standardization of orthodontic accessories, such as their constituent alloy and/or their manufacturing processes.

CONCLUSIONS

Based on the results of this study, it can be concluded that:

» There was no standardization in the manufacturing process of orthodontic brackets belonging to the groups DYN/3M, STD/MO and Ni-Free/MO, which showed a significant increase in the average height of their brackets slots;

» Regarding the wire sizes, the DYN/3M group presented a greater height than that specified by the manufacturers, unlike MO group;

» The Ni-Free/MO bracket group showed less homogeneity of the metal matrix, followed by STD/MO and DYN/3M groups, respectively.

REFERENCES

1. Sistkovsky R. Loss of anterior torque control due to variations in bracket slot and wire archwire dimensions. J Clin Orthod. 1999;33(9):508-10.
2. Kusy RP, Whitley JQ. Friction between different wire bracket configuration and materials. Semin Orthod. 1997;3(3):166-77.
3. Nanda RS, Gosh J. Biomechanical considerations in sliding mechanics. In: Nanda RS, Biomechanics in clinical orthodontics. Philadelphia: WB Saunders Company; 1999. cap. 10, p. 188-217.
4. Kuroe K, Tajiri T, Nakayama T, Nagakubo C, Kubota S, Matsuda T, et al. Frictional forces with friction free Edgewise brackets. J Clin Orthod. 1994;28(6):347-51.
5. Lee S, Chang Y. Effects of recycling on the mechanical properties and the surface topography of nickel-titanium alloy wires. Am J Orthod Dentofacial Orthop. 2001;120(6):654-63.
6. Dolci GS, Menezes LM, Souza RM, Dedavid B. Biodegradação de bráquetes ortodônticos: avaliação da liberação iônica in vitro. Rev Dental Press Ortod Ortop Facial. 2008;13(3):77-84.
7. Anusavice KJ. Constituição das ligas. In: Philips – Materiais Dentários. 10ª ed. Rio de Janeiro: Guanabara Koogan; 1996. cap 15, p. 193-204.
8. Assad-Loss TF, Cavalcante LM, Neves RM, Mucha JN. Avaliação dimensional de slots de bráquetes metálicos. Rev Flum Odont.

2010;15(1):45-51.

9. Cash AC, Good SA, Curtis RV, McDonald F. An evaluation of slot size in orthodontic brackets – Are standards as expected? Angle Orthod. 2004;74(4):450-3.
10. Leal RS. Comparação do atrito in vitro em bráquetes estéticos convencionais e autoligados [dissertação]. São Bernardo do Campo (SP): Universidade Metodista de São Paulo; 2009.
11. Vaughan JL, Ducanson MG, Nanda RS, Currier GF. Relative kinetic frictional forces between sintered stainless steel brackets and orthodontic wires. Am J Orthod Dentofacial Orthop. 1995;107(1):20-7.
12. Frank CA, Nicolai RJ. A comparative study of frictional resistances between orthodontic bracket and arch wire. Am J Orthod. 1980;78(6):593-609.
13. Baker KL, Nieberg G, Weimer AD, Hanna M. Frictional changes in force values caused by saliva substitution. Am J Orthod Dentofacial Orthop. 1987;91(4):316-20.
14. Kapila S, Angolkar PJ, Ducanson MG, Nanda RS. Evaluation of friction between edgewise stainless steel brackets and orthodontic wires for four alloys. Am J Orthod Dentofacial Orthop. 1990;98(2):117-26.
15. Kapur R, Sinha MB, Nanda RS. Comparison of frictional resistance in titanium and stainless steel brackets. Am J Orthod Dentofacial Orthop. 1999;116(3):271-4.
16. Sória ML. Avaliação da corrosão de bráquetes metálicos [dissertação]. Porto Alegre (RS): PUCRS; 2003.
17. Menezes LM, Souza RM, Dolci GS, Dedavid B. Biodegradação de braquetes ortodônticos: análise por microscopia eletrônica de varredura. Dental Press J Orthod. 2010;15(3):48-51.
18. Pratten DH, Popli K, Germane N, Gunsolley JC. Frictional resistance of ceramic and stainless steel orthodontic brackets. Am J Orthod Dentofacial Orthop. 1990;98(5):398-403.
19. Omana HM, Moore RN, Bagby MD. Frictional properties of metal ceramic brackets. J Clin Orthod. 1992;26(7):425-32.
20. Saunders CR, Kusy RP. Surface topography and frictional characteristics of ceramic brackets. Am J Orthod Dentofacial Orthop. 1994;106(1):76-87.
21. Kim H, Johnson JW. Corrosion of stainless steel, nickel-titanium, coated nickel-titanium, and titanium orthodontic wires. Angle Orthod. 1999;69(1):39-44.
22. Azevedo CRF. Characterization of metallic piercings. Eng Failure Anal. 2003;10(3):255-63.
23. Chappard D, Degasne I, Hure G, Legand E, Audan M, Basle MF. Image analysis of roughness by texture and fractal analysis correlate with contact profilometry. Biomater. 2003;24(8):1399-407.
24. Sernetz F. Normung kieferorthopädischer Produkte—Macht das Sinn? J Orofac Orthop 2005;66:307-18.
25. Deutsches Institut fur Normung e.V. DIN 13971-2: 2000-01 Kieferorthopadische Produkte.
26. Astrid J, Margit P, Frank W. Bracket slot and archwire dimensions: manufacturing precision and third order clearance. J Orthod. 2010;37(4):241-9.

Four chemical methods of porcelain conditioning and their influence over bond strength and surface integrity

João Paulo Fragomeni Stella[1], Andrea Becker Oliveira[1], Lincoln Issamu Nojima[2], Mariana Marquezan[3]

Objective: To assess four different chemical surface conditioning methods for ceramic material before bracket bonding, and their impact on shear bond strength and surface integrity at debonding. **Methods:** Four experimental groups (n = 13) were set up according to the ceramic conditioning method: G1 = 37% phosphoric acid etching followed by silane application; G2 = 37% liquid phosphoric acid etching, no rinsing, followed by silane application; G3 = 10% hydrofluoric acid etching alone; and G4 = 10% hydrofluoric acid etching followed by silane application. After surface conditioning, metal brackets were bonded to porcelain by means of the Transbond XP system (3M Unitek). Samples were submitted to shear bond strength tests in a universal testing machine and the surfaces were later assessed with a microscope under 8 X magnification. ANOVA/Tukey tests were performed to establish the difference between groups (α = 5%). **Results:** The highest shear bond strength values were found in groups G3 and G4 (22.01 ± 2.15 MPa and 22.83 ± 3.32 Mpa, respectively), followed by G1 (16.42 ± 3.61 MPa) and G2 (9.29 ± 1.95 MPa). As regards surface evaluation after bracket debonding, the use of liquid phosphoric acid followed by silane application (G2) produced the least damage to porcelain. When hydrofluoric acid and silane were applied, the risk of ceramic fracture increased. **Conclusions:** Acceptable levels of bond strength for clinical use were reached by all methods tested; however, liquid phosphoric acid etching followed by silane application (G2) resulted in the least damage to the ceramic surface.

Keywords: Orthodontic brackets. Ceramics. Orthodontics.

[1] Professor, Centro de Estudos Odontológicos Meridional (CEOM), Postgraduate program, Passo Fundo, Rio Grande do Sul, Brazil.
[2] Professor, Universidade Federal do Rio de Janeiro (UFRJ), Department of Pediatric Dentistry and Orthodontics, Rio de Janeiro, Rio de Janeiro, Brazil.
[3] Postdoc resident, Universidade Federal do Rio de Janeiro (UFRJ), Department of Pediatric Dentistry and Orthodontics, Rio de Janeiro, Rio de Janeiro, Brazil. Dentist, Universidade Federal de Santa Maria (UFSM), Department of Restorative Dentistry, Santa Maria, Rio Grande do Sul, Brazil.

» The authors report no commercial, proprietary or financial interest in the products or companies described in this article.

Mariana Marquezan
Rua Dr. Alberto Pasqualini, 70/809, Santa Maria/RS, Brazil - CEP 97015-010
Email: marianamarquezan@gmail.com

INTRODUCTION

The advent of adhesive systems has changed the technique of placing orthodontic appliances,[1] thus enabling brackets to be bonded to anterior teeth and in the intermediate part of the arch, thereby replacing the system of bands previously used. This fact has overcome the main disadvantages of the multi-banded appliance, such as poor esthetics, clinical time spent on placement and need for individual tooth separation.

The quest for an esthetic smile and the extensive use of the bracket bonding technique aroused adult patients' interest in orthodontic treatment.[2] However, this context has posed a challenge to the bonding technique: the presence of artificial surfaces, since many adult patients have restorations that were performed with material such as composite resins, amalgams, gold, acrylic resin and/or porcelain.[2,3] The demand for esthetics and technological advancements have caused the types of restorative material capable of accepting bracket bonding to increase, and a great variety of composites and ceramic systems are now available.[4,5] Porcelain plays an important role in restorative systems, and it is used in veneers, inlays, onlays, full crowns and bridges. Porcelain good color stability provides an esthetic advantage over other restorative material; however, it is highly friable and its clinical repair does not yield satisfactory results.[2,6]

An adequate bonding technique implies that the bracket will support masticatory and orthodontic forces without being detached during treatment, thereby preserving the integrity of the tooth or restorative surface to be maintained after debonding.[3] Surface conditioning is one of the most important factors in bracket bonding to the underlying artificial restorative surface. Ceramic surface conditioning can be performed by mechanical methods, such as increasing surface roughness by means of diamond burs, and air abrasion with aluminum oxide or silica; and chemical methods, such as acid etching, either with or without subsequent silane application.[7-10]

The choice between methods should take bracket bond strength and preservation of the ceramic surface after debonding into account. Adequate bond strength itself is not enough, if at the end of treatment the veneer or crown is damaged to the point where it needs to be replaced. However, preservation of the restorative work should not hamper adhesion or lead to successive rebonding. Therefore, appropriate bond strength should be allied to surface preservation.

It has been noted that chemical surface conditioning methods cause less damage to porcelain.[3,10,11,12] Among the chemical methods assessed, the highest bond strength was observed when hydrofluoric acid was used, with or without subsequent silane application.[3,4,6,10,13-17] However, the latter is capable of removing the glaze out of porcelain surface. Etching with 37% phosphoric acid followed by silane application was suggested as an alternative to hydrofluoric acid, but the acid should not be rinsed off between steps.[18] This acid has the advantage of being routinely used in-office, in addition to being less aggressive to oral tissues and not removing the porcelain glaze.[18]

Therefore, the aim of this study was to assess four different chemical conditioning methods for porcelain surface before bracket bonding, as well as assess their impact over bond strength and surface integrity after debonding.

MATERIAL AND METHODS

This research had an experimental *in vitro* study design. Fifty-two feldspathic porcelain cylinders of the VITA VM13 system, (Wilcos do Brasil, Petrópolis/RJ, Brazil), 2.2 mm high and 10.4 mm wide, with glazed surfaces, were used in this study (Fig 1A).

The ceramic cylinders were inserted into PVC tubes filled with self-curing acrylic resin. During embedment, the ceramic samples were pressed against a wax sheet so that they remained stationary. Subsequently, the PVC tubes were placed near the ceramic disks, taking care to ensure that the samples remained centered. Finally, self-curing acrylic resin was poured into the tubes. Samples were ready for the experiment immediately after the acrylic resin was polymerized (Fig 1B).

All samples were polished with a rubber cup and fluoride-free pumice for 10 seconds, sprayed with water, and then dried with compressed oil-free air stream. They were randomly divided into four groups (n = 13), each one containing the number of samples obtained by sample size calculation for mean differences (α = 5%, study power = 80%), using data provided by Wang et al.[12] Each experimental group underwent a different surface conditioning process (Table 1).

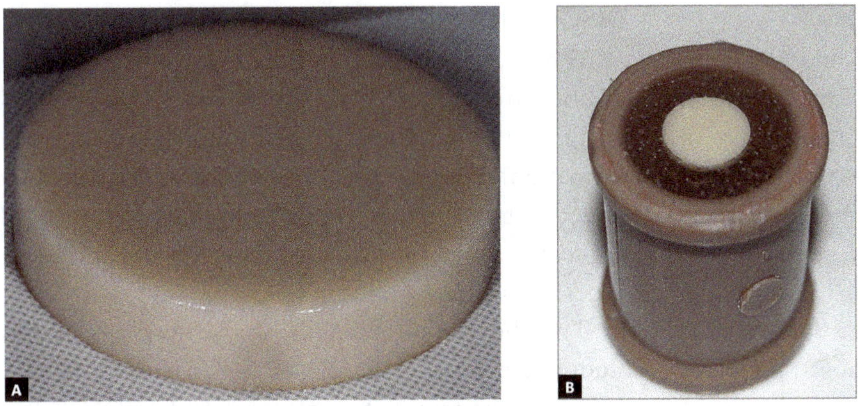

Figure 1 - A) Feldspathic ceramic cylinder; B) Sample ready for the experiment.

Table 1 - Experimental group distribution according to each surface conditioning method.

Group	Surface conditioning method
G1	37% gel phosphoric acid etching for one minute (FGM, SC, Brazil), followed by water rinsing for another minute and air drying procedure. Silane application for one minute (Dentsply, Petrópolis, RJ, Brazil).
G2	37% liquid phosphoric acid etching for one minute (Reliance, Itasca, IL, USA), removal of excess acid with gentle air drying, followed by silane application for another minute (Dentsply, Petrópolis, RJ, Brazil). Surface was thoroughly washed and dried (Swartz,[18] 2003).
G3	10% hydrofluoric acid etching for one minute (FGM, Joinville, SC, Brazil), followed by thorough washing and drying of surface.
G4	10% hydrofluoric acid etching for one minute (FGM, Joinville, SC, Brazil), followed by washing and drying of surface and application of silane for one minute (Dentsply, Petrópolis, RJ, Brazil).

The adhesive system used in this study was Transbond XT Light Cure Orthodontic Adhesive (3M Unitek, Monrovia, California, USA). After concluding the process of surface conditioning for each sample, adhesive was applied to the entire orthodontic bracket base. Standard Edgewise metal brackets for maxillary central incisors, with 80-micron mesh base (Morelli, Sorocaba/SP, Brazil), were chosen because their flat base allowed stable positioning on the samples. Each bracket was bonded to the center of the sample by means of applying a pressure of 260 gf. After bracket bonding, the adhesive was light-cured for 40 seconds (10 seconds on each bracket edge) using a calibrated LED Orthodontic Light activating device (Foshan Yunsheng Medical Instrument, Guangdong, China).

Each sample was submitted to shear bond strength test performed by a universal testing machine (EMIC DL2000, São José dos Pinhais, Brazil) at a speed of 0.5 mm/sec. The force per unit of area required to debond brackets was converted into megapascal (MPa) and named "shear bond strength." After debonding, the adhesive remnant index (ARI) was assessed under 10 x magnification (binocular optical microscope Nikon Eclipse E600, Nikon Corporation, Tokyo, Japan). Scores ranged from 0 to 3: 0 = absence of adhesive remnants; 1 = less than half of adhesive remnants; 2 = more than half of adhesive remnants; 3 = all adhesive remnants attached to the sample.[19]

A similar method was used to assess the damage caused to the ceramic surface. To this end, ceramic surface damage index (CSDI) was formulated, in which: 0 = no damage to the surface; 1 = absence of glaze on ceramic surface; 2 = presence of glaze and crack on ceramic surface; 3 = absence of glaze and presence of crack on ceramic surface; 4 = fractured ceramic surface.

Statistical analyses were performed by means of SPSS version 16 (SPSS Inc., Chicago, Illinois, USA). Data were displayed in tables and submitted to descriptive analysis. Variables were checked for normality and homogeneity by means of Shapiro-Wilk and Levene tests, respectively; with significance level set at 0.05. Once normal and homogenous distribution of variables was established, analysis of variance (ANOVA) was performed to establish the difference between groups, followed by Tukey's multiple comparisons test.

RESULTS

Table 2 displays descriptive analysis and ANOVA/ Tukey tests results for the differences found in mean bond strength values. The ARI values are displayed in Table 3, whereas CSDI results are shown in Table 4.

Groups G3 and G4, etched with hydrofluoric acid, yielded the highest shear bond strength values. The lowest values were found in G2 in which etching was performed with liquid phosphoric acid and subsequent silane application without previously rinsing the acid.

The group in which the porcelain surface was found to be best preserved was G2 which presented no fractures.

DISCUSSION

When orthodontic brackets are bonded to the enamel surface, bonding relies on adhesive penetration into the previously etched tooth surface and on formation of resin tags. In material with artificially glazed surfaces, such as porcelain, there is no such tag formation;[20] for this reason, it demands different types of surface conditioning.

The shear bond strength results obtained in this study were 22.83 MPa, 22.02 MPa, 16.42 MPa and 9.29 MPa, pertaining to surfaces etched with 10% hydrofluoric acid and subsequent silane application (G4), 10% hydrofluoric acid alone (G3), 37% gel phosphoric acid and subsequent silane application (G1), and 37%

Table 2 - Shear bond strength values.

Groups	Mean bond strength (MPa)	Standard deviation	Maximum value	Minimum value	Statistical difference*
G1	16.42	3.61	22.49	9.43	a
G2	9.29	1.95	13.99	7.21	b
G3	22.01	2.15	26.62	17.98	c
G4	22.83	3.32	27.66	16.51	c

*Different letters suggest statistically significant differences as regards ANOVA/Tukey tests with significance level set at 0.05.

Table 3 - ARI and fracture distribution per group.

	ARI				
	0 With ceramic fracture	0 Without ceramic fracture	1	2	3
G1 - n (%)	5 (38.46%)	5 (38.46%)	3 (23.07%)	0 (0%)	0 (0%)
G2 - n (%)	0 (0%)	9 (81.81%)	2 (18.18%)	0 (0%)	0 (0%)
G3 - n (%)	2 (16.66%)	6 (50%)	2 (16.66%)	0 (0%)	2 (16.66%)
G4 - n (%)	5 (38.46%)	2 (15.38%)	1 (7,.69%)	0 (0%)	5 (38.46%)

Table 4 - Ceramic surface damage index (CSDI).

	Ceramic surface damage index				
	0 = none	1 = absence of glaze	2 = presence of glaze and crack	3 = absence of glaze and presence of crack	4 = fracture
G1 - n (%)	3 (23.07%)	1 (7,69%)	4 (30.76%)	0 (0%)	5 (38.46%)
G2 - n (%)	6 (54.54%)	0 (0%)	5 (45.45%)	0 (0%)	0 (0%)
G3 - n (%)	1 (8.33%)	0 (0%)	0 (0%)	9 (75%)	2 (16.66%)
G4 - n (%)	5 (38.46%)	0 (0%)	0 (0%)	3 (23.07)	5 (38.46%)

liquid phosphoric acid and subsequent silane application without previously rinsing the acid (G2), respectively. As regards hydrofluoric acid etching, silane application was found to be unnecessary for direct bonding, which corroborates previous findings,[6,21] since similar shear bond strength results were found.

When hydrofluoric acid was compared with phosphoric acid, higher shear bond strength values were found for the former, as previously observed.[11,12,16] In spite of lower shear bond strength results being shown for phosphoric acid in comparison to hydrofluoric acid, the results proved to be clinically acceptable, and within the range of 6 to 8 Mpa established by Reynolds.[22] It has been previously reported that phosphoric acid etching with subsequent silane application yields satisfactory clinical results in ceramic surface conditioning.[11,12,18,23,24,25] According to Swartz,[18] the use of liquid phosphoric acid and subsequent silane application without previously rinsing the acid causes acid and silane to interact on the ceramic surface. Thus, liquid acid must be used because if a gel etchant is applied, silane will be unable to reach the ceramic surface and react with it.

Phosphoric acid may be an alternative to hydrofluoric acid, since the latter is highly toxic and corrosive.[11] Etching with 37% phosphoric acid for one minute will not scratch the porcelain, it will only clean the surface; and when used in association with silane, it reaches acceptable bond strength levels.[8,11,12,16,23-26] Considering that phosphoric acid is routinely used in dental practice and knowing that its use in association with silane yields acceptable bond strength results for bracket bonding, this acid could be the first choice of material to be used for this procedure.[26]

ARI evaluation showed evidence of a marked concentration of samples that scored 0, with or without associated ceramic fracture; that is, a trend towards complete removal of adhesive together with the bracket under shear stress. Score 3 is considered the safest, in which adhesive remains completely attached to the sample after bracket debonding. Rotating burs are required to remove adhesive present after debonding, which should be done carefully in order to prevent removal of the glaze layer responsible for maintaining porcelain integrity and isolating cracks and porosities. It is imperative to maintain the material surface integrity; therefore, roughness should be avoided.[24]

CSDI showed that the least damage was observed in G2, as suggested by Swartz.[18] Conversely, G4 was ranked highest in terms of percentage of fractured samples, supporting previous findings that claim more ceramic damage when hydrofluoric acid and silane are used in association.[11,13,27,28,29] In spite of that, other authors have stated that surface etching with 10% hydrofluoric acid for 60 seconds and subsequent silane application represents no risk to the ceramic structure.[12]

When shear bond strength, ARI and CSDI values were analytically compared, the following was noted: G1 showed intermediate bond strength values meeting clinical requirements, absence of adhesive remnants on most of the sample surface, and moderate (presence of glaze and cracks on the surface) to slight (absence of glaze) damage to the ceramic surface; G2 showed the lowest shear bond strength values, although it also achieved minimal clinical requirements, the highest rate of surface preservation with 54.54% of samples left intact and 45.45% with only slight damage (presence of glaze and crack), and none of the samples fractured despite the high concentration of samples with score 0 in ARI; G3 showed good shear bond strength values, but with a high rate of surface damage, with 16.66% of samples presenting fractures, and 75% of them presenting cracks and lack of glaze; G4 also showed high bond strength values, but similarly to G3, there were high levels of surface fracture (38.46%) and lack of glaze and cracking in 27.07% of cases.

Whenever preparing porcelain surfaces for bracket bonding, one should take all aforementioned characteristics into account. Thus, liquid phosphoric acid with subsequent silane application without previously rinsing the acid (G2), as described by Swartz,[18] seems to have yielded the best combination of results in terms of ARI, CSDI and shear bond strength values. This method was initially described over 10 years ago, but has not been widely used in *in vitro* studies or in the orthodontic practice.

One of the limitations of the present study is related to sample storage. The high shear bond strength results and surface damage may be related to lack of thermal cycling which, according to the literature, can increase shear bond strength and ceramic damage.[14,30] Future research should perform thermal cycling of samples before shear bond strength testing.

The results of this research should be considered for clinical application with caution, as it is a laboratory study. Clinical tests are also rendered necessary.

CONCLUSIONS

The highest shear bond strength values were obtained when hydrofluoric acid was used, with or without subsequent silane application (G3 and G4); whereas the lowest values were found when surfaces were etched with liquid phosphoric acid with subsequent drying and silane application (G2). However, all surface conditioning methods seem to result in acceptable bond strength levels.

Liquid phosphoric acid and subsequent silane application (G2) caused the least damage to the ceramic surface. As regards hydrofluoric acid etching, subsequent silane application seemed to have increased the risk of ceramic surface fracture.

REFERENCES

1. A critique of bond strength testing in orthodontics. Br J Orthod. 1994;21(1):33-43.
2. Winchester L. Direct orthodontic bonding to porcelain: an in vitro study. Br J Orthod. 1991;18(4):299-308.
3. Akova T, Yoldas O, Toroglu MS, Uysal H. Porcelain surface treatment by laser for bracket-porcelain bonding. Am J Orthod Dentofacial Orthop. 2005;128(5):630-7.
4. Türk T, Saraç D, Saraç YS, Elekdağ-Türk S. Effects of surface conditioning on bond strength of metal brackets to all-ceramic surfaces. Eur J Orthod. 2006;28(5):450-6.
5. Leinfelder KF. Porcelain esthetics for the 21st century. J Am Dent Assoc. 2000;131 Suppl:47S-51S.
6. Schmage P, Nergiz I, Herrmann W, Ozcan M. Influence of various surface-conditioning methods on the bond strength of metal brackets to ceramic surfaces. Am J Orthod Dentofacial Orthop. 2003;123(5):540-6.
7. Matinlinna JP, Lassila LV, Ozcan M, Yli-Urpo A, Vallittu PK. An introduction to silanes and their clinical applications in dentistry. Int J Prosthodont. 2004;17(2):155-64.
8. Ajlouni R, Bishara SE, Oonsombat C, Soliman M, Laffoon J. The effect of porcelain surface conditioning on bonding orthodontic brackets. Angle Orthod. 2005;75(5):858-64.
9. Goyal S. Silanes: Chemistry and applications. J Indian Prosthodont Soc. 2006;6:14-8.
10. Gillis I, Redlich M. The effect of different porcelain conditioning techniques on shear bond strength of stainless steel brackets. Am J Orthod Dentofacial Orthop. 1998;114(4):387-92.
11. Bourke BM, Rock WP. Factors affecting the shear bond strength of orthodontic brackets to porcelain. Br J Orthod. 1999;26(4):285-90.
12. Wang H, Xiong F, Zhenhua L. Influence of varied surface texture of dentin porcelain on optical properties of porcelain specimens. J Prosthet Dent. 2011;105(4):242-8.
13. Chung CH, Brendlinger EJ, Brendlinger DL, Bernal V, Mante FK. Shear bond strengths of two resin-modified glass ionomer cements to porcelain. Am J Orthod Dentofacial Orthop. 1999;115(5):533-5.
14. Huang TH, Kao CT. The shear bond strength of composite brackets on porcelain teeth. Eur J Orthod. 2001;23(4):433-9.
15. Harari D, Shapira-Davis S, Gillis I, Roman I, Redlich M. Tensile bond strength of ceramic brackets bonded to porcelain facets. Am J Orthod Dentofacial Orthop. 2003;123(5):551-4.
16. Larmour CJ, Bateman G, Stirrups DR. An investigation into the bonding of orthodontic attachments to porcelain. Eur J Orthod. 2006;28(1):74-7.
17. Imakami MB, Valle-Corotti KM, Carvalho PEG, Scocate ACRN. Evaluation of shear strength of lingual brackets bonded to ceramic surfaces. Dental Press J Orthod. 2011;16(3):87-94.
18. Swartz ML. Reliable porcelain bonding. Clin Impress. 2003;12(2):22-3.
19. Artun J, Bergland S. Clinical trials with crystal growth conditioning as an alternative to acid-etch enamel pretreatment. Am J Orthod. 1984;85(4):333-40.
20. Smith GA, McInnes-Ledoux P, Ledoux WR, Weinberg R. Orthodontic bonding to porcelain: bond strength and refinishing. Am J Orthod Dentofacial Orthop. 1988;94(3):245-52.
21. Zachrisson BU. Orthodontic bonding to artificial tooth surfaces: clinical versus laboratory findings. Am J Orthod Dentofacial Orthop. 2000;117(5):592-4.
22. Reynolds IR. A review of direct orthodontic bonding. Br J Orthod. 1975;2(3):171-8.
23. Whitlock BO 3rd, Eick JD, Ackerman RJ Jr, Glaros AG, Chappell RP. Shear strength of ceramic brackets bonded to porcelain. Am J Orthod Dentofacial Orthop. 1994;106(4):358-64.
24. Nebbe B, Stein E. Orthodontic brackets bonded to glazed and deglazed porcelain surfaces. Am J Orthod Dentofacial Orthop. 1996;109(4):431-6.
25. Pannes DD, Bailey DK, Thompson JY, Pietz DM. Orthodontic bonding to porcelain: a comparison of bonding systems. J Prosthet Dent. 2003;89(1):66-9.
26. Aboush YE. Removing saliva contamination from porcelain veneers before bonding. J Prosthet Dent. 1998;80(6):649-53.
27. Cochran D, O'Keefe KL, Turner DT, Powers JM. Bond strength of orthodontic composite cement to treated porcelain. Am J Orthod Dentofacial Orthop. 1997;111(3):297-300.
28. Falkensammer F, Freudenthaler J, Pseiner B, Bantleon HP. Influence of surface conditioning on ceramic microstructure and bracket adhesion. Eur J Orthod. 2012;34(4):498-504.
29. Ramos TF, Lenza MA, Reges RR, Freitas G. Influence of ceramic surface treatment on shear bond strength of ceramic brackets. Indian J Dent Res. 2012;23(6):789-94.
30. Zachrisson YO, Zachrisson BU, Büyükyilmaz T. Surface preparation for orthodontic bonding to porcelain. Am J Orthod Dentofacial Orthop. 1996;109(4):420-30.

31

Comparative study on direct and indirect bracket bonding techniques regarding time length and bracket detachment

Jefferson Vinicius Bozelli[1], Renato Bigliazzi[1], Helga Adachi Medeiros Barbosa[2], Cristina Lucia Feijo Ortolani[3], Francisco Antonio Bertoz[4], Kurt Faltin Junior[3]

Objective: The aim of this study was to assess the time spent for direct (DBB - direct bracket bonding) and indirect (IBB - indirect bracket bonding) bracket bonding techniques. The time length of laboratorial (IBB) and clinical steps (DBB and IBB) as well as the prevalence of loose bracket after a 24-week follow-up were evaluated. **Methods:** Seventeen patients (7 men and 10 women) with a mean age of 21 years, requiring orthodontic treatment were selected for this study. A total of 304 brackets were used (151 DBB and 153 IBB). The same bracket type and bonding material were used in both groups. Data were submitted to statistical analysis by Wilcoxon non-parametric test at 5% level of significance. **Results:** Considering the total time length, the IBB technique was more time-consuming than the DBB ($p < 0.001$). However, considering only the clinical phase, the IBB took less time than the DBB ($p < 0.001$). There was no significant difference ($p = 0.910$) for the time spent during laboratorial positioning of the brackets and clinical session for IBB in comparison to the clinical procedure for DBB. Additionally, no difference was found as for the prevalence of loose bracket between both groups. **Conclusion:** the IBB can be suggested as a valid clinical procedure since the clinical session was faster and the total time spent for laboratorial positioning of the brackets and clinical procedure was similar to that of DBB. In addition, both approaches resulted in similar frequency of loose bracket.

Keywords: Corrective orthodontics. Orthodontic brackets. Dental bonding. Dental detachment.

[1] Associate Professor, Department of Orthodontics, Paulista University (UNIP).
[2] MSc in Orthodontics, UNIP.
[3] Full professor, Department of Orthodontics Paulista University (UNIP).
[4] Full professor, Department of Orthodontics, State University of São Paulo (UNESP).

» The authors report no commercial, proprietary or financial interest in the products or companies described in this article.

Renato Bigliazzi
Faculdade de Odontologia de Araçatuba
Rua José Bonifácio, 1193 – Araçatuba/SP – CEP: 16.015-050
E-mail: bigliazzir@hotmail.com

INTRODUCTION

Bonding accessories on tooth surface revolutionized Orthodontics,making the clinical results easier and more reliable. It solved some of the difficulties encountered in orthodontic banding procedures; such as professional skills, patient's discomfort resulting from separators and banding, risk to periodontal diseases and cavities, better esthetic acceptance, material cost and the time spent to make and insert the bands.[1,2,3] Thus, directly bonding accessories on the enamel became the most common technique used by orthodontists considering that effective bracket bonding is essential for appropriate orthodontic mechanics. This approach also reduces treatment length and avoids rebonding caused by inappropriate positioning and/or loose bracket.[4] On the other hand, precise bracket bonding relies on the professional's experience and accuracy of bonding procedures.

Aiming at improving precision and attaining excellence in orthodontic procedures, Silverman et al[5] developed the indirect bracket bonding (IBB) technique. In this approach, the brackets are previously positioned on casts with water-soluble or intermediary adhesives, and then transferred to the mouth by means of an individual tray. For these authors, the direct bracket bonding (DBB) technique is time-consuming and the correct positioning of the brackets is difficult to achieve clinically.

Thus, the aim of this *in vivo* study was to compare the direct and indirect (tray transferred with fusible glue[6]) bracket bonding techniques regarding the time spent for laboratorial (IBB) and clinical (IBB and DBB) steps and its correlation for the IBB as well as the prevalence of loose bracket.

MATERIAL AND METHODS

Patient selection and study design

Seventeen patients (7 men and 10 women) with a mean age of 21 years, who required orthodontic treatment, were selected for the present prospective study conducted at the college of Dentistry of Paulista University - UNIP/SP from March to June, 2008. Treatment lasted for 2 years. Each subject signed a written informed consent before entering the cohort which was approved by the Paulista University-UNIP/SP Institutional Review board (number 122/05 CEP/ICS/UNIP).

Upper and lower dental casts of each patient were obtained after impression with irreversible hydrocolloid (Jeltrate, Dentsply, Brazil) manipulated according to the manufacturer's instructions. The impressions were rinsed with water for 1 minute, air-dried and then poured with dental stone (Dentsply, Brazil). After stone crystallization (40 minutes), the casts were removed from the impression trays and trimmed. The IBB technique requires working casts with minor irregularities.

Laboratorial step – Fabrication of transferring trays

All laboratorial procedures were conducted by the same operator according to an accurate methodology. Table 1 presents all the acronyms used in this study for laboratorial and clinical steps timings.

The tooth long axis and the gingival-occlusal height of the brackets tubes were determined manually in all patients for correct bracket positioning. The time spent during this procedure was measured by the software Palmaryclock® v. 23 (Palmarysoft 2002-2004) downloaded into Palm Tungsten T device (Palm® - Brazil) and recorded (TL1 – Time spent to determine the height and tooth long axis in the maxilla and mandible during laboratorial step).

The study by Aguirre et al[7] was used as reference to determine the protocol for the IBB technique conducted in the present study. The arches were divided into two sections: upper and lower right side (DBB) and upper and lower left side (IBB), and these sides were chosen based on the fact that they enabled direct visualization of bracket bonding, since a right-handed operator conducted the research by himself. The bonding procedure was initiated at the left central incisor and finished at the left second premolar in both the maxilla and mandible. Water-soluble glue was used and any excess material draining from the brackets base was removed. The Morelli® (0.018 x 0.030-in, Bioprogressive technique) metallic brackets were selected for treating all patients.

The time spent for bonding the brackets on the working casts was also measured and recorded (TL2, time spent for bonding the brackets in maxillary and mandibular casts). However, the time spent for clinical bonding was measured for each tooth individually and then summed up to obtain the total time for

Table 1 - Acronyms used for different laboratorial and clinical time

TL1	Time spent to determine the height and tooth long axis during laboratorial step in maxilla and mandible
TL2	Time spent for bracket bonding in the cast in maxilla and mandible
TL3	Time spent for fabrication of transferring trays in maxilla and mandible
TLt	Total laboratorial time in maxilla and mandible
TCI1	Time spent with IBB during clinical step in maxilla and mandible
TCI2	Time spent for removal and cleaning of the IBB area in maxilla and mandible
TCIt	Total clinical time for IBB in maxilla and mandible
TCD1	Time spent with DBB in maxilla and mandible
TCD2	Time spent for cleaning of the DBB area in maxilla and mandible
TCDt	Total time for DBB in maxilla and mandible
TPBt	Time spent for laboratorial positioning of the brackets

bonding performed in each hemi-arch. To make the transferring tray (Figs 1 and 2),hot melt adhesive (slightly fluid) was applied to each bracket and to the vestibular surface of each tooth, following the same bonding sequence for the model, in other words, the bonding started from tooth #21 to #25, then from #31 up to #35. After that, additional glue was inserted on the incisal and occlusal surfaces of the teeth in order to make a less flexible and harder tray. The time spent for making the transferring trays was also measured and recorded (TL3, time spent for fabrication of the upper and lower transferring trays).

After solidification of the silicone glue (hot melt glue), the casts were hydrated for 1 minute so that the glue could be dissolved and, then, the brackets were transferred with the transferring trays, concluding the laboratorial step of the IBB approach. The total laboratorial time included the time spent for bracket bonding and fabrication/cleaning of the transferring trays (TLt – total laboratorial time for maxilla and mandible), which means that TLt=TL1+TL2+TL3.

Clinical step

The IBB technique was conducted at the upper and lower left side while the right side was selected for the DBB technique (Fig 3). The procedure was timed after prophylaxis (pumice and rubber tip) and enamel etching performed with 37% of phosphoric acid (RMO) following the manufacturer's instructions since the time spent for this initial step was similar for both techniques. The self-curing resin (paste + liquid – No Mix) Mono Lock 2 (RMO®) was selected for bonding.

For IBB, the etched teeth and transferring trays were dried in order to maintain the chemical and physical properties of the adhesive system. Then, the activator of the bonding material (liquid) was applied on the enamel and brackets mesh positioned into the transferring tray. After that, resin (paste) was inserted on the brackets mesh that was positioned at the hemiarch of the patient.

The whole process from application of the activator (liquid) on enamel to positioning of the transferring tray

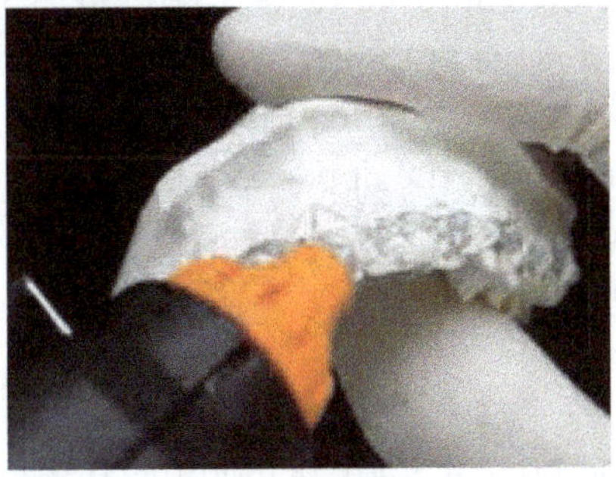

Figure 1 - Fabrication of the transferring tray.

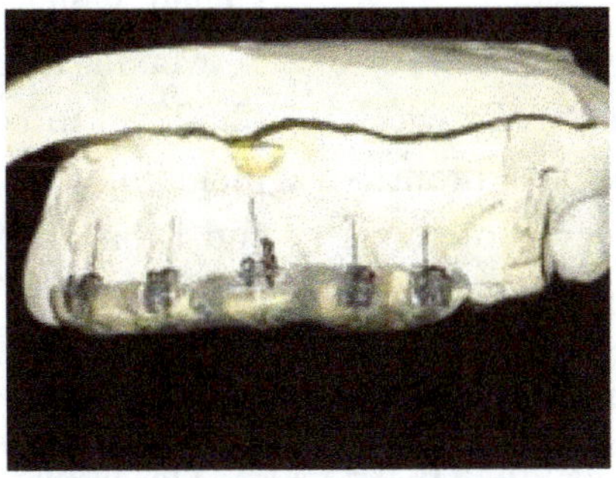

Figure 2 - Transferring trays with ideal dimension and thickness.

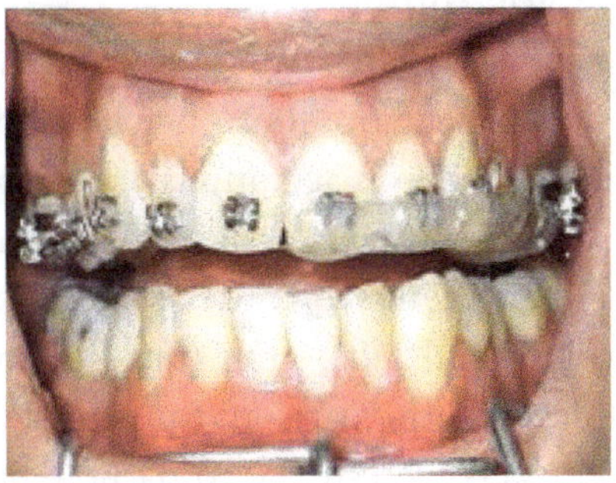

Figure 3 - Example of brackets bonded by means of DBB and IBB techniques in the maxilla

was timed and recorded (TCI1 – time spent for clinical session of IBB technique in maxilla and mandible).

The DBB approach was conducted in sequence, from the right central incisor to the right second premolar in both jaws. The whole process of the direct technique was timed (TCD1 – time spent with the DBB technique in maxilla and mandible). The bonding steps were similar to those of the IBB approach: Drying of the etched teeth, application of activator on enamel and bracket mesh, insertion of resin on brackets mesh, and positioning it on the teeth. The positioning respected the height of each tooth (Boone bracket positioning gauge).

After DBB, the removal and cleaning of the IBB area was conducted. The transferring tray and the excess resin were removed using the tip of the rubber band insertion tool and a bur for enamel (3M Unitek – California), respectively. This step was also timed and recorded (TCI2 – time spent for removal and cleaning of the IBB area in maxilla and mandible).

The total clinical time for the IBB approach was represented by the time spent for IBB and cleaning step (TCIt – total clinical time spent for IBB technique in maxilla and mandible), which means TCIt = TCI1+TCI2.

The cleaning of the DBB area was also conducted using a bur to remove excess resin on the enamel surface (3M Unitek – California). This process was also timed and recorded (TCD2 – time spent for cleaning of the DBB area in maxilla and mandible).

The total clinical time for the DBB approach was represented by the time spent for DBB (tooth by tooth) and cleaning step (TCDt – total clinical time spent for DBB technique in maxilla and mandible), which means TCDt = TCD1+TCD2.

After the clinical step, the patient was submitted to correction of dental positioning through orthodontic mechanics.

Follow-up

The patients were evaluated every 4 weeks in order to have the loose brackets assessed. A 24-week follow-up was accomplished, representing 6 monthly appointments. All detachments were noted on each patient's record taking into account the side (right and left), arch (maxilla and mandible), date (day/month/year), and position (tooth). The loose brackets were replaced by new brackets bonded according to the DBB technique.

Statistical analysis

The Wilcoxon non-parametric test was applied for comparison between the periods, since assumption of data normality was rejected. A significance level of 5% was used in all tests.

RESULTS

Based on the statistical analysis carried out, the following results were obtained.

Evaluation of time spent for bracket bonding with DBB and IBB techniques

Considering the total time spent with IBB (TLt+TCIt) and DBB (TCDt) in both jaws, the Wilcoxon test revealed significant difference ($p < 0.001$) between the groups, which means that IBB was more time-consuming than DBB (Table 2 and Fig 4). However, when only the clinical step was considered, a statistically significant difference ($p < 0.001$) was also observed, but IBB (TCIt) was less time-consuming than DBB (TCDt) (Table 3 and Fig 5).

There was no significant difference ($p = 0.910$) for the time spent during laboratorial positioning of the brackets (TPBt = TL1+TL2) and clinical step with IBB (TCIt) in comparison to the clinical time with DBB (TCDt) (Table 4 and Fig 6).

Total number of brackets detached with IBB and DBB techniques

After bracket bonding performed with IBB and DBB approaches in both jaws, a 24-week follow-up was conducted for all patients in order to check potential loose bracket. A total of 304 brackets were inserted, including 151 brackets with DBB technique (70 brackets in maxilla and 81 in mandible) and 153 brackets with IBB (72 brackets in maxilla and 81 in mandible). At the end, a total of 18 brackets were detached, which represents 5.92% (Table 5 and Fig 7).

Maxilla exhibited a lower number of loose brackets (22.22%) in comparison to the mandible (77.78%), including 4 detachments in the upper arch (3 for IBB and 1 for DBB) and 14 occurrences in the lower arch (8 for IBB and 6 for DBB).

DISCUSSION

The results of the present study demonstrated that the total time spent with the IBB technique (laboratorial

Table 2 - Total time spent with IBB (TLt+TClt) and DBB (TCDt), in both arches.

Time	n	Mean ± SD	Minimum	Maximum	Median
IBB (TLt+TClt)	17	1167,20 ± 239,39	961	1913	1092,00
DBB (TCDt)	17	892,73 ± 116,21	646	1057	914,00

Time in seconds.

Table 3 - Total time spent with IBB (TLt+TClt) and DBB (TCDt) in both arches, for clinical steps.

Time	n	Mean ± SD	Minimum	Maximum	Median
IBB (TClt)	17	380,13 ± 47,59	315	489	376,00
DBB (TCDt)	17	892,73 ± 116,21	646	1057	914,00

Time in seconds.

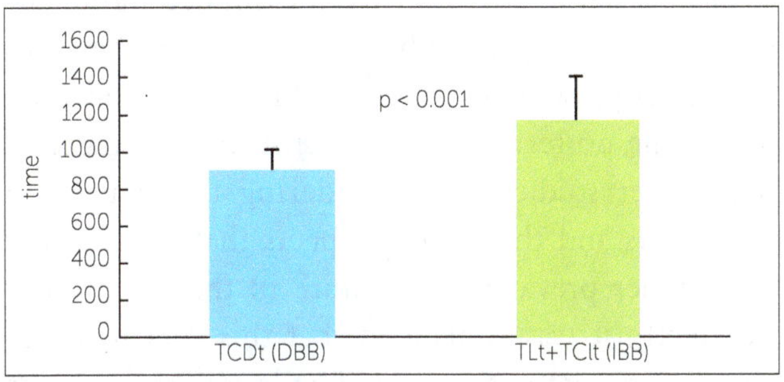

Figure 4 - Comparison of the time spent with IBB (TLt+TClt) and DBB (TCDt) in the maxilla and the mandible.

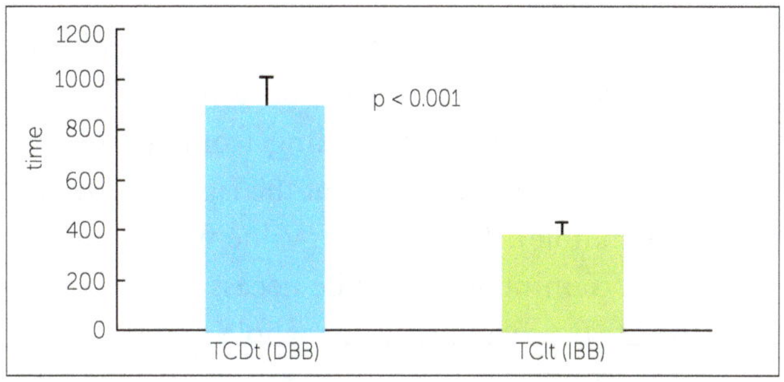

Figure 5 - Comparison of the time spent with IBB (TClt) and DBB (TCDt) in the maxilla and the mandible during clinical step.

Table 4 - Total time spent for laboratorial and clinical steps with IBB (TPBt+TClt) and DBB (TCDt).

Time	n	Mean ± SD	Minimum	Maximum	Median
IBB (TPBt+TClt)	17	885,87 ± 149,31	720	1296	842,00
DBB (TCDt)	17	892,73 ± 116,21	646	1057	914,00

Time in seconds

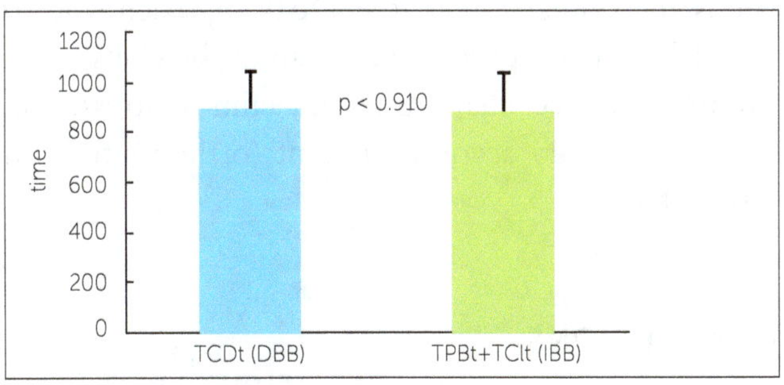

Figure 6 - Comparison of the time spent during laboratorial and clinical steps with IBB (TPBt+TClt) and DBB (TCDt).

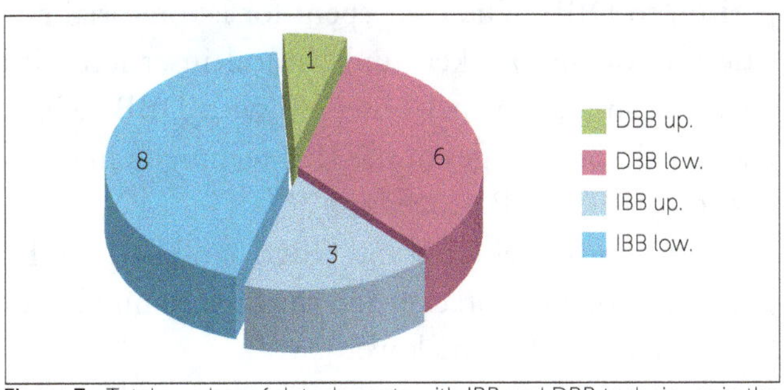

Figure 7 - Total number of detachments with IBB and DBB techniques in the maxilla and the mandible.

Table 5 - Distribution of the total number of loose brackets in maxilla and mandible regarding time and teeth.

		Months						
Technique	tooth	1	2	3	4	5	6	Detachment
IBB	25							0
	24					1		1
	23					1		1
	22							0
	21			1				1
DBB	11							0
	12					1		1
	13							0
	14							0
	15							0
IBB	35	1						1
	34	1						1
	33	2						2
	32	1						1
	31	2	1					3
DBB	41				1			1
	42			1				1
	43	2						2
	44							0
	45				1		1	2
Detach.		9	1	2	2	3	1	18

and clinical steps) was significantly longer than that with the DBB approach, which is in agreement with other authors[3,6-9]. The mean total time for IBB (TLt+TCIt) was 1167.20 seconds, nearly 19.46 minutes to conclude the process from the central incisor to the second premolar at the left side (maxilla and mandible). If this value were doubled, a total of 38.92 minutes would be spent to complete de IBB procedure in the whole mouth.

As for the DBB technique, a mean time of 892.73 seconds was used to complete the process (TCDt), nearly 14.88 minutes for bonding from the central incisor to the second premolar at the right side (maxilla and mandible). Again, if this value were double, a total of 29.76 minutes would be necessary to accomplish the DBB procedure in the whole mouth.

Thus, the time spent with both IBB and DBB techniques in the present study was shorter than that reported by other researches.[7,9] In this sense, the IBB procedure can be considered faster due to being considered as an easy technique, demanding fewer laboratorial steps and being clinically applied with ease.

With regard to the clinical phase, the present study revealed that the IBB technique was significantly less time-consuming than the DBB.[8-11] A mean of 380.13 seconds was necessary to complete the clinical procedure with the IBB (TCIt), representing about 6.33 minutes. Thus, based on the same analogy described previously, the procedure would be completed in 12.68 minutes for the whole mouth. Considering that the total time (laboratorial and clinical steps) for both jaws (maxilla and mandible) was 38.92 minutes, the laboratorial phase represents 67.50% of the IBB technique. However, trained assistants could carry out some of these procedures (fabrication and cleaning of the transferring tray), reducing the difference between IBB and DBB approaches.[11]

As for DBB, the mean total time in both jaws was 29.76 minutes, longer than time used to perform the clinical step with IBB (12.68 minutes). Thus, the IBB is advantageous in comparison to the DBB since it reduces chair-time for bracket bonding, minimizes clinical stress and increases patient's comfort.[11]

It is important to highlight that the time spent to make the working casts was not considered since it can be obtained at the same session in which diagnostic casts are made or even at a dental radiology center. However, the other laboratorial steps could not be disregarded.

As for loose brackets, the results demonstrated a value of 5.92% during a 24-week follow-up, which was similar to previous studies.[7,9,12-13] It has been suggested that there is no statistically significant difference between the IBB and DBB techniques regarding the retention of brackets bonded to human enamel.[14,15,16]

In this sense, the lower teeth exhibited more failures than the upper teeth.[7,17,18,19] However, the anterior teeth presented more detachments in comparison to the posterior teeth, which is in disagreement with other studies.[17-20] Considering the analysis of the results and the clinical aspects that could result in a higher prevalence of failure in the lower anterior teeth, it was concluded that this data was specific for the present sample. The loose brackets may have been caused by failure during initial impression or positioning (DBB), failure during laboratorial step (IBB), poor tooth polishing, failure during acid etching, poor control of humidity, several contaminations (saliva and blood), improper occlusion (contact with orthodontic accessories), repeated trauma (hard food), and enamel quality.[21]

Considering the literature and the present results, it was observed that the IBB technique is advantageous in comparison to the DBB approach due to easy laboratorial procedure, accurate brackets positioning, reduced chair-time and clinical stress, and multidisciplinary accomplishment (orthodontist and assistants).

CONCLUSIONS

The total time spent with the DBB technique was shorter than that with the IBB approach. However, the clinical step took less time with IBB in comparison to DBB. The time spent for laboratorial positioning of the brackets and clinical insertion with IBB was similar to that observed with DBB, which justifies the advantages of the IBB technique in comparison to the DBB procedure.

Both approaches (IBB and DBB) exhibited similar prevalence of loose bracket and the highest number of failures occurred in the lower jaw.

REFERENCES

1. Reynolds IR. A review of direct orthodontic bonding. Br J Orthod. 1975;2(3):171-8.
2. Wertz RA. Beginning bonding – state of the art. Angle Orthod 1980;50(3):245-7.
3. Thomas RG. Indirect bonding: simplicity in action. J Clin Orthod. 1979;13(2):93-106.
4. Brandt S, Servoss JM, Wolfson J. Practical methods of bonding, direct and indirect. J Clin Orthod. 1975;9(10):610-35.
5. Silverman E, Cohen M, Gianelly A, Dietz V. A universal direct bonding system for both metal and plastic brackets. Am J Orthod Dentofacial Orthop. 1972;62(3):235-44.
6. White LW. A new and improved indirect bonding technique. J Clin Orthod. 1999;33(1):17-23.
7. Aguirre MJ, King GJ, Waldron JM. Assessment of bracket placement and bond strength when comparing direct bonding and indirect bonding techniques. Am J Orthod. 1982;82(4):269-76.
8. Fried KH, Newman GV. Indirect bonding with a no-mix adhesive. J Clin Orthod. 1983;17(6):414-7.
9. Scholz RP. Indirect bonding revisited. J Clin Orthod. 1983;17(8):529-36.
10. Reichheld S, Ritucci R, Gianelly A. An indirect bonding technique. J Clin Orthod. 1990;24(1):21-4.
11. Hickham JH. Predictable indirect bonding. J Clin Orthod. 1993;27(4):215-7.
12. Beech DR, Jalaly T. Clinical and laboratory evaluation of some orthodontic direct bonding systems. J Dent Res. 1981;60(6):972-7.
13. Miles PG, Weyant RJ. A comparison of two indirect bonding adhesives. Angle Orthod. 2005;75(6):1019-23.
14. Yi GK, Dunn WJ, Taloumis LJ. Shear bond strength comparison between direct and indirect bonded orthodontic brackets. Am J Orthod Dentofacial Orthop. 2003;124(5):577-81.
15. Thiyagarajah S, Spary DJ, Rock WP. A clinical comparison of bracket bond failures in association with direct and indirect bonding. J Orthod. 2006;33(3):198-204.
16. Deahl ST, Salome N, Hatch JP, Rugh JD. Practice-based comparison of direct and indirect bonding. Am J Orthod Dentofacial Orthop. 2007;132(6):738-42.
17. Knoll M, Gwinnet AJ, Wolff MS. Shear strength of brackets bonded to anterior and posterior teeth. Am J Orthod Dentofacial Orthop. 1986;89(6):476-9.
18. Sondhi A. Efficient and effective indirect bonding. Am J Orthod Dentofacial Orthop. 1999;115(4):352-9.
19. Linklater RA, Gordon PH. Bond failure patterns in vivo. Am J Orthod Dentofacial Orthop. 2003;123(4):534-9.
20. Langlade M. Terapêutica ortodôntica. 3ª ed. São Paulo: Ed. Santos; 1992.
21. Kinch AP, Taylor H, Warltier R, Oliver RG, Newcombe RG. A clinical trial comparing the failures rates of directly bonded brackets using etch times of 15 or 60 seconds. Am J Orthod Dentofacial Orthop. 1988;94(6):476-83.

Evaluation of the influence of dental bleaching with 35% hydrogen peroxide in orthodontic bracket shear bond strength

Marcus Vinicius Neiva Nunes do Rego[1], Roanselli Marllon Lima dos Santos[2], Leanne Matias Portela Leal[3], Carlos Gustavo Silva Braga[4]

Objective: The purpose of this study was to evaluate, *in vitro*, the bond strength of brackets bonded to premolars previously subjected to bleaching with a 35% hydrogen peroxide. **Methods:** Twenty one healthy premolars were selected and randomly divided into three groups (n = 7). Group I (G1) included teeth that were not submitted to bleaching. The enamel surfaces of Groups II (G2) and III (G3) were submitted to a bleaching process with 35% hydrogen peroxide (Whiteness HP Maxx). On Group II (G2), after bleaching, the teeth were stored for 24 hours in distilled water at 98.6 °F, and then, premolar metallic brackets were bonded using Transbond XT (3M) resin. Group III (G3) was submitted to the same procedure seven days after bleaching. After bonding, all teeth were stored in distilled water at 98.6 °F for 24 hours. All groups were submitted to a traction test using an EMIC DL2000 universal testing machine at a speed of 0.5 mm/min. **Results and Conclusion:** The bracket resistance to debonding was compared between the groups by the Kruskal-Wallis nonparametric test ($p < 0.05$) and it was verified that the bleaching agent significantly reduced bracket adhesion when bonded 24 hours after bleaching. However, seven days after bleaching, there was no significant difference on the resistance to debonding among groups G1 (19,52 kgf) and G3 (18,44 kgf), meaning that it is necessary to wait longer after bleaching to bond brackets.

Keywords: Orthodontic brackets. Dental bleaching. Tensile strength.

[1] Professor and Chairman, Specialization Course in Orthodontics, NOVAFAPI.
[2] Graduated in Dentistry, NOVAFAPI.
[3] Professor, Specialization Course in Orthodontics, NOVAFAPI.
[4] Specialist in Orthodontics, NOVAFAPI.

» The author reports no commercial, proprietary or financial interest in the products or companies described in this article.

Marcus Vinicius Neiva Nunes do Rego
Av. Lindolfo Monteiro, 1030, Bairro de Fátima, Teresina/PI – Brazil
CEP: 64.049-440 – E-mail: mrego@novafapi.com.br

INTRODUCTION

Based on the current beauty standards, where beautiful is to have white and aligned teeth, the search for esthetic treatment is the desire of most patients that seek for a dental treatment.[9]

Dental bleaching is the most popular esthetic treatment with the purpose of modifying tooth color. Among the bleaching agents, hydrogen peroxide is the most used for treating intrinsic staining of healthy teeth, presenting or not endodontic treatment. Hydrogen peroxide presents several concentrations and periods of application.[10,20]

There are evidences in the literature that the utilization of bleaching agents can interfere on the bond strength of orthodontic brackets. Prietsch[14] concluded that dental bleaching with a 35% hydrogen peroxide reduces bond strength after 24 hours, suggesting that a period of seven days should be waited after bleaching. On the other hand, Matta[11] concluded that the bleaching agent with a 10% carbamide peroxide increases significantly the mechanical bond strength of orthodontic brackets, and that the elapsed time from the end of the bleaching treatment to the bonding of the orthodontic brackets did not interfere on the mechanical bond strength when it was performed after 24 hours or one week.

However, according to Bishara et al,[3] bleaching with a 10% carbamide peroxide does not interfere on bond strength of dental enamel. Thus, despite researches reporting the effect of bleaching agents to the dental enamel, it is noticed that there is no consensus about the real interference on bond strength of orthodontic brackets.

Therefore, due to the increasing demand of adult patients for orthodontic treatment, associated to increasing care for dental esthetic, it is relevant to perform an evaluation of the influence of bleaching with a 35% hydrogen peroxide on the bond strength of orthodontic brackets.

MATERIAL AND METHODS

To perform the present study, twenty one healthy human teeth (premolars) were stored in distilled water at 98.6 °F for 24 hours. The teeth were, then, randomly divided into three groups (n=7), according to waiting period post-bleaching (24 hours and 7 days) (Table 1).

Table 1 - Description of the sample according to the procedures performed in each group.

Groups (n = 7)	Procedures	
	Bleaching	Bonding
G1	No	24 hours
G2	Yes	24 hours
G3	Yes	7 days

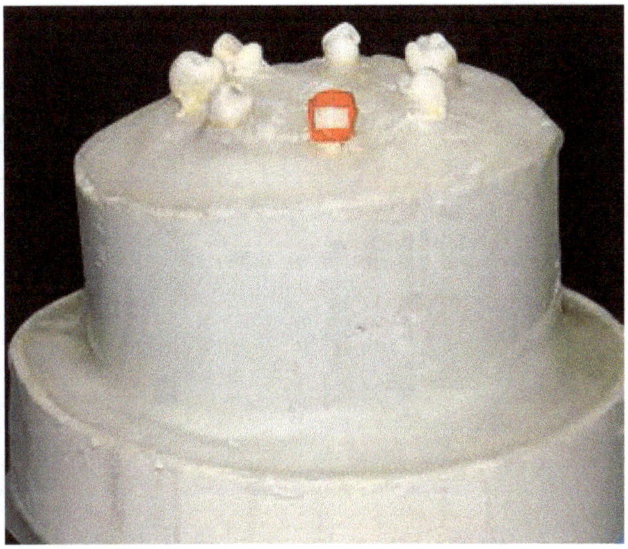

Figure 1 - Mounting the teeth with acrylic resin to the PVC bases.

Using self curing acrylic resin, each tooth was mounted in two PVC bases with different diameters, so that the buccal surface of each tooth formed a 90 degree angle with the acrylic base (Fig 1). This was necessary to standardize the traction tests in the universal testing machine.

Group I (G1) or Control group included the teeth that were not submitted to bleaching. For this group bracket bonding was performed according to the same protocol adopted for the experimental groups. The enamel surfaces of Group II (G2) and III (G3) were submitted to bleaching with 35% hydrogen peroxide (Whiteness HP Maxx). The bleaching agent was applied for three times and activated by an halogen light, according to instructions from the manufacturer.

For Group II (G2), after bleaching, the teeth were stored for 24 hours in distilled water at 98.6 °F, then, the area to be bonded to the bracket in each tooth was bounded by a mask made from adhesive tape[11] (Fig 2A). After setting the mask, a prophylaxis with rubber cup and pumice paste and water was performed during 10 second for each tooth (Fig 2B), rinsing and drying (Fig 2C), with subsequent etching with 37% phosphoric acid for 15 seconds (Fig 2D), followed by rinsing for 10 seconds and drying for 10 seconds[11] (Fig 2E). Metallic brackets (Abzil) for premolars were bonded using the same amount of Transbond XT (3M) resin light cured for 40 seconds. All accessories were bonded at the same cervical distance, using a Boone gauge (Morelli) with a 4.0 mm distance (Figs 2F to 2M).

Group III (G3) was also submitted to the same procedures above described, but in this group the bonding was performed seven days after bleaching. After bracket bonding, all teeth were stored in distilled water at 98.6 °F for 24 hours. Then, all groups were submitted to the traction test using an EMIC DL2000 universal testing machine at a speed of 0.5 mm/min.[5] In this test the resistance values were obtained in kgf (kilogram-force) and registered by a printer attached to the machine (Fig 3A).

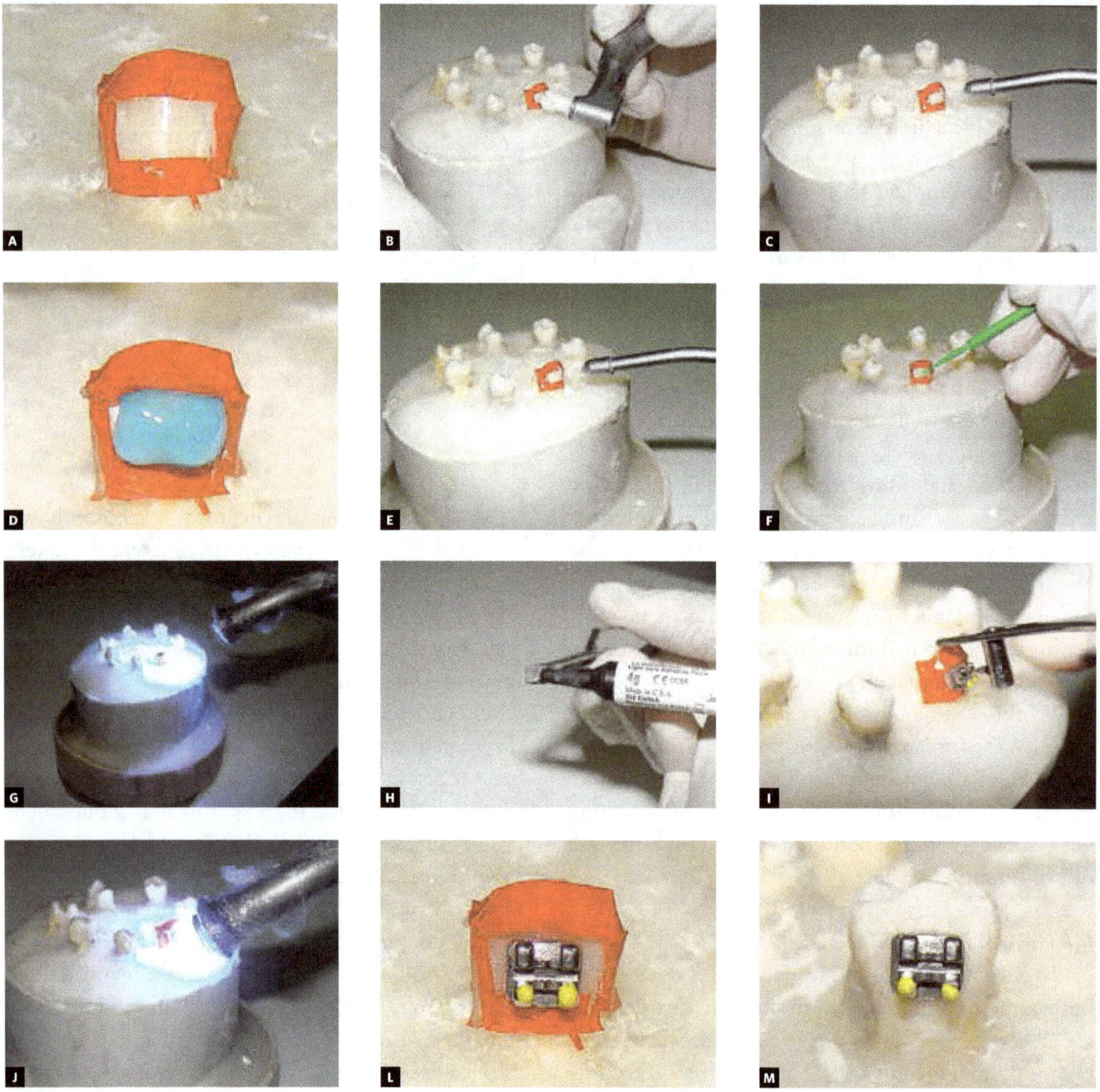

Figure 2 - **A)** Setting the mask. **B)** Prophylaxis (10s each tooth). **C)** Rinsing and drying. **D)** Acid conditioning (15s). **E)** Rinsing and drying (10s each tooth). **F)** Applying the primer. **G)** Photopolymerization of the primer. **H)** Applying the resin on the bracket base. **I)** Checking the distance of the accessory (4.0 mm). **J)** Photopolymerization. **L)** Bracket attached before removal of the mask. **M)** Bracket attached after removal of the mask.

Then, a descriptive analysis of the mean and standard deviation for the tensile resistance (kgf) was performed for all groups.

The influence of 35% hydrogen peroxide bleaching agent on the bonding strength of orthodontic brackets was evaluated comparing the traction force (kgf) results necessary to debond the accessories.

The Kruskal-Wallis nonparametrical test, with significance level of 5% ($p < 0.05$), using the SPSS 13.0 was applied.

RESULTS

The results (Table 2 and Fig 4) showed that there was a statistically significant reduction on the bond strength when compared to the Control group (19.52 kgf) and to the group where bonding was performed 24 hours after bleaching (12.31 kgf). When the bracket debonding strength was confronted with the Control group and the group where bonding was performed seven days after bleaching (18.44 kgf), it was noticed that there was no statistically significant differences.

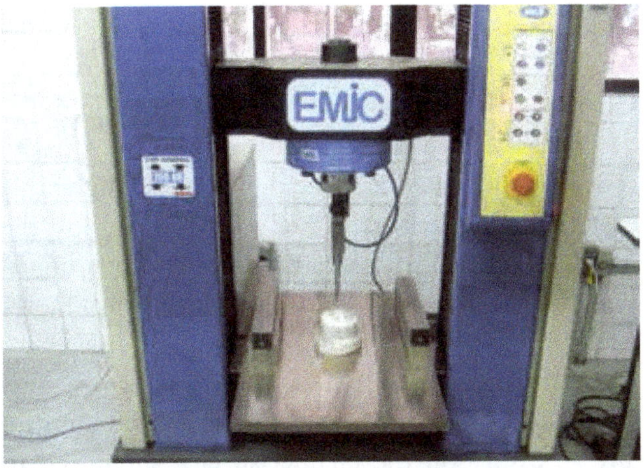

Figure 3 - Emic DL2000 universal testing machine.

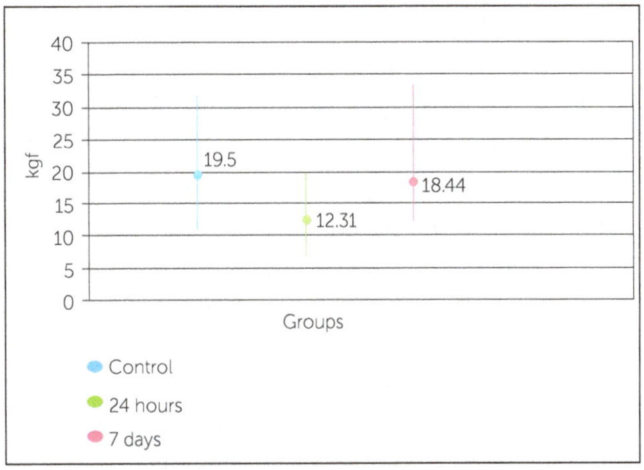

Figure 4 - Mean values and standard deviation of bond strength (kgf).

Table 2 - Bond strength values (kgf) obtained for each group according to tensile test.

Group	N	Minimum	Maximum	Mean	Standard Deviation
control	7	11.67	32.74	19.52[a]	6.537
24 hours	7	8.01	18.17	12.31[b]	3.240
7 days	7	11.42	35.78	18.44[a,b]	9.722

Kruskal Wallis nonparametrical test $p < 0.05$. Distinct letters (a/b) represent that there was statistical difference.
Control X 24 hours – p = 0.025*. Control X 07 days – p=0.098. 24 hours X 07 days – p = 0.338.

Table 3 - Evaluation of the influence of bleaching agents on the bonding strength of orthodontic brackets, according to existent studies.

Author	Type of tooth	Bleaching agent	Test	Resistance
Matta, Maia, Chevitarese[11]	Bovine	10% carbamide peroxide	Shear	Increase
Prietsch et al[14]	Bovine	35% hydrogen peroxide	Shear	Decrease
Uysal et al[21]	Humans	35% hydrogen peroxide	Shear	No alteration
Dishman et al[6]	Humans	25% hydrogen peroxide	-	Decrease
Quintella[16]	Humans	35% hydrogen peroxide	Shear	Decrease
Miles et al[12]	Humans	10% carbamide peroxide	Traction	Decrease
Homewood, Tyes, Woods[7]	Humans	Hydrogen peroxide	Shear	No alteration
Van der Vyver et al[22]	-	Hydrogen peroxide	-	Decrease
Bishara et al[2]	Humans	10% carbamide peroxide and 25% hydrogen peroxide	Traction	No alteration
Bello, Souza[1]	Humans	10% carbamide peroxide	Traction	Increase
Kraether, Souza[8]	Humans	10% carbamide peroxide	Traction	Increase

DISCUSSION

According to the literature on the influence of bleaching agents on the bonding strength of orthodontic brackets, there is still some doubt if these substances interfere negatively on bonding strength or not, since in some works there is a reduction on the adhesion, in others there is an increase and yet in some others there is no alteration (Table 3). A careful observation of these studies allows to number a series of variables that can explain the great variation in the results, such as: Type of bleaching agent, bleaching technique, type of enamel (human or bovine) and type of debonding tests (traction or shear).

The values obtained from the present study indicate a decrease on the bond strength of orthodontic brackets immediately after bleaching. These results were confirmed by others works,[6,12,14,16,22] which also obtained a reduction on the bond strength depending on the waiting period post-bleaching. However, some authors[1,8,11] presented different results and obtained an increase on the bond strength. The results found by Homewood et al,[7] Uysal et al[21] and Bishara et al[2] showed no alteration on adhesion.

The reduction of bond strength can be explained by a significant decrease on the calcium/phosphorus relation on the enamel bleached with hydrogen peroxide, affecting adversely the dental hard tissues.[17] Another reason for this decrease on the adhesion can be the fast decomposition of the residual bleaching agent, releasing oxygen into the porosities on the tooth surface. This oxygen has the capacity to inhibit the polymerization of the resinous material used in the procedures of bracket bonding, compromising the conversion degree of monomer to polymer and consequently, the union of the material with the enamel structure.

Therefore, the results of the present study suggest a waiting period of about seven days after bleaching to bond any accessory on the enamel surface, in order to minimize possible adverse effects of bleaching to adhesion.

CONCLUSION

From the results obtained in this *in vitro* study, it can be concluded that the dental bleaching with a 35% hydrogen peroxide, reduced significantly the bond strength of orthodontic brackets when bonding was performed 24 hours post-bleaching. However, after seven days from bleaching, differences were not noticed on bond strength, being recommended a longer waiting period when bonding of any accessory on the enamel surface submitted to bleaching agents is necessary.

REFERENCES

1. Bello DRM, Souza MAL. A influência do branqueamento dental, in vitro, na colagem de brackets com cimento de ionômero de vidro modificado por resina. Ortod Gaúcha. 2000;4(2):87-100.
2. Bishara SE, Oonsombat C, Soliman MM, Ajlouni R, Laffoon JF. The effect of tooth bleaching on the shear bond strength of orthodontic brackets. Am J Orthod Dentofacial Orthop. 2005;128(6):755-60.
3. Bishara SE, Sulieman AH, Olson M. Effect of enamel bleaching on the bonding strength of orthodontic brackets. Am J Orthod Dentofacial Orthop. 1993;104(5):444-7.
4. Bishara SE, VonWald L, Olsen ME, Laffoon JF, Jakobsen JR. Effect of light-cure time on the initial shear bond strength of a glass-ionomer adhesive. Am J Orthod Dentofacial Orthop. 2000;117(2):164-8.
5. Cal Neto JOAP, Miguel JAM. Uma análise dos testes in vitro de força de adesão em Ortodontia. Rev Dental Press Ortod Ortop Facial. 2004;9(4):44-51.
6. Dishman MV, Covey DA, Baughan LW. The effects of peroxide bleaching on composite to enamel bond strength. Dent Mater. 1994;10(1):33-6.
7. Homewood C, Tyas M, Woods M. Bonding to previously bleached teeth. Aust Orthod J. 2001;17(1):27-34.
8. Kraether J, Souza MAL. A influência do clareamento dental in vitro na colagem de brackets. Ortod Gaúch. 2002;6(1):6-16.
9. Marcondes M. Eficácia de dois métodos de clareamento dental e sua influência sobre as propriedades físico-químicas e sobre a resistência à união de sistemas adesivos [dissertação]. Porto alegre (RS): Pontifícia Universidade Católica; 2006.
10. Matis BA, Cochran MA, Eckert G, Carlson TJ. The efficacy and safety of a 10% carbamide peroxide bleaching gel. Quintessence Int. 1998;29(9):555-63.
11. Matta ENR, Maia JAC, Chevitarese O. Influência do agente clareador peróxido de carbamida a 10% na resistência mecânica da colagem de brackets ortodônticos. Rev Dental Press Ortod Ortop Facial. 2005;10(2):69-74.
12. Miles PG, Pontier JP, Bahiraei D, Close J. The effect of carbamide peroxide bleach on the tensile bond strength of ceramic brackets: an in vitro study. Am J Orthod Dentofacial Orthop. 1994;106(4):371-5.
13. Patel MP, Pinzan A, Francisconi PA, Pinzan CRM, Ferreira KB. Estudo da resistência ao cisalhamento na colagem de acessórios ortodônticos com e sem homogeinização da resina superbond. J Bras Ortodon Ortop Facial. 2004;9(51):242-7.
14. Prietsch JR, Broilo JR, Spohr AM. Influência do clareamento dental com peróxido de hidrogênio na colagem de brackets ortodônticos: estudo in vitro. Ortod Gaúch. 2003;7(2):136-44.
15. Prietsch JR, Mainieri ET, Oshima HMS, Spohr AM. Colagem de bráquetes em cerâmica: revisão de literatura. Ortod Gaúch. 2005;9(2):142-8.
16. Quintella LPAS. Avaliação da força de adesão e tempos de espera na colagem de brackets ortodônticos, após clareamento dental com peróxido de hidrogênio 35 por cento: estudo "in vitro". Araçatuba; [s.n]; 2003. 135 p. ilus, tab.
17. Rotstein I, Dankner E, Goldman A, Heling I, Stabholz A, Zalkind M. Histochemical analysis of dental hard tissues following bleaching. J Endod. 1996;22(1):23-5.

18. Surmont P, Dermaut L, Martens L, Moors M. Comparison in shear bond strength of orthodontic brackets between five bonding systems related to different etching times: an in vitro study. Am J Orthod Dentofacial Orthop. 1992;101(5):414-9.
19. Tavares CA, Zanini LK, Borges L. Estudo clínico comparativo da retentividade de brackets ortodônticos. Rev SOB. 1998;3(6):225-8.
20. Tytley KC, Torneck CD, Smith DC. The effect of concentrated hidrogen peroxide solutions on the surface morphology of human tooth enamel. J Endod. 1988;14(2):69-74.
21. Uysal T, Basciftci FA, Usümez S, Sari Z, Buyukerkmen A. Can previously bleached teeth be bonded safely? Am J Orthod Dentofacial Orthop. 2003;123(6):628-32.
22. Van der Vyver PJ, Lewis SB, Marais JT. The effect of bleaching agent on composite/enamel bonding. J Dent Assoc S Afr. 1997 Oct;52(10):601-3.

Permissions

All chapters in this book were first published in DPJO, by Dental Press International; hereby published with permission under the Creative Commons Attribution License or equivalent. Every chapter published in this book has been scrutinized by our experts. Their significance has been extensively debated. The topics covered herein carry significant findings which will fuel the growth of the discipline. They may even be implemented as practical applications or may be referred to as a beginning point for another development.

The contributors of this book come from diverse backgrounds, making this book a truly international effort. This book will bring forth new frontiers with its revolutionizing research information and detailed analysis of the nascent developments around the world.

We would like to thank all the contributing authors for lending their expertise to make the book truly unique. They have played a crucial role in the development of this book. Without their invaluable contributions this book wouldn't have been possible. They have made vital efforts to compile up to date information on the varied aspects of this subject to make this book a valuable addition to the collection of many professionals and students.

This book was conceptualized with the vision of imparting up-to-date information and advanced data in this field. To ensure the same, a matchless editorial board was set up. Every individual on the board went through rigorous rounds of assessment to prove their worth. After which they invested a large part of their time researching and compiling the most relevant data for our readers.

The editorial board has been involved in producing this book since its inception. They have spent rigorous hours researching and exploring the diverse topics which have resulted in the successful publishing of this book. They have passed on their knowledge of decades through this book. To expedite this challenging task, the publisher supported the team at every step. A small team of assistant editors was also appointed to further simplify the editing procedure and attain best results for the readers.

Apart from the editorial board, the designing team has also invested a significant amount of their time in understanding the subject and creating the most relevant covers. They scrutinized every image to scout for the most suitable representation of the subject and create an appropriate cover for the book.

The publishing team has been an ardent support to the editorial, designing and production team. Their endless efforts to recruit the best for this project, has resulted in the accomplishment of this book. They are a veteran in the field of academics and their pool of knowledge is as vast as their experience in printing. Their expertise and guidance has proved useful at every step. Their uncompromising quality standards have made this book an exceptional effort. Their encouragement from time to time has been an inspiration for everyone.

The publisher and the editorial board hope that this book will prove to be a valuable piece of knowledge for researchers, students, practitioners and scholars across the globe.

List of Contributors

Francilena Maria Campos Santos Dias
MSc in Orthodontics, Universidade Ceuma, São Luís, Maranhão, Brazil

Célia Regina Maio Pinzan-Vercelino
Assistant professor, Universidade Ceuma, Department of Orthodontics, São Luís, Maranhão, Brazil

Rudys Rodolfo de Jesus Tavares
PhD in Oral Rehabilitation, Universidade de São Paulo (USP), School of Dentistry, Bauru, São Paulo, Brazil

Júlio de Araújo Gurgel
PhD in Orthodontics, Universidade Ceuma, São Luís, Maranhão, Brazil

Fausto Silva Bramante
Associate Professor, Master's Program in Odontology, Universidade Ceuma, São Luís, Maranhão, Brazil

Melissa Nogueira Proença Fialho
MSc in Orthodontics, Universidade Ceuma, São Luís, Maranhão, Brazil

Delmo Santiago Vaitsman
Adjunct professor, Department of Analytical Chemistry, LaDA - IQ/UFRJ

Fernanda Alves Rodrigues Britto
Master's student in Orthodontics, Centro Universitário Hermínio Ometto (UNIARARAS), Araras, São Paulo, Brazil

Adriana Simoni Lucato, Heloisa Cristina Valdrighi and Sílvia Amélia Scudeler Vedovello
Professor, Centro Universitário Hermínio Ometto (UNIARARAS), Postgraduate program, Department of Orthodontics, Araras, São Paulo, Brazil

Bruna Coser Guignone and Ludimila Karsbergen Silva
MSc in Orthodontics, Pontifícia Universidade Católica de Minas Gerais (PUC Minas), Belo Horizonte, Minas Gerais, Brazil

Rodrigo Villamarim Soares and Emilio Akaki
Associate professor, Pontifícia Universidade Católica de Minas Gerais (PUC Minas), Belo Horizonte, Minas Gerais, Brazil

Marcelo Coelho Goiato
Full professor, Universidade Estadual Paulista Júlio de Mesquita Filho (UNESP), Araçatuba, São Paulo, Brazil

Matheus Melo Pithon
Adjunct professor of Orthodontics, Universidade Estadual do Sudoeste da Bahia (UESB), Jequié, Bahia, Brazil

Dauro Douglas Oliveira
Director of Orthodontics Program, Pontifícia Universidade Católica de Minas Gerais (PUC Minas), Belo Horizonte, Minas Gerais, Brazil

Leonard Euler Andrade Gomes do Nascimento
Visiting professor, Federal University of Piauí (UFPI)

Margareth Maria Gomes de Souza
Full professor, Department of Pediatric Dentistry and Orthodontics, Federal University of Rio de Janeiro (UFRJ)

Lucianne Cople Maia
Full Professor, Department of Pediatric Dentistry and Orthodontics, UFRJ

Liliana Avila Maltagliati
MSc and PhD in Orthodontics, Bauru School of Dentistry, University of São Paulo (USP)

Yasushi Inoue Myiahira
MSc in Orthodontics, School of Dentistry, Methodist University of São Paulo (UMESP)

Liana Fattori
Professor, Specialization Course in Orthodontics, Straight-Wire Group of Rio de Janeiro

Leopoldino Capelozza Filho and Mauricio Cardoso
Professor, Graduation and Post-Graduation Program and MSc in Orthodontics, Sacred Heart University

Lúcio Henrique Esmeraldo Gurgel Maia and Hibernon Lopes Filho
PhD resident of Orthodontics, Federal University of Rio de Janeiro (UFRJ)

Antônio Carlos de Oliveira Ruellas and Mônica Tirre de Souza Araújo
Associate professor, Department of Pediatric Dentistry and Orthodontics, UFRJ

Tarulatha R. Shyagali
Professor, Darshan Dental College and Hospital, Department of Orthodontics and Dentofacial Orthopedics, Udaipur, India

Deepak P. Bhayya
Professor, Darshan Dental College and Hospital, Loyara, Department of Pediatric and Preventive Dentistry, Udaipur, India

Chandralekha B. Urs
Former professor and head, Vaidehi Dental College and Hospital, Department of Orthodontics and Dentofacial Orthopedics, Bangalore, India

Shashikala Subramaniam
Professor, KGM Dental College and Hospital, Department of Orthodontics and Dentofacial Orthopedics, Kolar, India

Érika Mendonça Fernandes Franco
Graduate student, Faculdade Ingá (UNINGÁ), Department of Orthodontics, Maringá, Paraná, Brazil

Fabrício Pinelli Valarelli, Rodrigo Hermont Cançado and Karina Maria Salvatore de Freitas
Professor, Faculdade Ingá (UNINGÁ), Department of Orthodontics, Maringá, Paraná, Brazil

João Batista Fernandes
Mechanical Engineer, Universidade Federal de Itajubá (UNIFEI), Itajubá, Minas Gerais, Brazil

Cibele Braga de Oliveira
MSc in Orthodontics, State University of São Paulo (UNESP)

Luiz Guilherme Martins Maia
Professor, Department of Orthodontics, UNIT/SE

Ary Santos-Pinto and Luiz Gonzaga Gandini Júnior
Full professor, Department of Orthodontics, State University of São Paulo (UNESP)

José Rino Neto
Associate Professor, Department of Orthodontics, School of Dentistry, University of São Paulo (FOUSP)

Gilberto Vilanova Queiroz
MSc and PhD in Orthodontics, FOUSP

João Batista de Paiva
Full Professor, Department of Orthodontics, FOUSP

Rafael Yagüe Ballester
Full Professor, Department of Dental Materials, FOUSP

Renato Parsekian Martins
Adjunct professor, Universidade Estadual Paulista Julio de Mesquita Filho (UNESP), School of Dentistry, Department of Orthodontics, Araraquara, São Paulo, Brazil

Sergei Godeiro Fernandes Rabelo Caldas
Adjunct Professor, Universidade Federal do Rio Grande do Norte (UFRN), Department of Dentistry, Natal, Rio Grande do Norte, Brazil

Alexandre Antonio Ribeiro
Professor, Universidade Potiguar (UnP) and Associação Brasileira de Odontologia (ABO), Specialization course in Orthodontics, Natal, Rio Grande do Norte, Brazil

Luís Geraldo Vaz
Professor, Universidade Estadual Paulista Julio de Mesquita Filho (UNESP), School of Dentistry, Department of Prosthesis and Dental Material, Araraquara, São Paulo, Brazil

Roberto Hideo Shimizu
Professor, Universidade Tuiuti do Paraná (UTP), School of Dentistry, Curitiba, Paraná, Brazil

Lídia Parsekian Martins
Professor, Universidade Estadual Paulista Julio de Mesquita Filho (UNESP), School of Dentistry, Department of Orthodontics and Pediatric Dentistry, Araraquara, São Paulo, Brazil

Guilherme Caiado Sobral
MSc in Orthodontics, School of Dentistry – University of Araras (UNIARARAS)

Mário Vedovello Filho and Viviane Veroni Degan
Professor, Department of Orthodontics, UNIARARAS

Milton Santamaria Jr
Professor, Postgraduate program in Orthodontics, UNIARARAS

Ione Helena Vieira Portella Brunharo and Cristiane Canavarro
Assistant professor, Department of Orthodontics, FOUERJ

Angela Rita Pontes Azevedo
Doctorate student in Orthodontics, UFRJ

Carlos Nelson Elias
Assistant professor, Military Institute of Engineering (IME)

Luciana Borges Retamoso
PhD in Dental Materials, Catholic University of Rio Grande do Sul (PUCRS)

Cátia Cardoso Abdo Quintão
Adjunct professor, Department of Orthodontics, FOUERJ

Grace Kelly Martins Carneiro
Master's student in Orthodontics, Faculdade e Centro de Pesquisas São Leopoldo Mandic, Campinas, São Paulo, Brazil

Juliano Alves Roque
Assistant professor, Faculdade e Centro de Pesquisas São Leopoldo Mandic, Department of Orthodontics, Campinas, São Paulo, Brazil

Aguinaldo Silva Garcez Segundo
Professor, Faculdade e Centro de Pesquisas São Leopoldo Mandic, Department of Orthodontics, Campinas, São Paulo, Brazil

Hideo Suzuki
Head of the Master's program in Orthodontics, Faculdade e Centro de Pesquisas São Leopoldo Mandic, Department of Orthodontics, Campinas, São Paulo, Brazil

José Maurício da Rocha
MSc in Orthodontics, Adjunct professor, Department of Orthodontics - School of Dentistry – Federal University of Juiz de Fora (FO/UFJF)

Marco Abdo Gravina
PhD in Dentistry, State University of Rio de Janeiro (UERJ)
MSc in PhD in Orthodontics, State University of Rio de Janeiro (UERJ)
Associate professor of Orthodontics, School of Dentistry, and professor of the graduate program in Orthodontics, UFJF
Adjunct professor, Department of Orthodontics, UFJF

Marcio José da Silva Campos
Postdoc in Orthodontics and professor, FO/UFJF

Cátia Cardoso Abdo Quintão
PhD in Orthodontics and Adjunct professor of Orthodontic, UERJ

Robert Willer Farinazzo Vitral
Associate professor, Department of Orthodontics, FO/UFJF

Marcelo Faria da Silva
Private practice, Palmas, Tocantins, Brazil

Célia Regina Maia Pinzan-Vercelino and Júlio de Araújo Gurgel
Assistant Professor, Universidade Ceuma, Department of Orthodontics, São Luís, Maranhão, Brazil

Josiane Xavier de Almeida and Mauren Bitencourt Deprá
Graduated in Dentistry, Catholic University of Paraná (PUCPR)

Camila Ivini Viana Vieira
Private practice, Aracaju, Sergipe, Brazil

Sergei Godeiro Fernandes Rabelo Caldas
Assistant professor, Universidade Federal do Rio Grande do Norte (UFRN), Natal, Rio Grande do Norte, Brazil

Orlando Tanaka
Postdoc in Orthodontics, Saint Louis University and Federal University of Juiz de Fora
Full professor at PUCPR

Fábio Lourenço Romano
Professor, Universidade de São Paulo, Ribeirão Preto Dental School, Department of Pediatric Clinics, Ribeirão Preto/SP, Brazil

Giovanna Pessoti
Dental surgeon, Universidade de São Paulo, Ribeirão Preto Dental School, Ribeirão Preto/SP, Brazil

Rodrigo Galo
Professor, Universidade Federal dos Vales do Jequitinhonha e Mucuri, School of Biological and Health Sciences, Department of Dentistry, Diamantina/MG, Brazil

Jaciara Miranda Gomes-Silva and Marília Pacífico Lucisano
Dental surgeon, Universidade de São Paulo, Ribeirão Preto Dental School, Department of Pediatric Clinics, Ribeirão Preto/SP, Brazil

Maria Cristina Borsatto and Paulo Nelson-Filho
Full professor, Universidade de São Paulo, Ribeirão Preto Dental School, Department of Pediatric Clinics, Ribeirão Preto/SP, Brazil

Gladys Cristina Dominguez
Associate Professor, Department of Orthodontics and Pediatric Dentistry, School of Dentistry, São Paulo University (FOUSP), São Paulo, Brazil

André Tortamano
Professor, PhD, Department of Orthodontics and Pediatric Dentistry, FOUSP, São Paulo, Brazil

Luiz Vicente de Moura Lopes
PhD student, Department of Orthodontics, FOUSP, São Paulo, Brazil

Priscilla Campanatti Chibebe Catharino
MSc student, Department of Orthodontics, FOUSP, São Paulo, Brazil

Camillo Morea
Post-doctor in Orthodontics, USP

Aisha de Souza Gomes Stumpf
Assistant Professor, UFRGS

Carlos Bergmann
Professor of Materials Science, School of Engineering, UFRGS

José Renato Prietsch
Professor of Orthodontics, Dental School, UFRGS

Juliane Vicenzi
Assistant Professor, School of Engineering, UFRGS

Yong-Keun Lee
Director, Institute for Clinical Performance of Biomaterials (ICPB) and ETN Dental Clinic, Seoul, Korea

Yu Bin
Associate Professor, Chinese Academy of Sciences, State Key Laboratory of Multiphase Complex Systems, Institute of Process Engineering, Beijing, China

Gabriel Schmidt Dolci
Associate Professor, Department of Orthodontics, Brazilian Association of Dental Surgeons

Ana Maria Spohr
Associate Professor, Department of Dental Materials, PUC-RS

Eduardo Rigon Zimmer
PhD student, Department of Biochemistry, McGill University

Ernani Menezes Marchioro
Head, Department of Orthodontics, Brazilian Association of Dental Surgeons

Jefferson Vinicius Bozelli and Renato Bigliazzi
Associate Professor, Department of Orthodontics, Paulista University (UNIP)

Helga Adachi Medeiros Barbosa
MSc in Orthodontics, UNIP

Cristina Lucia Feijo Ortolani and Kurt Faltin Junior
Professor, Department of Orthodontics Paulista University (UNIP)

Francisco Antonio Bertoz
Professor, Department of Orthodontics, State University of São Paulo (UNESP)

Sergio Luiz Mota Júnior, Marcio José da Silva Campos, Marcelo Reis Fraga and Robert Willer Farinazzo Vitral
Universidade Federal de Juiz de Fora, Departamento de Odontologia Social e Infantil (Juiz de Fora/MG, Brazil)

Carina Abrantes Schmitberger
Universidade Federal de Juiz de Fora, Programa de Pós-graduação em Saúde (Juiz de Fora/MG, Brazil)

Juliana de Andrade Vitral
Universidade Federal de Juiz de Fora, Curso de Graduação em Arquitetura e Urbanismo, (Juiz de Fora/MG, Brazil)

Julia Sotero Vianna
Private practice, Rio de Janeiro, Rio de Janeiro, Brazil

Mariana Marquezan
Postdoc resident, Universidade Federal do Rio de Janeiro (UFRJ), Department of Pediatric Dentistry and Orthodontics, Rio de Janeiro, Rio de Janeiro, Brazil
Dentist, Universidade Federal de Santa Maria (UFSM), Department of Restorative Dentistry, Santa Maria, Rio Grande do Sul, Brazil

Thiago Chon Leon Lau
PhD resident, Universidade Federal do Rio de Janeiro (UFRJ), Rio de Janeiro, Rio de Janeiro, Brazil

Eduardo Franzotti Sant'Anna
Professor, Universidade Federal do Rio de Janeiro (UFRJ), Rio de Janeiro, Rio de Janeiro, Brazil

Sergio Luiz Mota Júnior
PhD Student in Health, Federal University of Juiz de Fora (UFJF)

Márcio José da Silva Campos
Post-Doctorate Student in Health, UFJF
Professor of the graduate program in Orthodontics, UFJF

José Maurício dos Santos Nunes Reis and Lídia Parsekian Martins
Assistant Professor, Universidade Estadual Paulista (UNESP), Department of Dental Material, School of Dentistry, Araraquara, São Paulo, Brazil

Marcelo Reis Fraga
MSc in Orthodontics, Pontifical Catholic University of Minas Gerais (PUCMG). Doctorate student in Health, UFJF. Professor of the graduate program in Orthodontics, UFJF

Robert Willer Farinazzo Vitral
Associate professor and program director of the graduate program in Orthodontics, UFJF

Tatyane Ribeiro Mesquita, Lídia Parsekian Martins and Renato Parsekian Martins
Universidade Estadual Paulista, Faculdade de Odontologia de Araraquara, Departamento de Clínica Infantil (Araraquara/SP, Brazil)

Luiz Geraldo Vaz
Professor, Universidade Estadual Paulista (UNESP), Department of Dental Material, School of Dentistry, Araraquara, São Paulo, Brazil

Renato Parsekian Martins
Private practice and part-time Faculty, Universidade Estadual Paulista (UNESP), Department of Pediatric Dentistry, School of Dentistry, Araraquara, São Paulo, Brazil

Camilla Ivini Viana Vieira
MSc, Universidade Estadual Paulista (UNESP), Department of Pediatric Dentistry, School of Dentistry, Araraquara, São Paulo, Brazil

João Paulo Fragomeni Stella and Andrea Becker Oliveira
Professor, Centro de Estudos Odontológicos Meridional (CEOM), Postgraduate program, Passo Fundo, Rio Grande do Sul, Brazil

Lincoln Issamu Nojima
Professor, Universidade Federal do Rio de Janeiro (UFRJ), Department of Pediatric Dentistry and Orthodontics, Rio de Janeiro, Rio de Janeiro, Brazil

Marcus Vinicius Neiva Nunes do Rego
Professor and Chairman, Specialization Course in Orthodontics, NOVAFAPI

Roanselli Marllon Lima dos Santos
Graduated in Dentistry, NOVAFAPI

Leanne Matias Portela Leal
Professor, Specialization Course in Orthodontics, NOVAFAPI

Carlos Gustavo Silva Braga
Specialist in Orthodontics, NOVAFAPI

Index

R

S

T

U

W

www.ingramcontent.com/pod-product-compliance
Lightning Source LLC
LaVergne TN
LVHW060558210926
848485LV00005B/1336